FABULOUS

Life

ELAINE KILGORE NEELY *ꝏ* PATRICIA NEELY-DORSEY

Contact Information: 1196 CR 681, Saltillo, MS. 38866   901-848-6800   magnoliagirl21@yahoo.com

ISBN: 9781960853080

Cover Photos (Back and Front) James Dorsey
Before and After Photos James Dorsey
Patricia's Fashion Photos James Dorsey
Fitness Photos ; Sophie Venzia
Picture and Poem graphics Debra Estep

Liberation's Publishing ~ 183 Cottrell St. West Point, MS. 39773

In Loving memory of

JAMES HENRY NEELY M.D.

SOUTHERN MAN

There's nothing like a Southern man,

He's a man that you should know;

He's one to whom you'll find no equal

Anywhere you go.

He has a sweet molasses talk

And a slow, smooth gliding walk.

He's got strong firm hands that let you know,

Real work is nothing new;

He has no problem with the fact,

That he should provide for you.

There are certain kinds of values

This man is sure to hold

His love of home and family

Is sure to not grow cold.

He'll deeply love his mother

It's a bond that's always there

All throughout his life this man

Will show her tender care.

He's one that you can count on,

To do the manly things;

He'll change the tire and check the oil

And fix the backyard swing.

But, underneath a tough exterior,

A gentle soul lies, too;

He's one who'll rock the baby,

And even cook a meal or two,

On Sundays he'll sit beside you singing,

On the same church pew.

There's nothing like a Southern man,

He's a rare and special kind;

If you look forever anywhere,

He's the best you'll ever find.

2008 Patricia Neely-Dorsey

I've always had a fondness for older people. For me, it was the women in my family that carried the strongest message on aging, especially around beauty. I can still see the creamy bright red lipstick that my glamorous grandmother applied with aplomb. Red lipstick was her legacy. My mother wore it dramatically. My sister wears it boldly and I wear it classically. By ten, I knew color and clothing were going to hold sway in my life, due to these fabulous women I saw wrapping themselves in fine fabrics, stylish clothing, brilliant colors and the attitude to pull it off. They were true influencers and my original style mentors. Not just memories, my grandmother, great aunt and mother provided me with a template, a platform and launching pad for a sense of color, personal style and beauty. They provided the foundation for appreciating that beauty lives long after 60 and an aging woman could still dress fashionably, creatively and colorfully. In my 50s I began thinking how I wanted to invest my time post retirement. Aging was my calling, while color and style was my passion. How could I marry the two?

In 2008, I started Color Style Studio that shifted to Greying Goddess, and ultimately The Art of Mindful Aging was born in 2011. In my commitment to the aging community, I have found information, influencers, teachers, mentors and friends on the social media giants, Facebook and Instagram. I met Patricia Neely-Dorsey, the co-author of this book, on Facebook who is doing a fabulous job of showcasing the beauty and benefits of dressing every day and looking our best. Patricia is an influencer and the poster woman for classic style and aging well! Beauty is not reserved for youth. Mature beauty has a regal glow, a deep awareness and knowledge of what our bodies need to look and feel beautiful. We have a lived experience and can call on that wisdom for guidance. We don't need to be Oprah Winfrey or J.Lo to talk about aging. The mere fact that we are alive and aging gives us all the permission we need. And the world needs to hear it from the everyday woman – the woman that so many can relate to and be inspired by.

Aging is no longer a personal problem to overcome; it is an anthem for courage, grit and pride as we move toward another stage of life, not alone, but with a legion of women standing behind us and in front of us. Aging is a form of grace and medicine" that is holy and worth preparing for. Let us not fear aging, but fear a society that doesn't support aging, especially in women. Why not leave a legacy that others will want to aspire to. Be Fabulous, Look Fabulous and Feel Fabulous at every age and stage of your life. Age with awe!

—Denise Lampron, Los Angeles, CA
May 18, 2023
The Art of Mindful Aging
Mature Beauty and Style

A GIRL SHOULD BE TWO THINGS: CLASSY AND FABULOUS."- COCO CHANEL

CONTENTS

Foreword

I HAVE SOME BIG BOOK NEWS!!!

On my 58th birthday (Feb 2022), I made the decision to embark on a fitness journey to get into my "best shape ever" by 60. I started going to a personal trainer (April 2022) Miss Fit: Sophie's Wellness Personal Training and adopted a plant based diet "Pretty much fully" by August 2022.

Mom watched and cheered me on every step of the way. (She has ALWAYS been my BIGGEST cheerleader!) After Mom saw the results, she was truly impressed. She said, we (not you) should do a book about the plant-based diet and healthy eating. (She has been a vegetarian for almost 40 years and has recently become a vegan.) I was BLOWN AWAY!!! We???!!! If you know my mother, you will know this is something HUGE!!!

My mother is a VERY private person! I could not ever imagine her wanting to put something WRITTEN-about herself-out into the world! Trust me...you would have to know her to KNOW what a HUGE deal this is ! I was super excited about the idea, but I was kind of dragging my feet because I really had no idea what I would want to put in the book, for my part, besides the few months of my fitness journey, some things about my plant based diet and some before and after photos. I didn't see that taking up any more than 10 or 12 pages. That would be more of a pamphlet or something! But, after I thought about it, I realized that so many friends over the years (at least 10 years) have been asking and telling me to write a book on my thrift shopping tips and finds. I really had no desire to do that. But, since Mom came up with this idea of a book, I thought it would be perfect material to throw in there!

You know I have a lot to say about being a Diva on a Dime and even more pictures!!! LOL!!!! People have been asking and asking me when I was going to write another book. I had no plans to do so WHATSOEVER...anytime soon or anytime later! It was a no for me.... But now, guess what folks... It's On!!!

WE are gonna do this!!! Woo Hoo!!!

Mom has been so excited about this and has been talking about and working on her part EVERY DAY for the past few months!!! I was so thrilled that this project was so mind and time consuming for her, because she has been deeply grieving the death of my dad, since he passed in 2020. They were married 66 years. Just the other day, I was telling her that Dad would be so amazed that she wants to do something like this!!! She agreed! The plan is to have it published by July 2023 The title???? FABULOUS...What else? Actually, Mom might have created a monster because I keep thinking of all kinds of things that I am going to throw into the pot! (pictures, poems, Facebook posts, childhood memories...it has gotten ridiculous!) Stay tuned and get your coins ready.

Patricia Neely-Dorsey   Taken from my Facebook Post announcing this project!   January 7, 2023 at 7:19 AM

For many years, on my social media pages I have been known for two slogans

Be You ! Do You ! SHINE!

Go Forth and Be Fabulous !

Fabulous

adjective

extraordinary, exceptionally good or unusual

splendid

extremely pleasing

wonderful

excellent , outstanding , marvelous superb, first- rate, first-class

spectacular, stunning , uncommon , impressive, remarkable

astonishing , astounding

phenomenal

Patricia Neely Dorsey

Being "Fabulous" or having a "Fabulous Life" is not about being arrogant or conceited .
It is about being confident in your own God given specialness, being proud of the uniqueness of You and feeling good in your own skin. You are proud of who and how you are and it shows.

"There is no passion to be found playing small — in settling for a life that is less than the one you are capable of living." There is NOTHING to be gained from settling for a version of you LESS than the quality of your potential."

-Nelson Mandela

Our deepest fear

Our deepest fear is not that we are inadequate.
Our deepest fear is that we are powerful beyond measure.
It is our light, not our darkness
That most frightens us.

We ask ourselves
Who am I to be brilliant, gorgeous, talented, fabulous?
Actually, who are you not to be?
You are a child of God.

Your playing small
Does not serve the world.
There's nothing enlightened about shrinking
So that other people won't feel insecure around you.

We are all meant to shine,
As children do.
We were born to make manifest
The glory of God that is within us.

It's not just in some of us;
It's in everyone.

And as we let our own light shine,
We unconsciously give other people permission
to do the same.
As we're liberated from our own fear,
Our presence automatically liberates others.

-Marianne Williamson
A Return to Love

FIT AND FABULOUS FOR LIFE

On my 58th birthday in 2022

I decided that I would embark on a journey to get into my best shape every by 60.

That also included the goal of a Six Pack By Sixty.

I started intermittent fasting in March.

I began looking for some type of fitness program that I could join.

I was most interested in strength training.

This is very important as one ages.

When I typed in strength training Tupelo Mississippi,

I ran across Fit Miss:

> March 2, 2022 10am
> Message to FitMiss Facebook Page
>
> I am interested in training sessions.
> How much do you charge?

Wed, Mar 2, 2022 at 9:05 PM

Hello Patricia! Thank you for reaching out. I would love to help you. Can you possibly share a little more about yourself and objectives? Are you currently active, overweight, do you have physical limitations, how's your health in general, what your schedule looks like, etc. I am on a completely full schedule right now, but I might have an opening in April, if your schedule very flexible? If your schedule permits some flexibility, I would be happy to schedule a consultation so we can get to know each other and reserve you a training spot. And to answer your questions and to make sure that what I do corresponds to what you are searching for, here's a brief description: I only do one-on-one training in a private studio, which catered directly to your fitness needs, objectives and budget. The studio is located in Tupelo in the gated part of Deer Park Estates neighborhood, around a lake, very private and beautiful, my fees start at $50/session.

Every session is 1 hour to 1h15 long and consists of rebounding, resistance training, HIIT, most of the strengthening moves are done on the BOSU and TRX, every session ends with a mix of yoga, Pilates and stretching. I am a fitness nutritionist and all programs include nutrition support, I can definitively guide you on all aspects of health. Thank you Patricia, I will be looking forward to hearing back from you. If you can respond by text, it would be appreciated.

-Sophie

Mar 4, 2022 at 2:21 AM

So sorry that I am late in responding . Somehow, I missed the message. I am so sorry that I am terrible with texting! I don't do it at all. So I do hope that this e-mail response will be fine. Again, so sorry for the inconvenience. I do most of my messaging on Facebook and otherwise am very technology challenged! I am very, very interested in getting started with training! My schedule is very flexible and I could start in April if you have an opening . I can come at any time. I am 58 years old . I am 5'6" .I weigh 175 bs. I am pretty sedentary. I do walk some. As far as nutrition , I have begun trying some intermittent fasting and have cut out eating a lot of meat. I am trying to stick with mostly tuna for meat. (my Mom has been a vegetarian for over 35 years) I want to lose weight, tone my body and gain strength and muscle to keep my body strong, mobile and flexible as I age. I do have good health at this time. I take no medications . I don't have any physical limitations , except for being out of shape. I would love to schedule a one on one consultation, whenever your time permits. If possible could you send the message back through Facebook or give me a call whenever you can.

P.S. Another thing I am working on is getting my sleep patterns regulated! During the pandemic and quarantine I started being awake in the early morning hours , getting up around one o'clock in the morning and going to sleep bed very early in the evening.

-Patricia

March 5, 2022

Good morning Patricia!

I understand your incentive to be the best version of your self and would definitely love to be part of your health journey as you look very motivated and understand the benefits of osmosis and that that everything needs to be all aligned with sleep, nutrition, exercise and mind to achieve your goal. My approach is very holistic and I love women who are receptive to this approach and open minded. Our environment and the standard American diet is destroying our health and microbiomes, which is leading to an epidemic of obesity. I usually do not consider women who are not interested in adjusting their diet and lifestyle, it is more than just exercise. As I mentioned I am at a completely full schedule but what intrigued me and made me consider you is your enthusiasm and that you mentioned doing intermittent fasting and talked about your sleep patterns. I would be happy to schedule a consultation and to add you on my waiting list for the next opening. I am out of town next week but would be happy to schedule to meet the week of the 14th. I will reach back that Monday to see what works best for both of us to meet and see if it is a good fit. Will be looking forward to meeting you Patricia. Thank you for reaching out again.

-Sophie

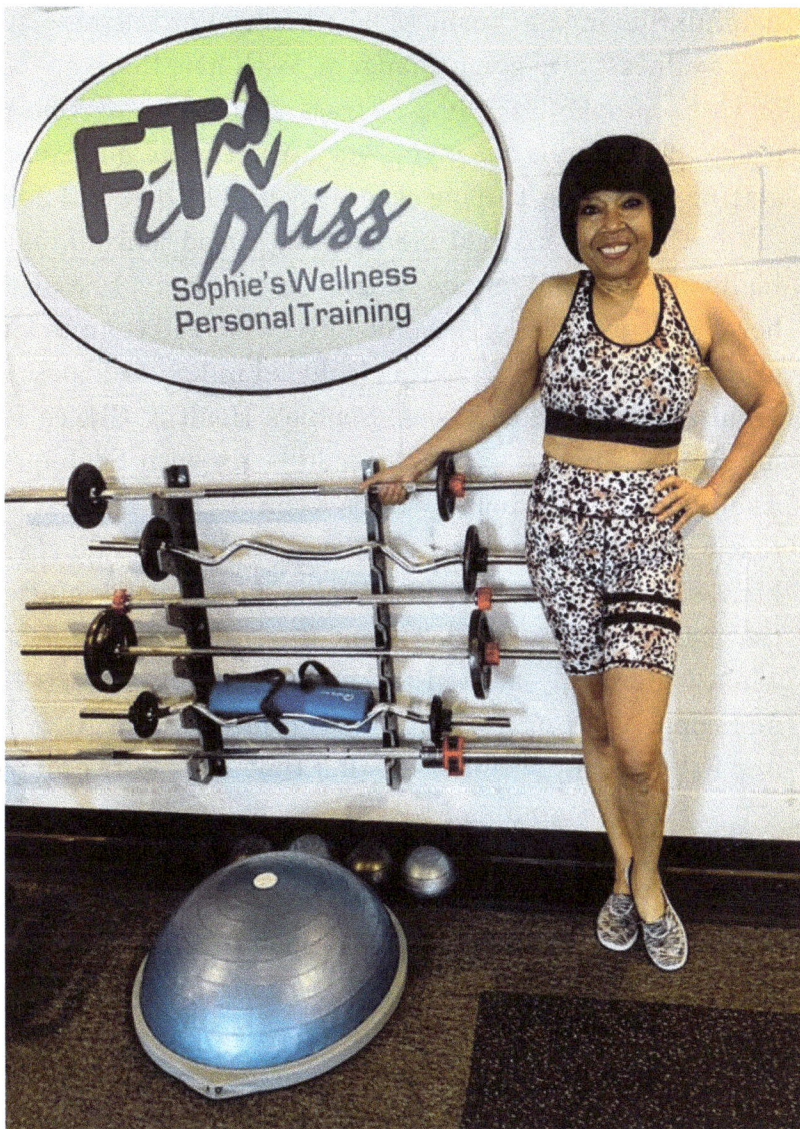

I started fitness training near the end of April with Sophie Vezina Fit Miss -Sophie's Wellness Personal Training Sophie is a certified personal trainer and fitness nutritionist . She is a   native French Canadian and has been living in the United States for over 20 years. I always thought it amusing how she would be speaking French with her husband before a training session and switch seamlessly to speaking English for our time together. She is a truly amazing woman . And, her body , at 50+ is all of the advertisement that she needs! At our first session, when she asked about goals. I said, " I want to look like that" and pointed at her. She chuckled. She probably was thinking that I had no idea what it really takes to look like that. She was right! Even after I had decided to be all in on the healthy eating , I would have two or three hot wings or a little piece of fried catfish or barbecue here or there.

I would always put that "little" part in there when I was explaining about what I had eaten, after the scale did not go down my required one pound that week. She would just shake her head and give me that stern schoolmarm disapproving look. I really finally started a truly almost fully plant based diet about three months in after I began with her .

Training with Sophie has been a total life changing experience. The knowledge that she has imparted is invaluable! Her rules and tips swirl around in my head all of the time and are very helpful! She means business, she knows her business and her wholistic approach to weight loss and wellness are game changers. With her, there are always frequent conversations on quality of sleep, proper breathing,   stress reduction etc. She puts special emphasis on nutrition and proper diet. As the old saying goes: You cannot out exercise a poor diet". It is so true! I would say getting to your best shape ever is about 80% diet and 20% exercise.

Of course, she had me keeping a food journal, as she does with all of her clients which I highly recommend on any weight loss journey! She also has a shake recipe that she encourages her clients to have for breakfast every day. I began to look forward to this shake every day. I am practically addicted to it! It is included in her cookbook, along with more of Sophie's healthy, personal recipes. The cookbook, Sophie's Healthy Choice Recipes, is available on Amazon. Each of my fitness training sessions would begin with Sophie going over my food journal pages for the week. There were so many rules when it came to meat and animal products as far as what kinds to eat like organic and grass fed etc. And she would always remind me not to eat meat within an hour of fruit. I would mess up that meat and fruit thing so much that I decided to just stop eating the meat, because I didn't want to see her face and hear the reprimand reinforcing that rule when I inevitably messed up. Elimination of meat really made all of the difference in the ease and consistency of my weight loss from then on! As for meat, I was eating mostly only chicken and fish (mainly sardines) by that time I began training with her .

In the beginning I was always balking against some advice or instructions she would give. It was usually something I just did not want to do. Finally, I came to the realization that she had the knowledge that I needed and wanted, and SHE was the expert, not me. On top of that, I was PAYING for that knowledge and expertise. I had to make a mental Note to Self: Just Do What the Lady Says! As time went along, I never had any problems with my food journals passing with flying colors, because I wasn't eating meat and I was doing intermittent fasting up to 20 hrs. a day, sometimes. So, there were not a lot of entries or meals to mess up!

OF COURSE, SHE HAD ME KEEPING A FOOD JOURNAL!

TODAY

DAILY FOOD LOG
AND CHECK LIST

MEAL #1 & TIME :

WEIGHT :

Lemon water ☐
Coffee or green tea ☐
Shake ☐
Other meal _____

MEAL #2 & TIME :

MEAL #3 & TIME :

CHECK LIST :

☐ ACV
☐ Kimchi or Sauerkraut
☐ Nutritional Yeast
☐ Legumes
☐ Exercise & Duration _____
Herbal Tea and Water ☐ ☐ ☐ ☐ ☐ ☐ ☐ ☐

HOW I FEEL:

_____
_____
_____

Sophie's Morning Shake

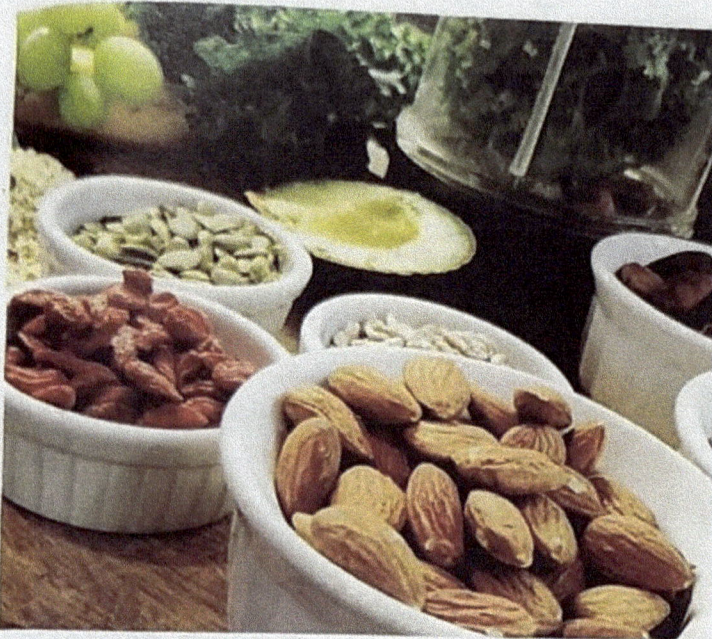

Ingredients

1	teaspoon Spirulina
1	tablespoon flax seeds
1	tablespoon pure cacao (beans or nibs)
1	tablespoon Goji berries
2	tablespoons raw Hemp hearts
1	handful fresh spinach
1	kale leaf
1	celery stalk
¼	cup frozen organic blueberries (or mixed berries)
¼	avocado or ½ banana
½	cup unsweetened almond milk (or coconut milk)
	water
	ice cubes (optional)
1	tablespoon chia seeds

THIS IS ONE OF MANY SHAKE RECIPES that can be made using a blender. I've been alternating the fruit in this one, but the grains, vegetables and supplements remain unchanged. This shake is always made with ALL organic ingredients. It will energize you, and it's substantial enough to keep you going all morning. I freeze the banana—the colder the shake, the better it is!

Directions:

Serves 1

Prep time: 5 min.

Calories: 468
Fat: 19g
Carbs: 55g
Protein: 23g

➤ Prepare and place all ingredients EXCEPT chia seeds into blender

➤ If desired, ice cubes may be added prior to blending to make the shake extra cold

➤ Fill with water up to fill line, and blend until perfe[...]

➤ Add chia seeds to the shake and mix manually—[...] chia will lose some of its properties

➤ Use a large milkshake straw and enjoy!

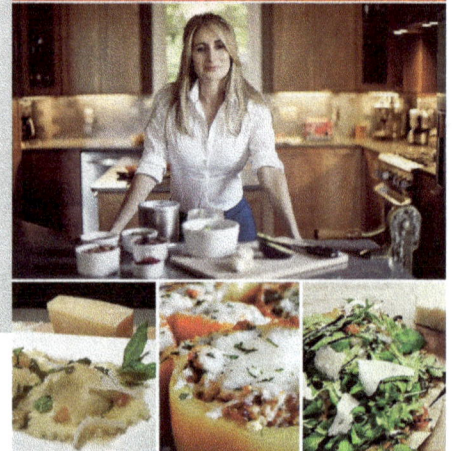

Sophie's Healthy Choice Recipes

Mom became very excited with the idea of me sharing my fitness journey in a book, because she became very impressed with it. That is how this book came about! She was so very pleased with my transformation week by week. Every morning before or after my training sessions , we would talk about my progress. She would go over the top with her praises, as she always does.

#MyBiggestCheerleader

My trainer's emphasis on nutrition made me want to learn more and more about how what we eat affects our bodies. One morning, as I was watching different You Tube videos on the benefits of a plant based diet , I heard Eric Adams (mayor of New York, although he was not the mayor at the time of that program) speaking at a conference on health issues , talking about the benefits of the vegan lifestyle and the amazing things that it had done in his life and his mother's life.

I was mesmerized by his presentation and the information that he shared I immediately told my mother about it . Of course she wanted to find out more information about him. I found that he had a book and ordered it for her.

After she read the book, she decided that day that she would become a vegan. Just like that! The name of the book is *Healthy At Last* She ,now, recommends the book , as a must read for everyone! She actually reads the book over and over like a reference book. One day, out of the blue, she said, we should write a book about our diets and the amazing things that a plant based diet can do.

 I am totally not cut from the same cloth as my mother ,when it comes to sticking to diet restrictions, even if they are self ‑imposed. I might eat the same things over and over again. But, I don't like anyone telling me I can't have something, even if that someone is me!

I might make up by mind to follow a certain diet , but, I am "subject" to fall off the wagon at any time!
And, if truth be told, sometimes I just wholeheartedly, stubbornly jump off the wagon!

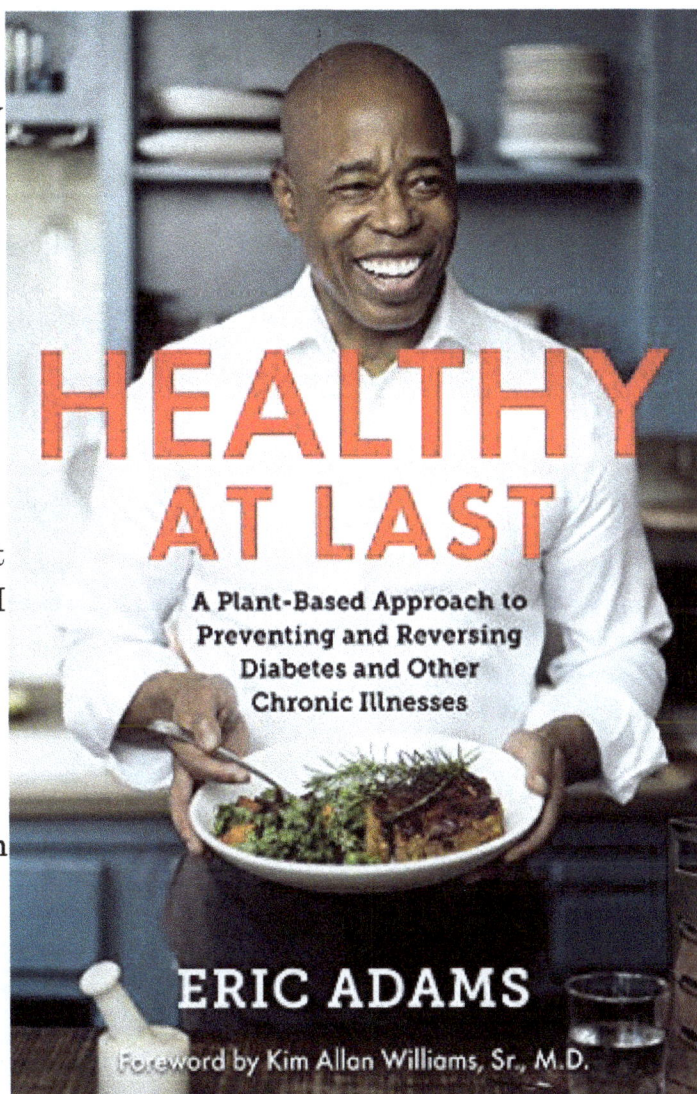

I can say that I am very much like mother in one way. We don't mind eating the things that we like over and over again, endlessly, without getting bored with them or seeking more variety. She eats basically the same 4 or 5 things EVERY day! Sweet potatoes, collard greens, black eyed peas, red peppers, and red onions arranged very attractively in different ways on her plate.

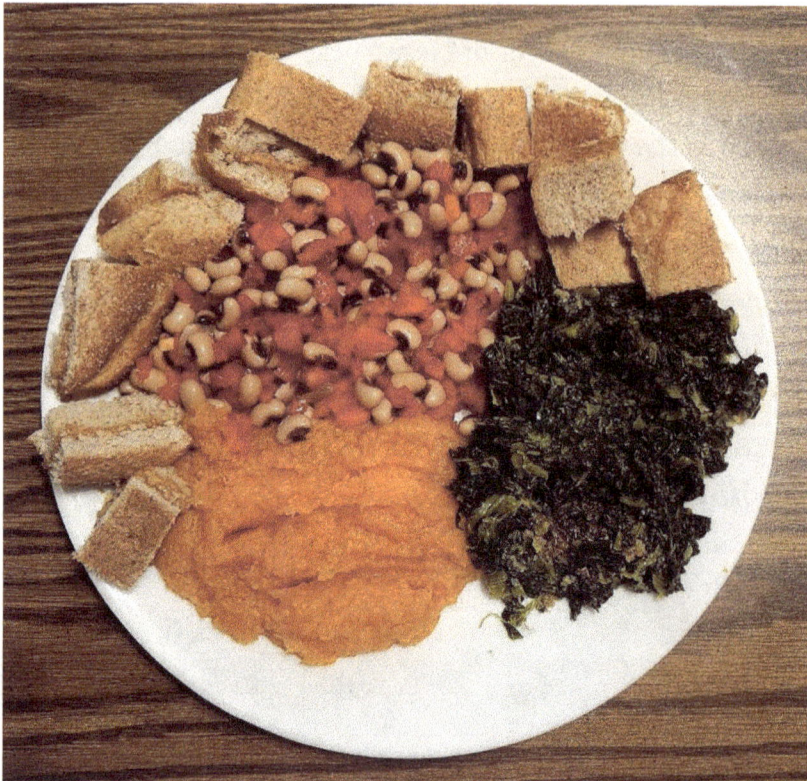

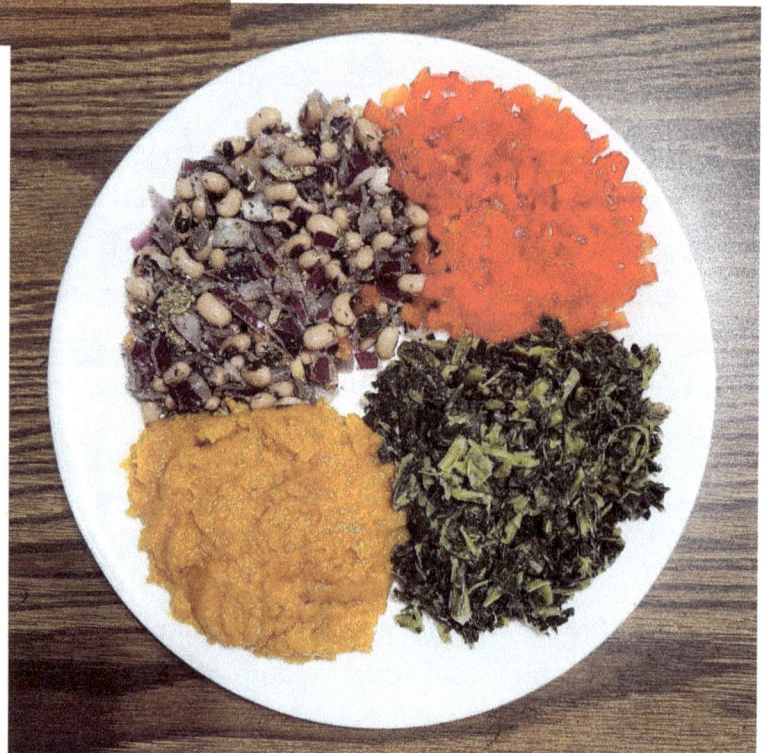

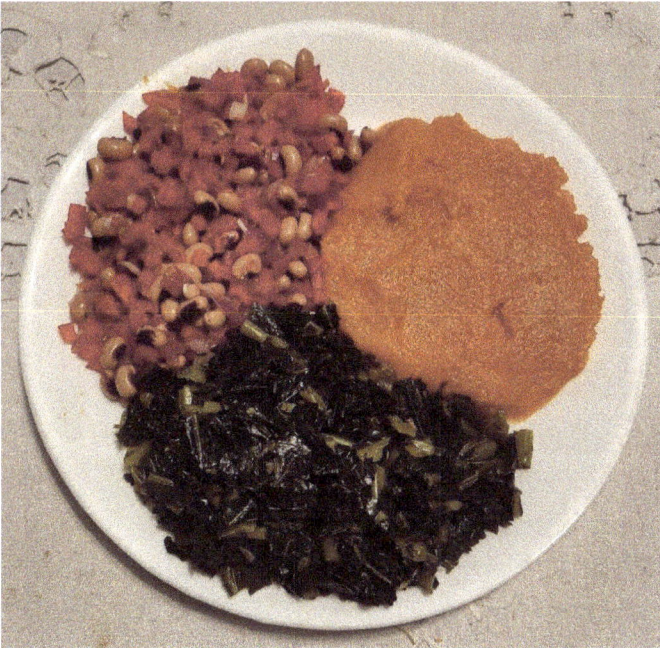

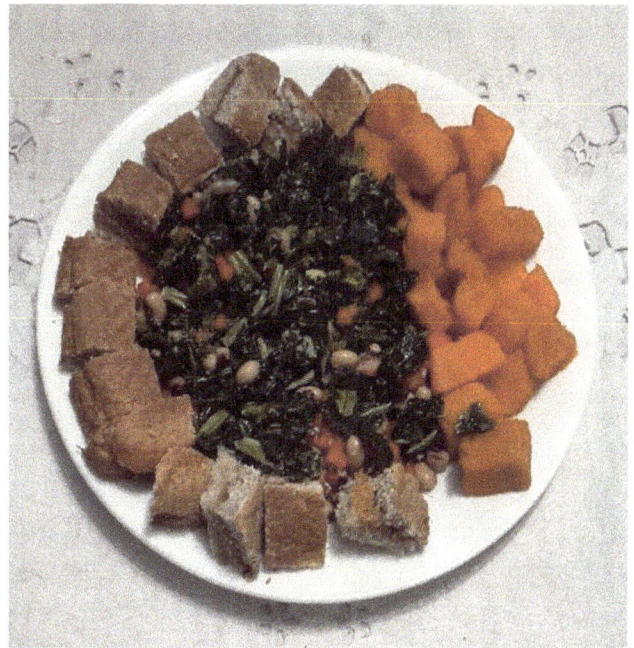

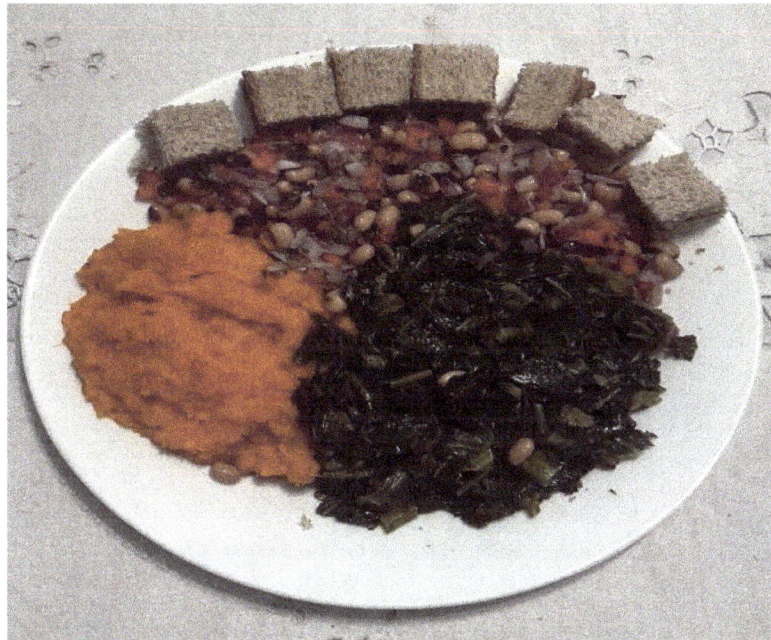

Please believe that I understand how hard it is to give up some of the food we Southerners love! We are ALL about the food ! Almost every activity or event is somehow centered around food. I absolutely did not know how obsessed I was with food until I published my first book and started reading some of my own poems over and over again! Almost every   other poem is about food. So, take heart. If I can do this healthy eating lifestyle thing anyone can!

There will be slips and falls along the way. Just get back up.

I have included a few of my poems to let you know that. I TOTALLY understand ! :)

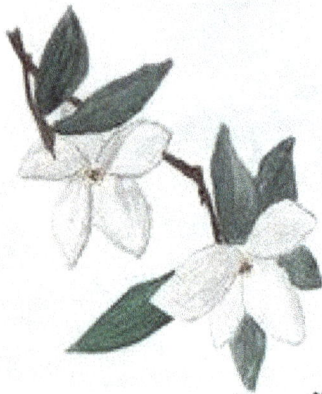

~ Southern Life ~

If you want a glimpse of Southern life,
Come close and walk with me;
I'll tell you all the simple things,
That you are sure to see.
You'll see mockingbirds and bumblebees,
Magnolia blossoms and dogwood trees,
Caterpillars on the step,
Wooden porches cleanly swept;
Watermelons on the vine,
Strong majestic Georgia pines;
Rocking chairs and front yard swings,
June bugs flying on a string;
Turnip greens and hot cornbread,
Coleslaw and barbecue;
Fried okra, fried corn, fried green tomatoes,
Fried pies and pickles, too.
There's ice cold tea that's syrupy sweet,
And cool, green grass beneath your feet;
Catfish nipping in the lake,
And fresh young boys on the make.
You'll see all these things
And much, much more,
In a way of life, that I adore.

Patricia Neely-Dorsey
Reflections of a Mississippi Magnolia-
A Life in Poems © 2008

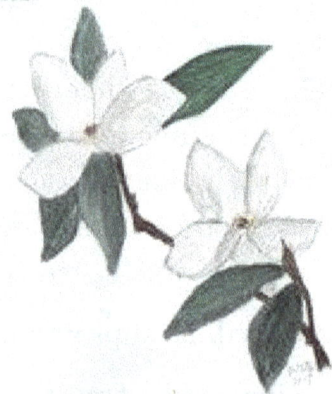

SOUL FOOD RESTAURANT

When you visit your favorite soul food
spot,
Along with your faithful friends,
What you'll eat any given day,
On your tastes it all depends.
The selections are quite varied
And the menu might read like this:
For breakfast Country Ham and Eggs,
With biscuits and cheese grits,
For Lunch : Neckbones, Catfish,
Smothered Chicken,
Pork Chops and Pigs Feet.
Everything looks so delicious,
And these are just the meats.
The vegetables you might enjoy,
include greens, squash, and black-eyed
peas;
Or you might want fried corn and pinto
beans,
Along with macaroni and cheese.
What ever it is that you decide,
It's sure to hit the spot,
It'll come to your booth,
Fresh and piping hot.
Be prepared to sit a spell,
Cause you won't want to move;
For you will have dined most
sumptuosly,
As your clean plate will prove.

Patricia Neely-Dorsey

My poem Soul Food Restaurant is included in a half credit fully online elective
course in African American History being used in the School District of Philadelphia , grades 9-12 (Philadelphia,
Pennsylvania)

SOUTHERN COMFORT
(Food)

It's been announced about our state,
That we are the fattest in the nation;
We always top the "unhealthy list,"
It's always seemed our station.
It's absolutely clear to me,
That the world would know just why;
If they'd ever been to South Pontotoc
Grocery,
And tried the Peach Fried Pie.
The food in our state's so good,
There's just no parallel;
If eating good cooking were against the
law,
We'd all certainly go to jail.
We've got some men who cook for us,
Like no woman ever could;
And passing up a plate of hot catfish,
Now, tell me one who would.
Yes, everything is filled with fat,
Or fried deeply in some grease;
And if our tea's not sweet enough,
We can hardly keep our peace.
We all want to "live our best life,"
Be healthy and all of that;
But, unfortunately in our fair state,
It's SO delicious getting fat.
2012 Patricia Neely-Dorsey

FELLOWSHIP SUNDAY
The Word
(God's Word that is)
The Bird
(Chicken that is)
Macaroni and Cheese
Potato Salad
Turnip Greens
Black-eyed Peas
Cornbread
Banana Pudding
Caramel Cake
Dressing
And did I say...
The Word?

Patricia Neely-Dorsey

COUNTRY BREAKFAST

A real country po'folk's breakfast
Is in these days quite rare,
It's certainly not your typical
Bacon and eggs type affair.
There'd be crispy fried chicken,
With all the parts there to eat;
The usual ones represented,
Plus the neck, back and feet.
There might be some country ham,
But not the thin sterile kind;
It's the thick, salty slices
From the smokehouse you'll find.
If you're lucky, there's rabbit,
From a recent hunt trip;
With juicy, brown gravy
That drips from your lips.
There would probably be rice,
With sugar and butter of course;
And big chunky biscuits
That could choke any horse.
What goes in the middle,
Is anyone's guess;
Some molasses or syrup
Would sure pass the test.
But, most want preserves
From the cook's vast store;
From the past summer's canning,
In flavors galore.
The milk would be powdered,
And straight from a box;
There's likely no juice,
'til opportunity knocks.
But, we all know one thing
That's sure to be had;
It's a jug full of Kool-AId,
And the flavor is
Red

Patricia Neely-Dorsey

Fitness Journey Story by my Trainer Sophie Vezina
FitMiss-Sophie's Wellness Personal Training

If she CAN do it – Everyone CAN

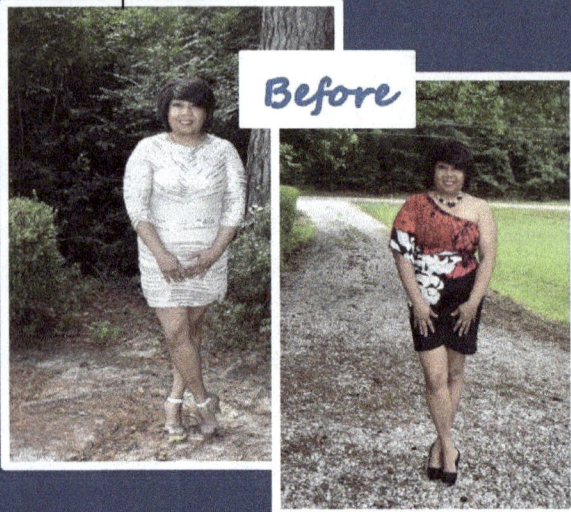

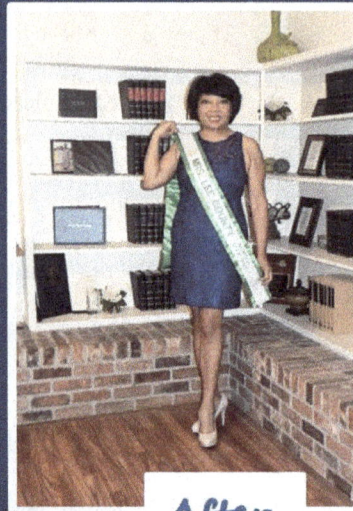

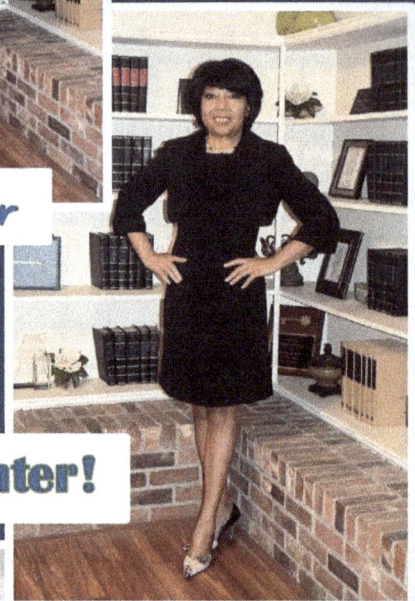

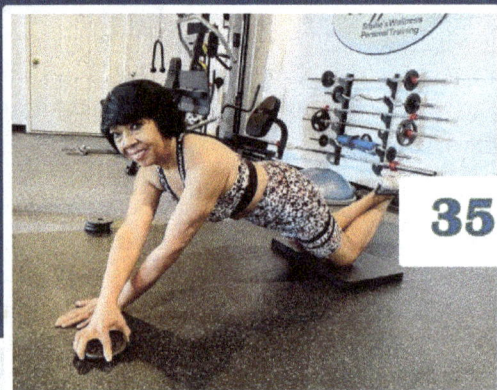

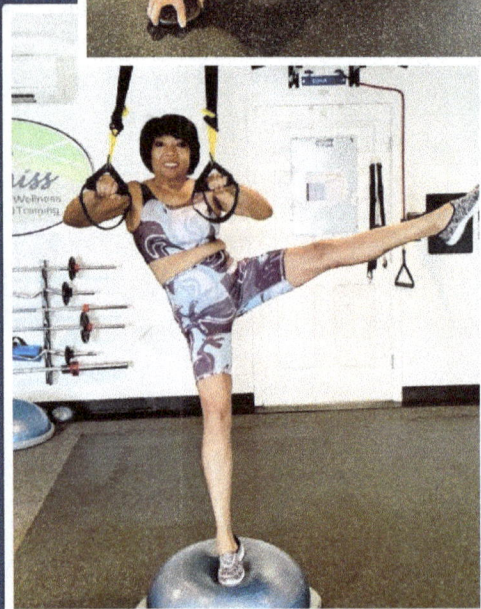

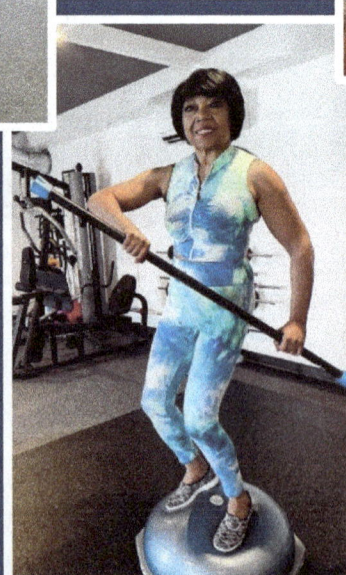

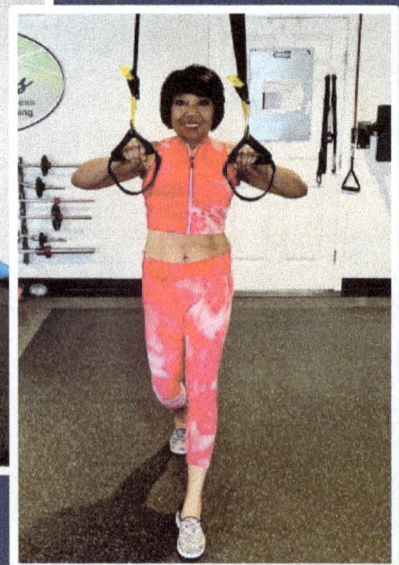

Before

After

35 pounds lighter!

-Sophie

How do I even begin to describe the unique and inspirational story of the beautiful, strong-willed, and intellectual woman that is Patricia? On April 20th, 2022 Patricia Neely-Dorsey began her transformative journey (coincidentally, she started by confessing that I would be writing a story of her in the near future)! "If I can do it, every woman can do it!" she told me... Now, 6 months later and 35 lbs. lighter, we are ready to share her story and inspire women of any age to undertake the same challenge!

Prior to meeting, I made sure to clearly emphasize my holistic approach to health and exercise, forewarning that nutrition plays as pivotal of a role in transforming both your body and your mind as exercise. Patricia confirmed that she was determined to participate in and apply any means necessary to reach her goals. Patricia's objective was to be the best version of herself possible before reaching 60, in two years, and in order to compete in the Miss Magnolia State pageant (Mrs. category) on November 20th, 2022. With a BMI of almost 28%, this was no small feat - but Patricia held up to her word. Though her aversion to exercising is undeniable, we did manage to make the best out of our sessions - though not without our fair share of conversations regarding pleasure and whether we wanted to continue our 1-hour sessions with a smile or a pout, ha!

Patricia (AKA Magnolia Girl) is undeniably more of a writer and poet than an athlete, and therefore we worked together to make the process of developing an interest in working out and learning new moves.

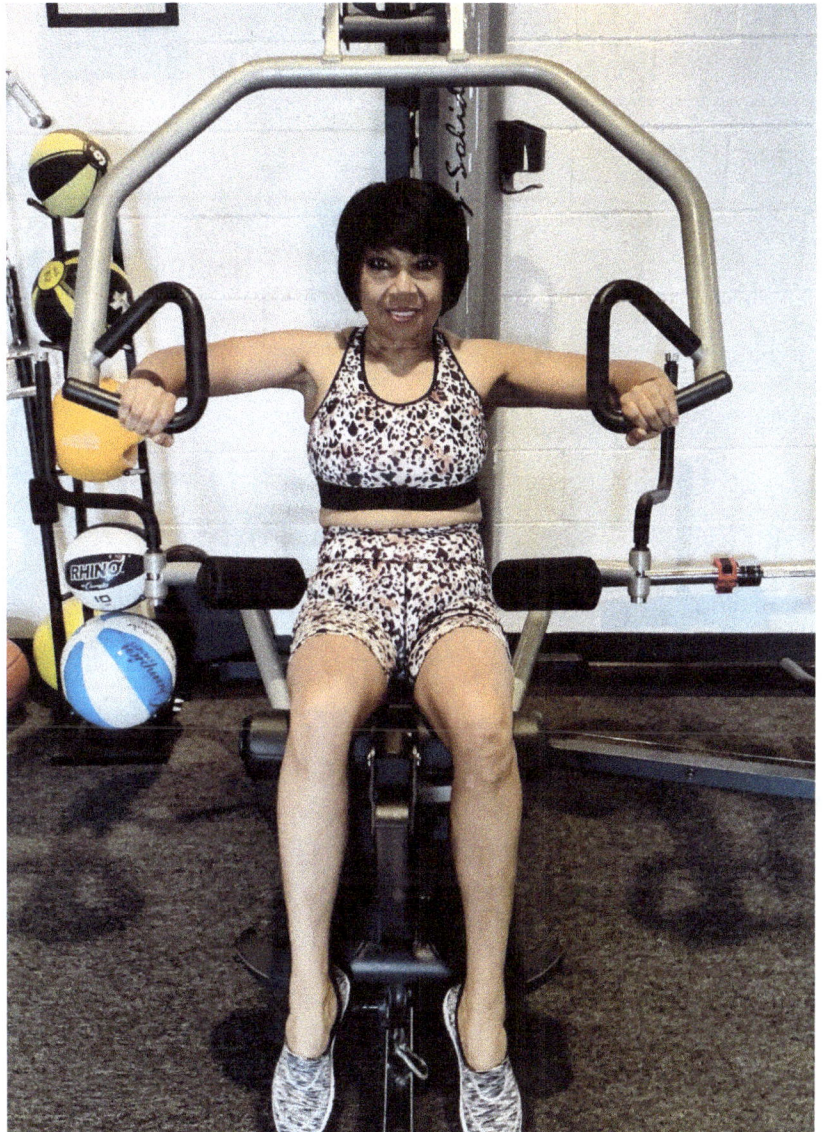

It's easy to target fitness routines for women to their personal abilities, strength and limitations - the hardest part is to make it enjoyable for someone who dislikes working out. I have to admit, Patricia became quite the comedian when asked if she shared my excitement in the new workouts and moves I prepared for her (her opinion? "How on earth can someone like exercising to start with?") But even through her disdain of working out, I struggled to get her to feel soreness from even the toughest of workouts - a strong woman indeed! In the end this turned out to be a blessing in disguise.

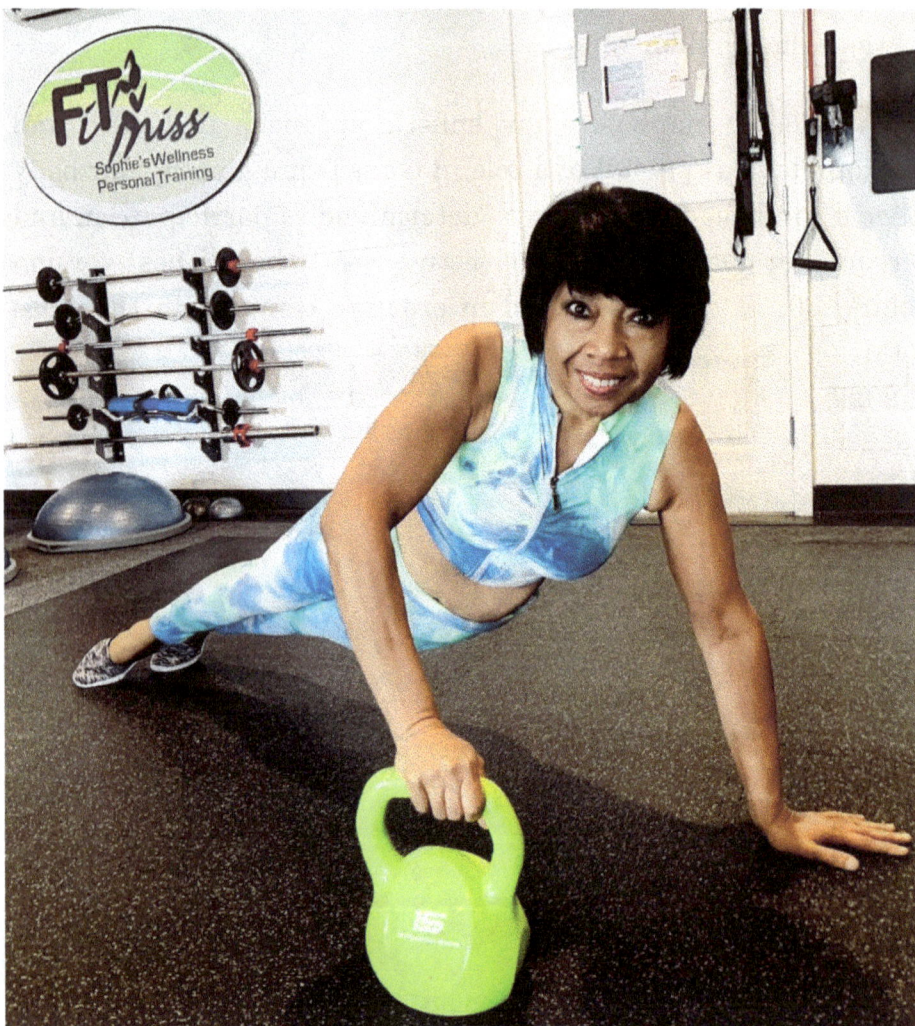

The few times she did feel sore provided her with the excitement and motivation needed to keep pushing through.

I soon realized that in order to succeed and to make the process more enjoyable there needed to be opportunities to disassociate in a sense: transport to a dreamy location, or be in a more mindful place. I tried like never before to tailor workouts that were focused on having fun and being less intimidating. The goal: make it challenging, but simple enough at the same time. Whenever I would see a half grin forming from a specific routine or move, my day would be made. Patricia's spirit and sense of humor is as unique as she is. She made me laugh for hours after leaving the studio. As I helped Patricia reach her goals, she also changed and challenged me. I took extra time to research the science behind determination and spirit, realizing that nothing is stronger than these factors when working towards overcoming your objectives.

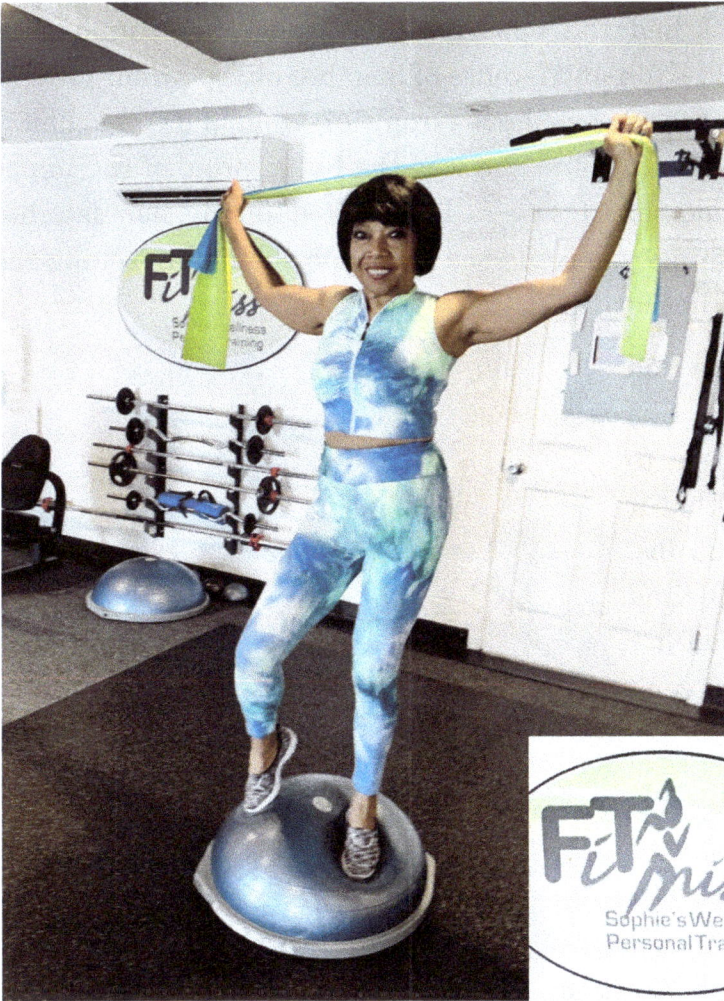

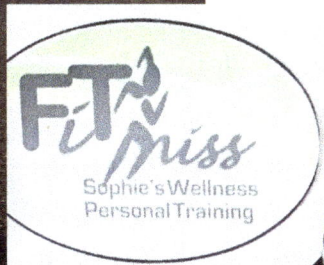

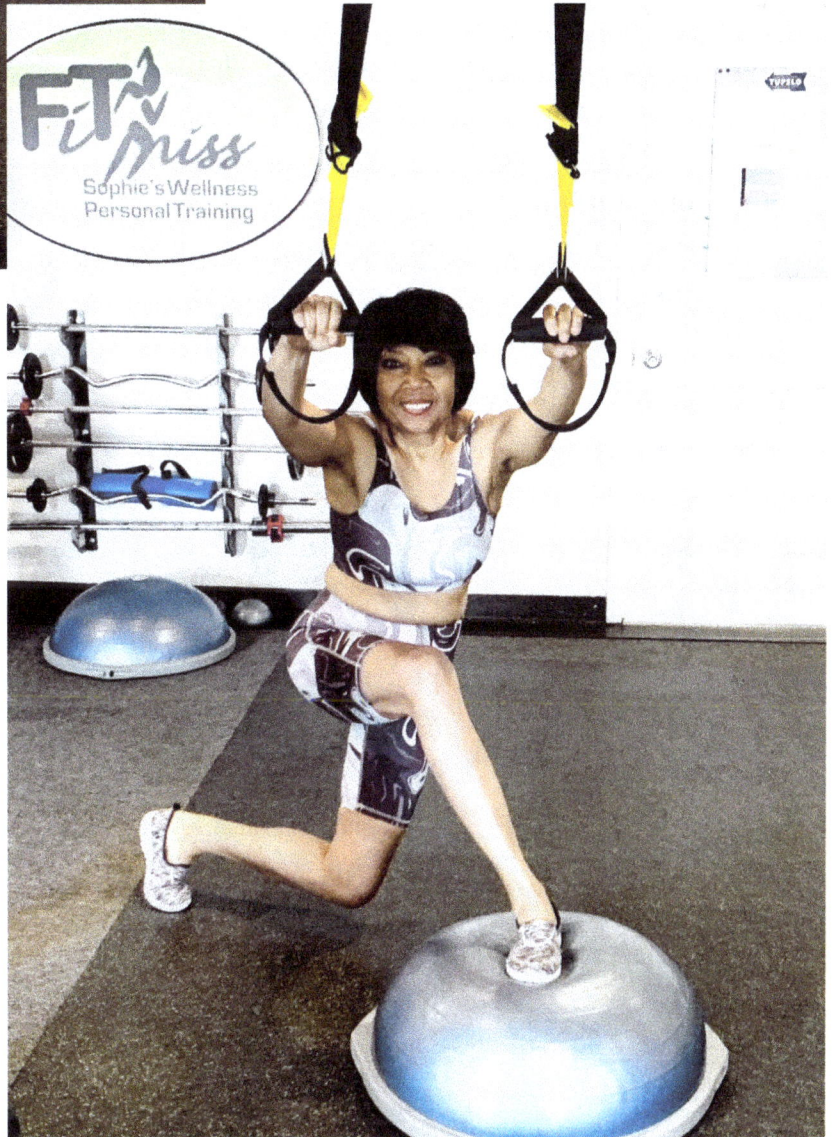

After a few months of training, I had the opportunity to meet her number one cheerleader: Patricia's mother, Mrs. Neely. Even at 87 years of age, her sharp mind, physical condition, alertness and curiosity made me realize how strong of an impact she had in Patricia's life. Being plant-based for almost 40 years, she was the living proof of the impact that our diet has on our health. The pride that I saw in her eyes watching her daughter during one of our sessions was heartwarming; you could see the pride she had in seeing that her daughter was finally taking control of her health.

Patricia's commitment, perseverance and determination are her strongest attributes. She had one goal, and she was going to prove to herself, and to all the skeptics out there, that it was possible – and did she ever! Now, 35 lbs. lighter, with a BMI of 22%, toned up, and stronger than ever before, she has reached her goal and is back to wearing clothes that haven't fit in over 10 years.

Continuing this journey will most definitely prove to be a work in progress, and not without its challenges, since Patricia loves food (anything palatable, really), to the point of writing a poem in her book (Reflections of a Mississippi Magnolia - A Life in Poems) about it. In it, she reflects on her roots and how ingrained it is to her culture, her being.

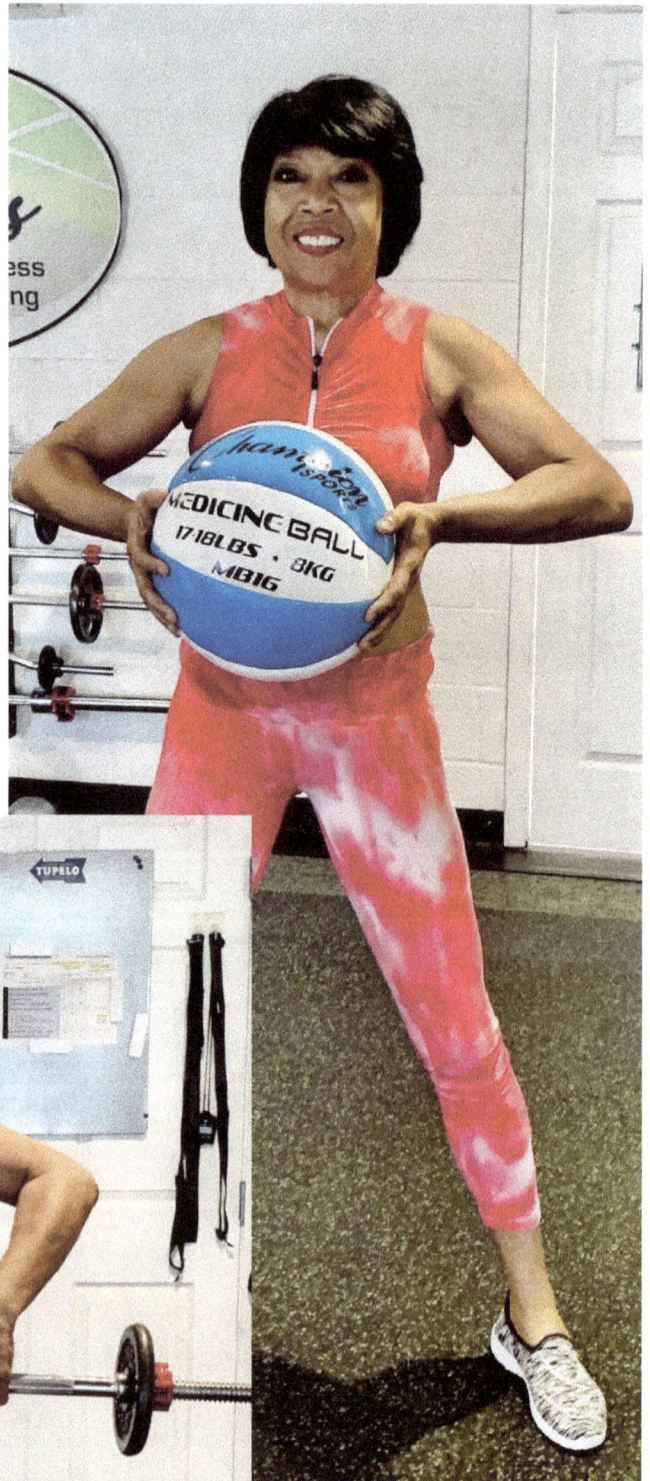

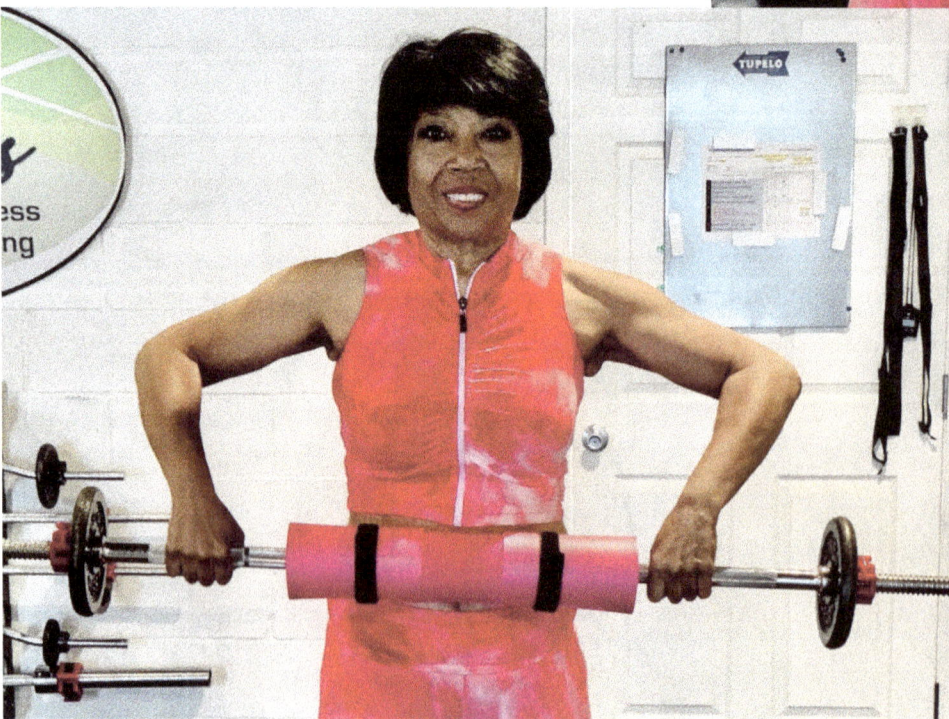

Food defines us, food brings us together, but it can also have a huge impact on our health. We are what we eat and it is not easy to go against what we have been taught and brought up with. However, with a few adjustments to her diet, adopting a more whole-food plant-based diet, and by incorporating some intermittent fasting, Patricia changed both her physique and her mood; her sleep is now better, her stress level lower. Her achievements should not be weighed solely in pounds – Patricia's improvement is in ALL areas of her life: physical, confidence, energy, vitality, wellbeing and self-love.

Thank you again to my "Magnolia Girl". Thank you for allowing me to be part of your journey, for allowing me to get to know the beautiful woman that you are, inside and out. We will all be your cheerleaders on November 20th, as well as beyond, as we all know the challenges you had to overcome. It is not easy to change your lifestyle, to set a goal and to obtain it, particularly in your late 50s. You transformed yourself in only 6 months, and (as promised) will spread the word that, "every woman can do it!"

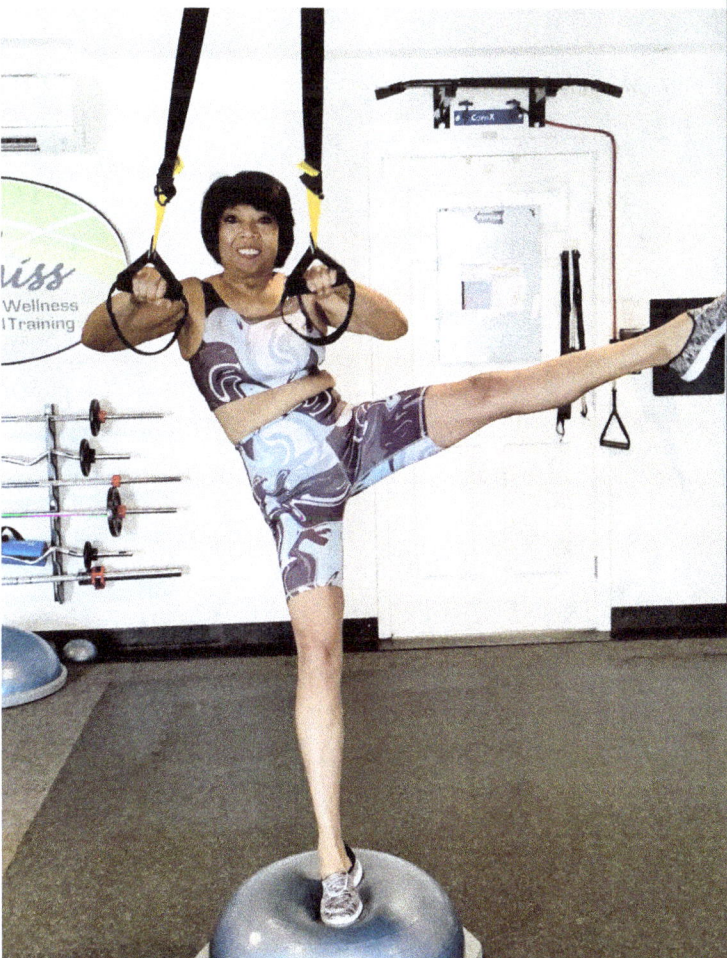

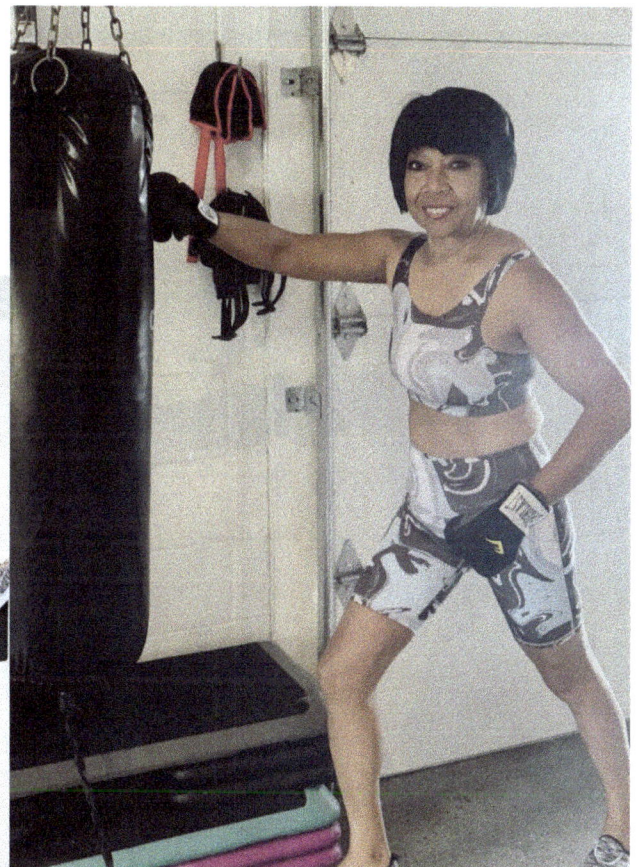

A picture is worth a thousand words.

I love sharing my fitness/weight loss/lifestyle journey. Even with all of the pictures that I take, I had no true perception of my size. I always say that if I can do it anyone can!
I love and still crave super fatty and super greasy foods! I love fat and grease ...Period.
I am not sure if I like the fatty strips on my steaks and pork chops more than the meat.
It's a close tie . But, I think the fat might win ! I like fat and grease oozing out of my food!
In my head , there is no such thing as too much bacon or too much grease.
I don't say it in past tense because I still like it...I just don't eat it.
In my before pictures, all of my poor choices are written all over my face ...literally .
I want to tell /show others what a difference a plant based diet, intermittent fasting and strength training have done to transform me !
The proof is in the pudding...I mean pictures.

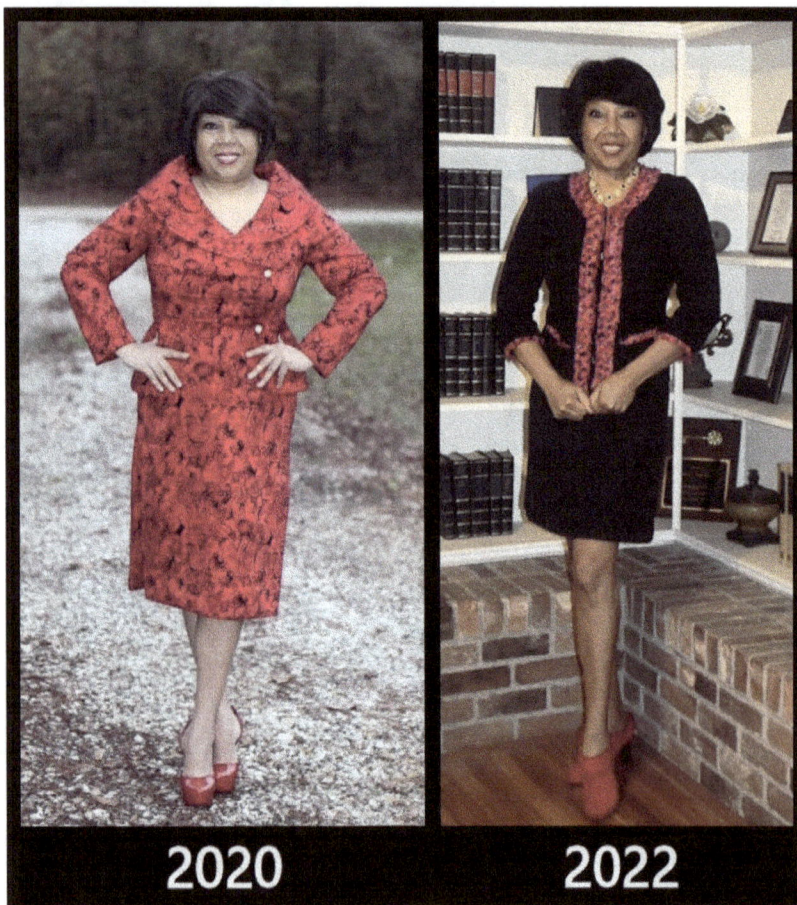

2020   2022

**WARNING:
HUGE PHOTO DUMP
COMING UP !!!**

Online friends and followers have been asking me for years (over 10) to do a book featuring my yard sale and thrift shop finds (including pictures and tips.) I kept telling them "No!" (with no intentions of doing so) This book is going to MORE than make up the years of waiting!:) You're welcome! (You can thank my Mom for this !) Note: 95% of all of the clothing pictures shown are from yard sales and thrift shops or online resale sites (mainly Poshmark) There is a sprinkling of items from ROSS , because it is a favorite place to find great bargains! I must give a shout out to Hubby, who has been my own personal shopper for the past several years. He is an expert on what I like!

I TAUGHT HIM VERY WELL ! :) These days , I just have to sit back and let the rewards of that FABULOUS training pour in ! (And, I do mean POUR!)

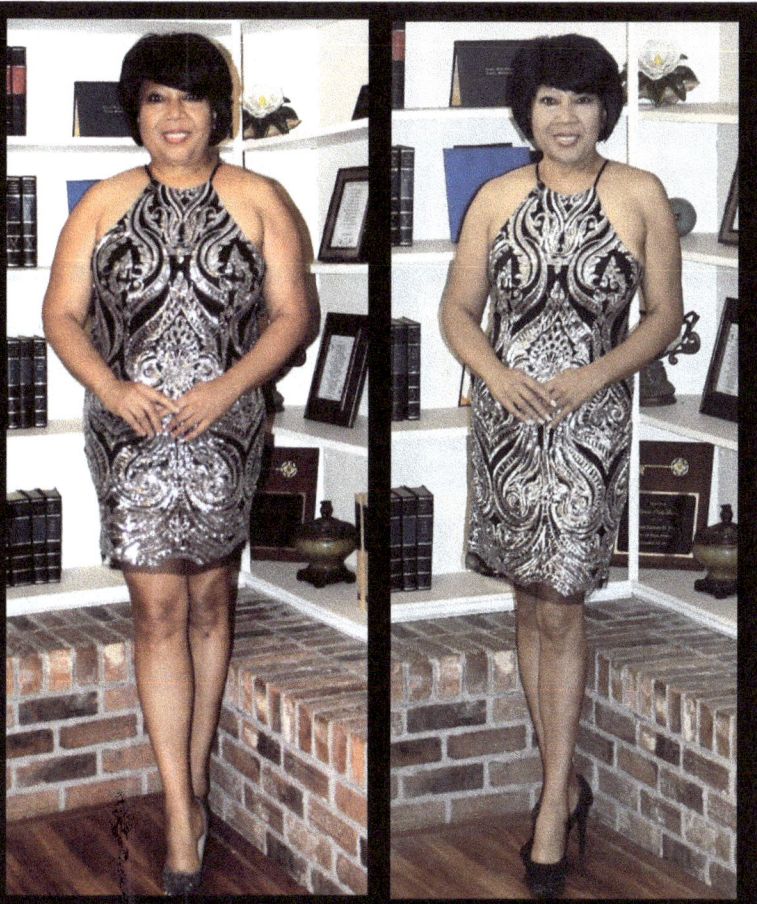

DEC 2021	DEC 2022

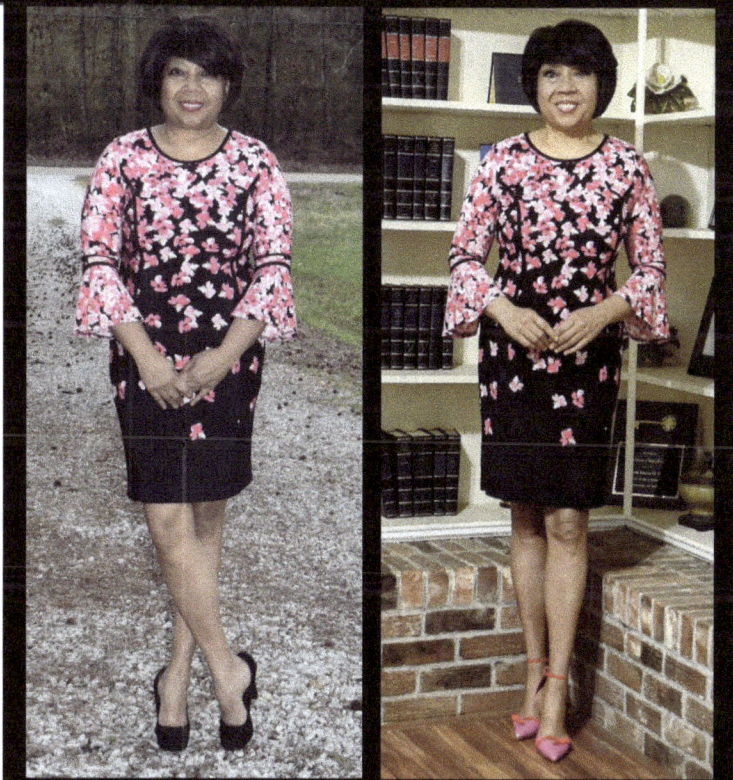

March 2020	April 2023

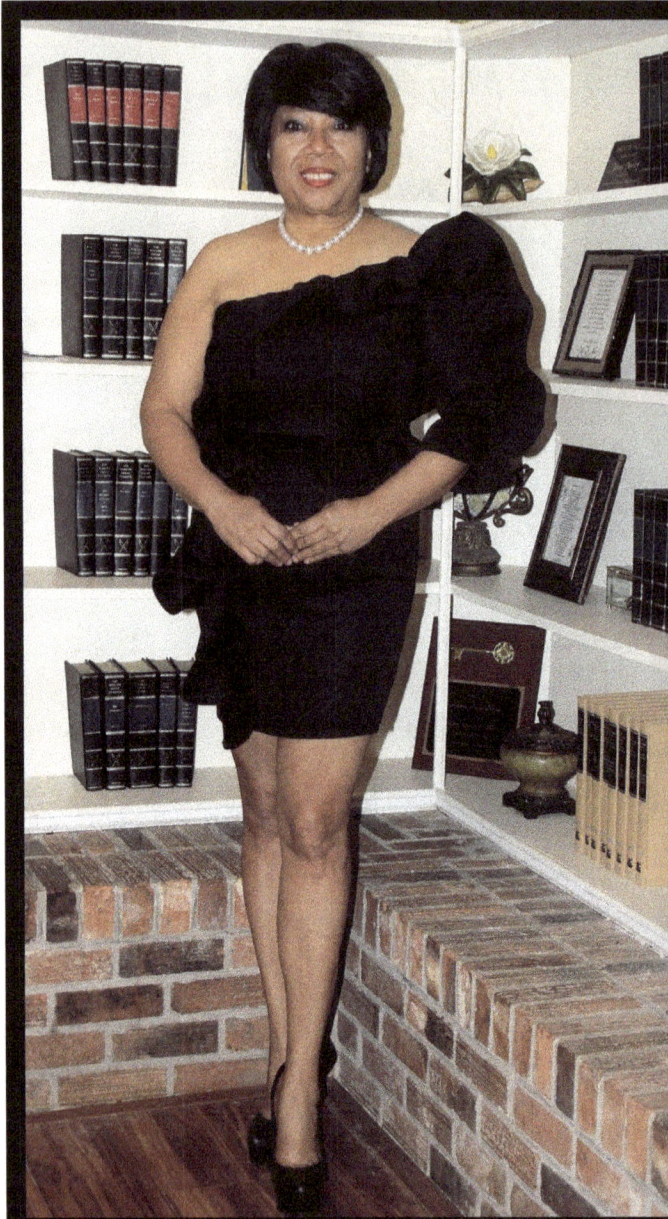

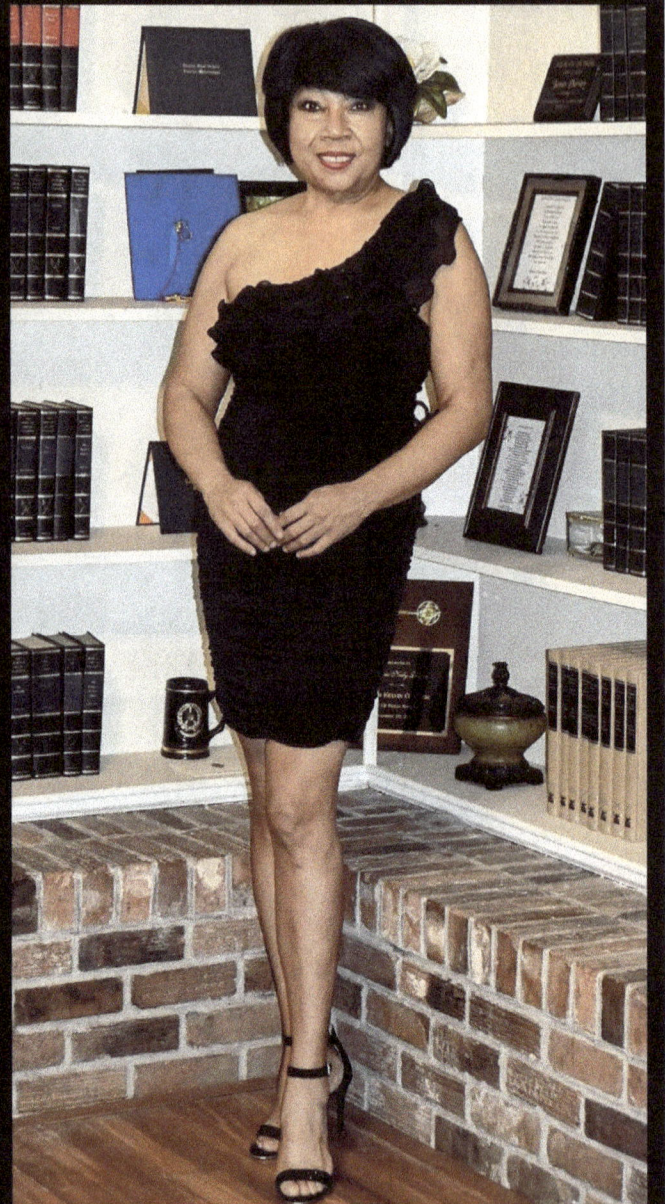

Feb 2022

Feb 2023

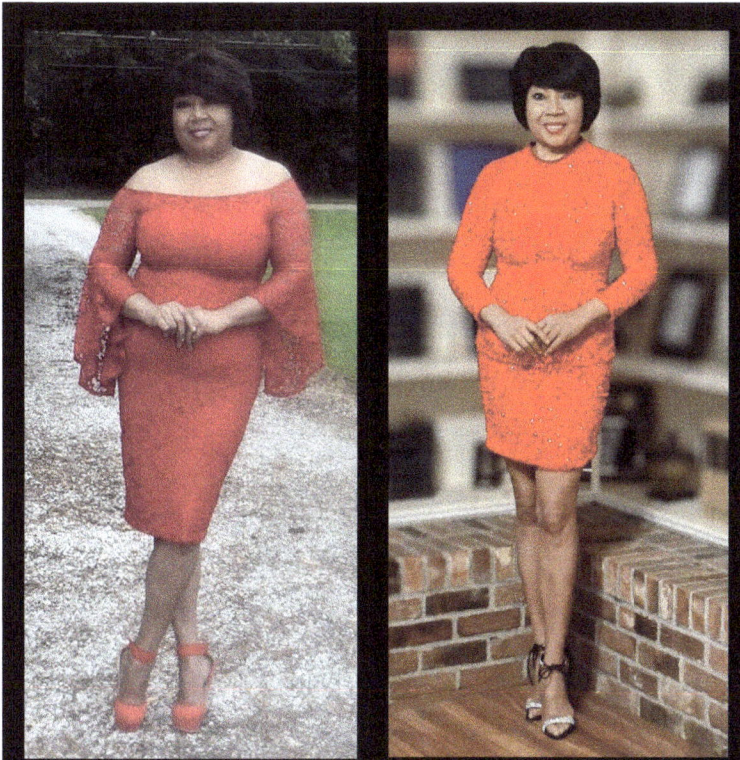

Aug 2020   Feb 2023

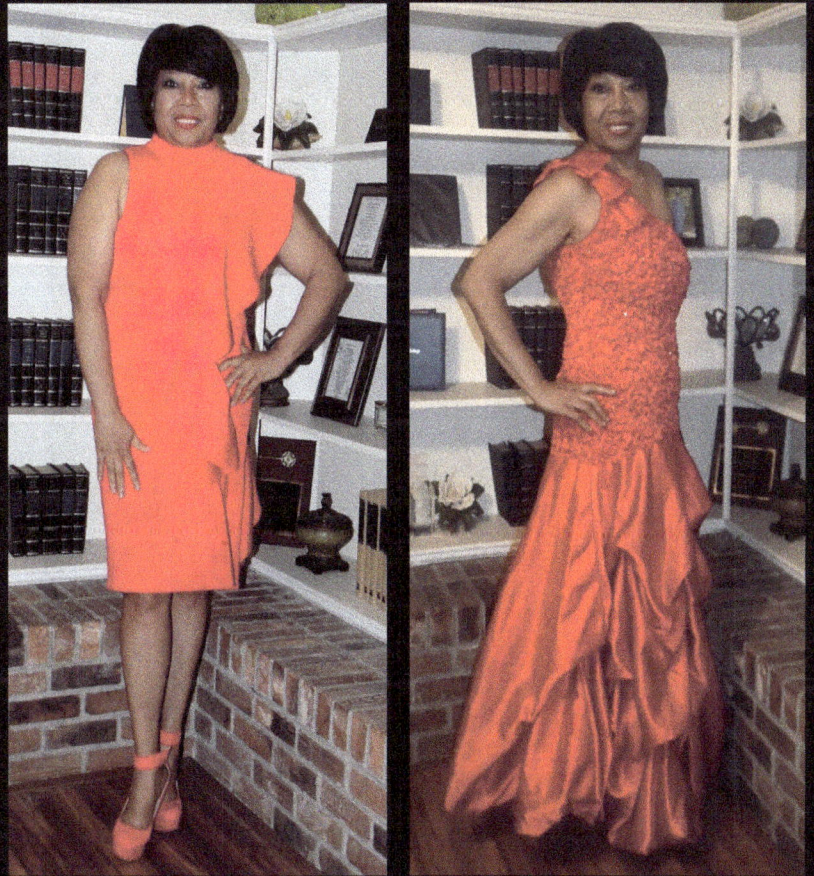

Feb 2022   Nov 2022

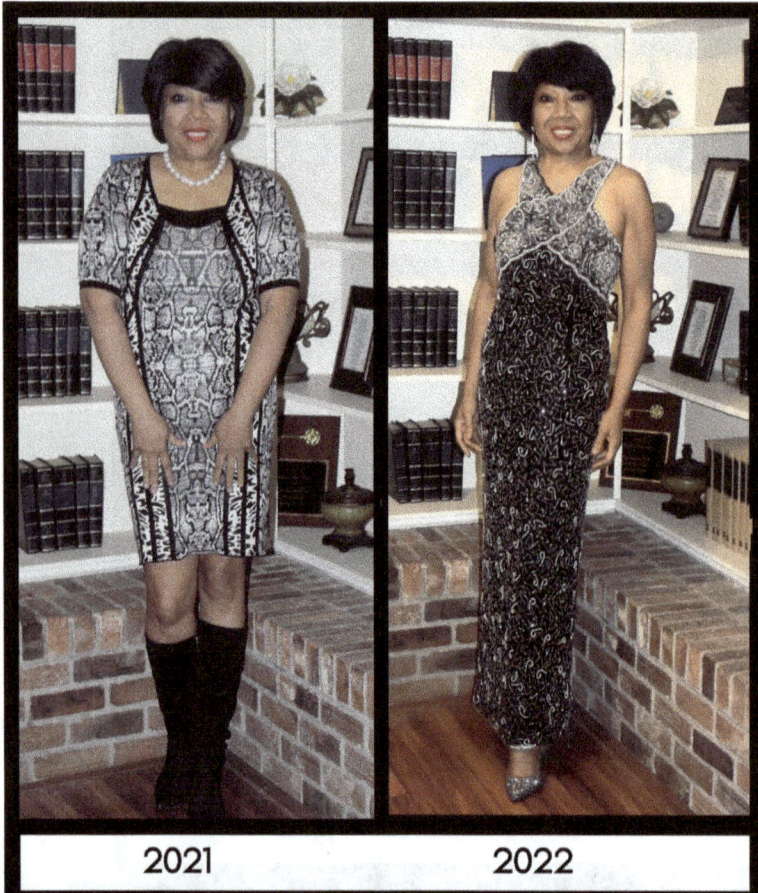

2021   2022

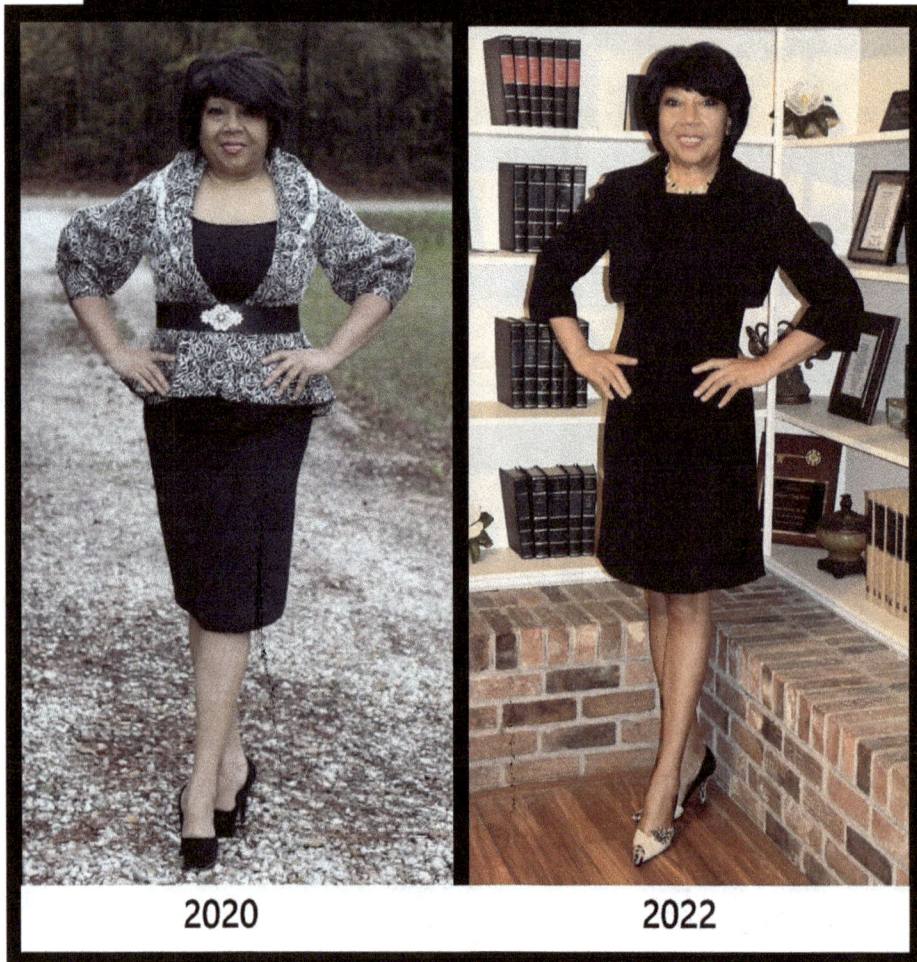

2020   2022

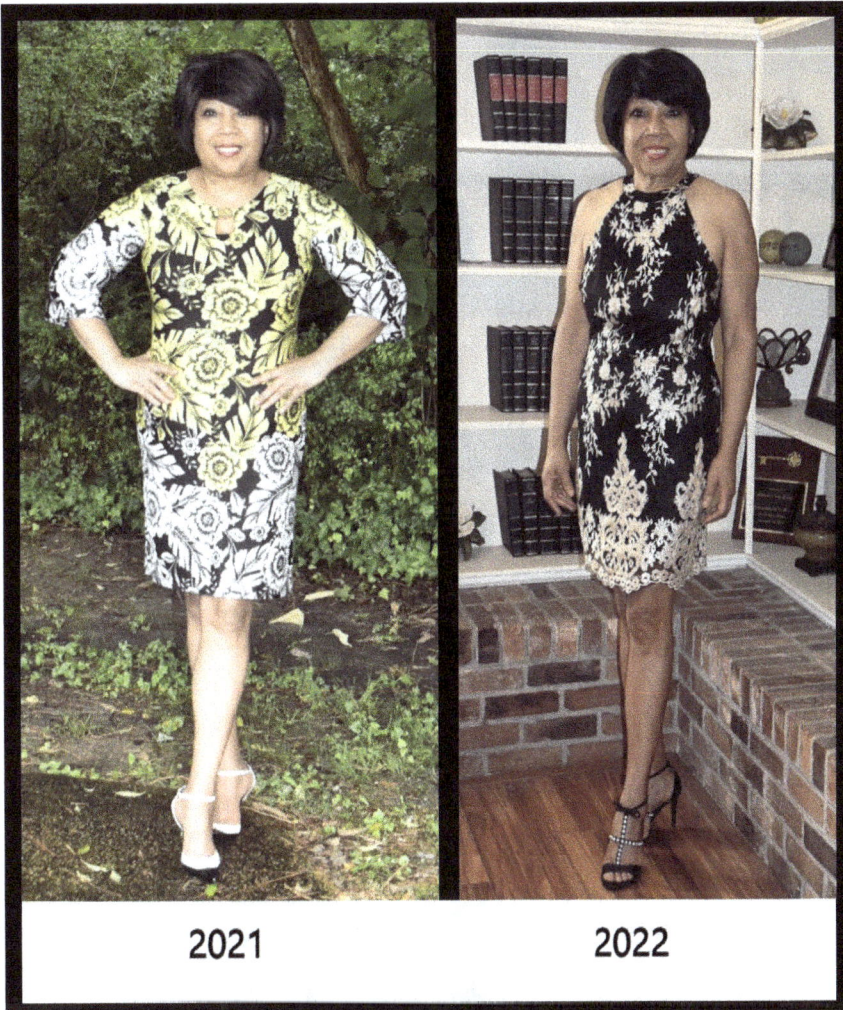

2021   2022

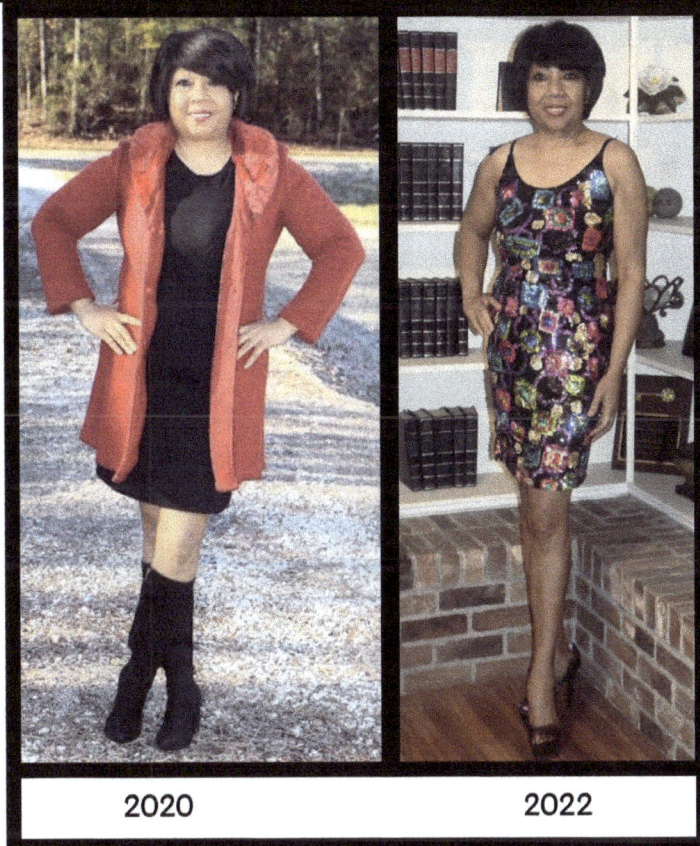

2020   2022

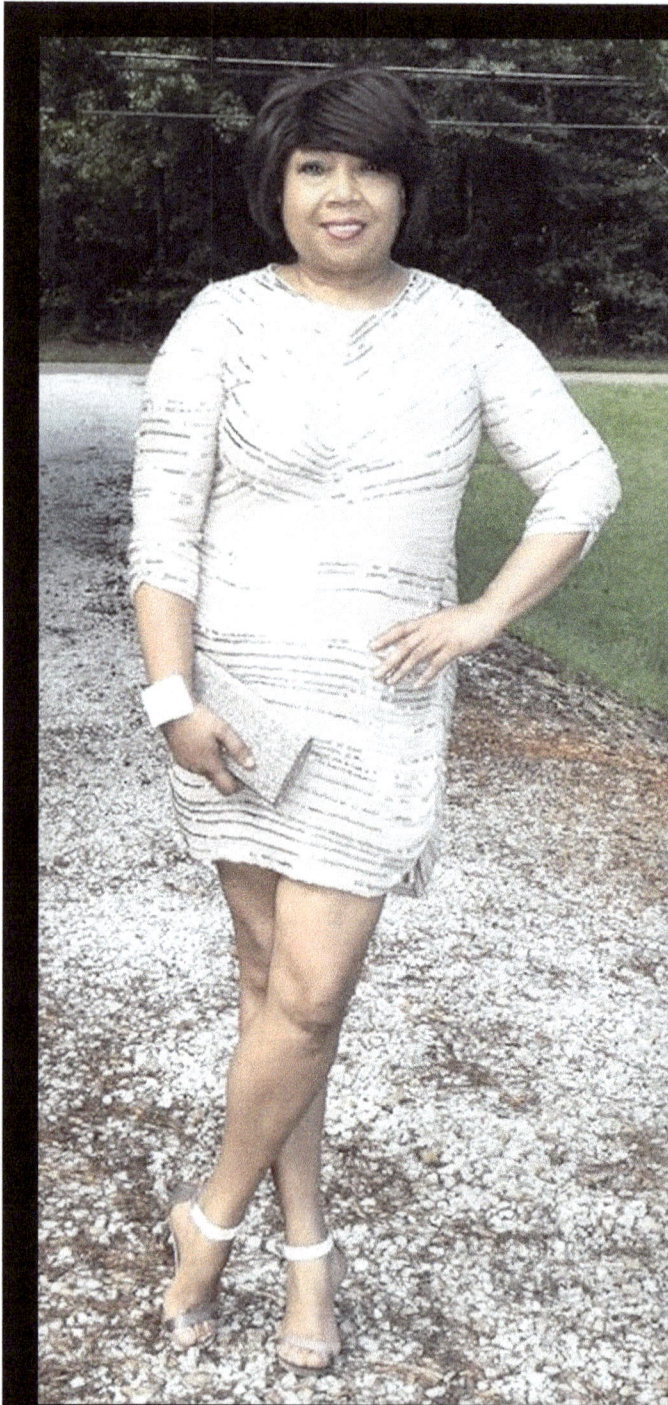

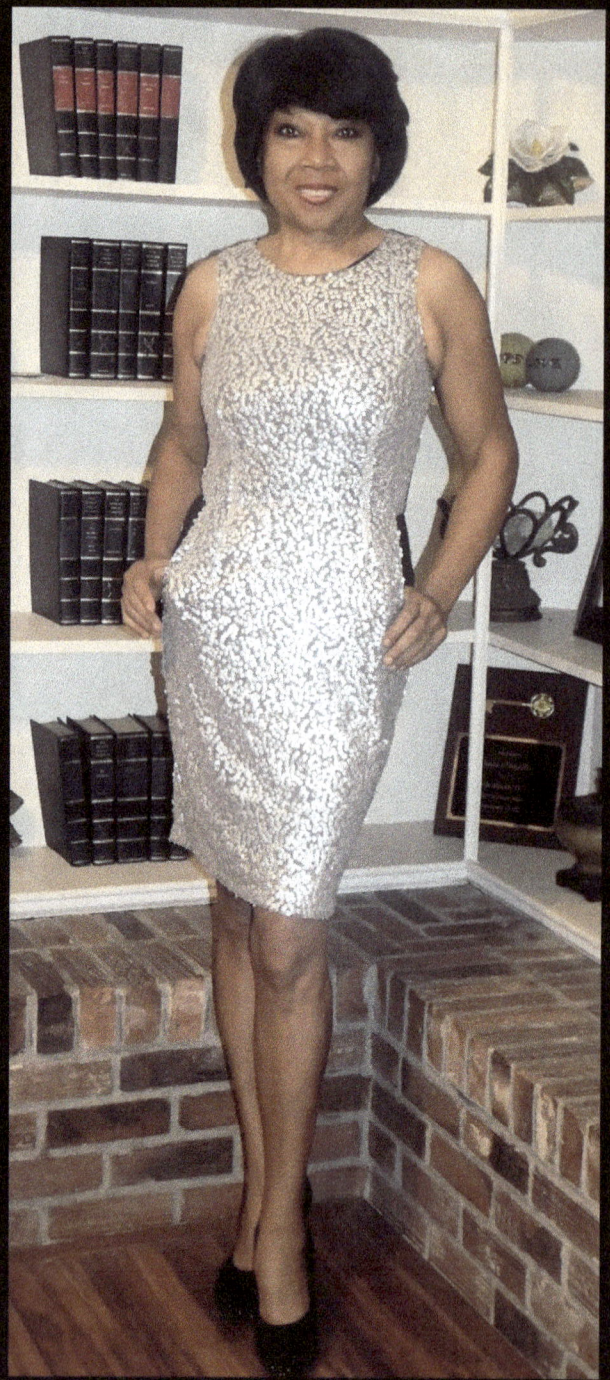

2020   2022

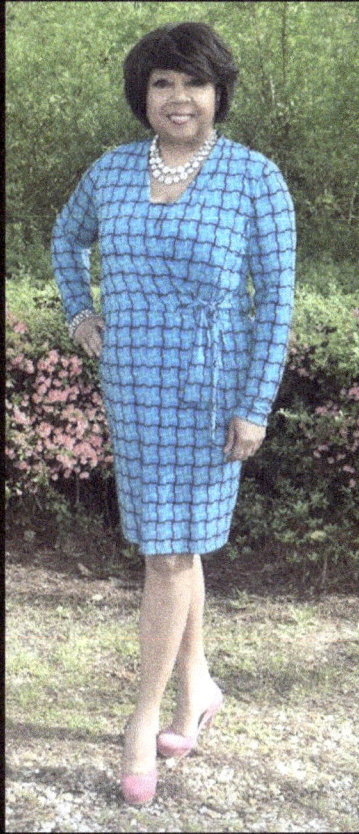

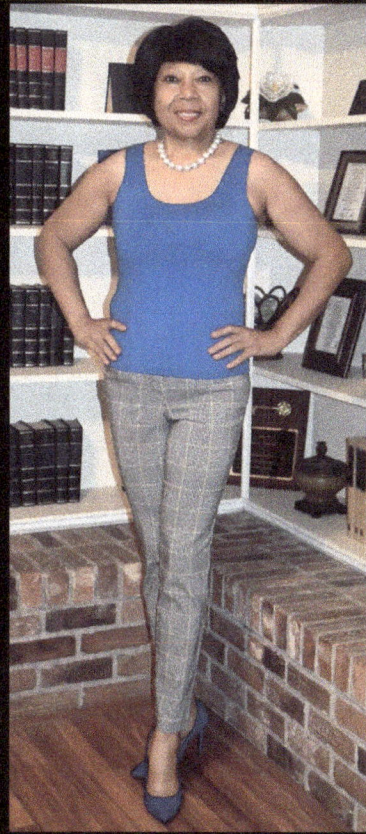

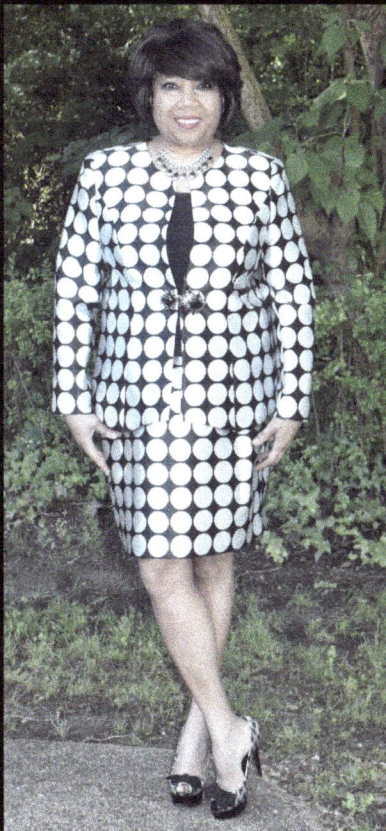

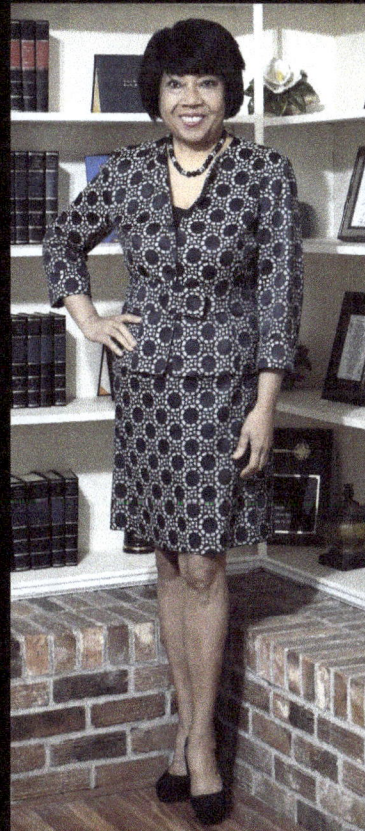

May 2020   March 2023

THE GOAL: BEST SHAPE EVER BY SIXTY

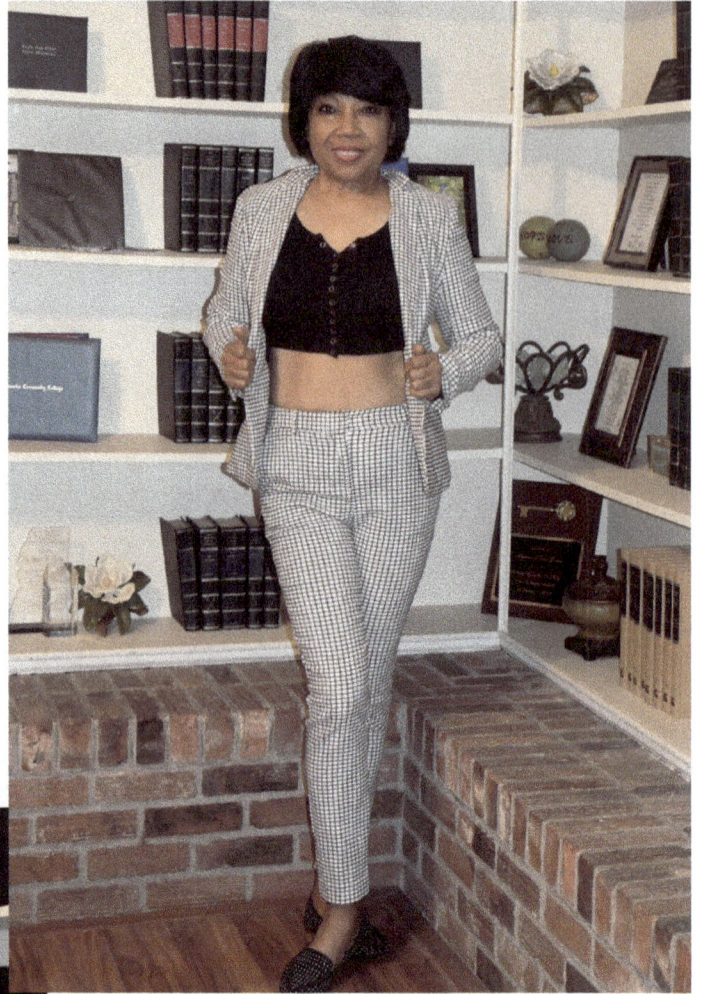

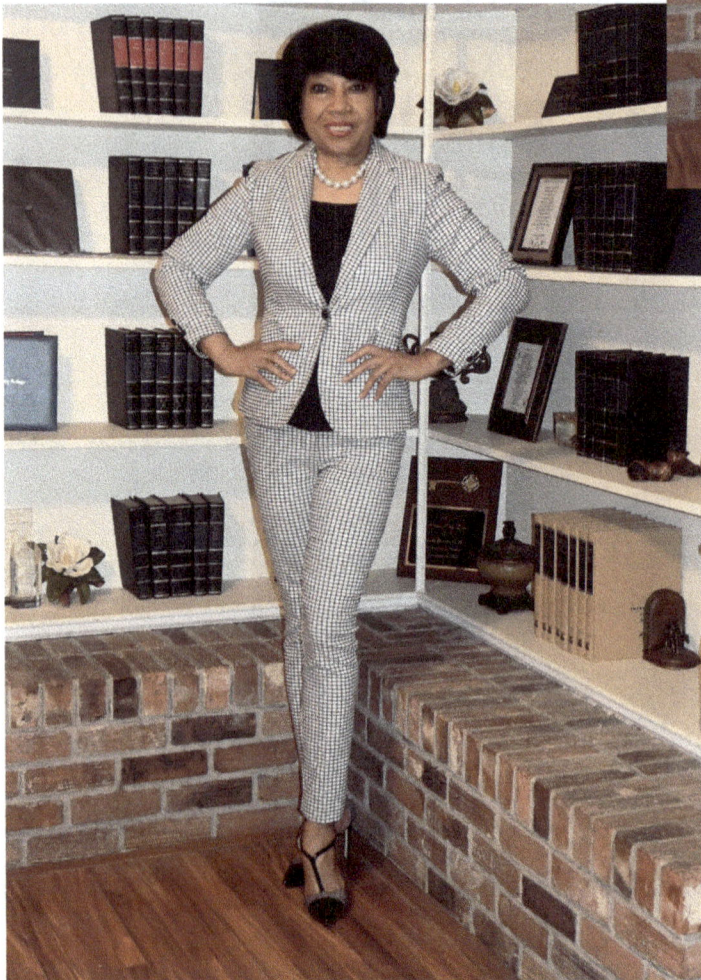

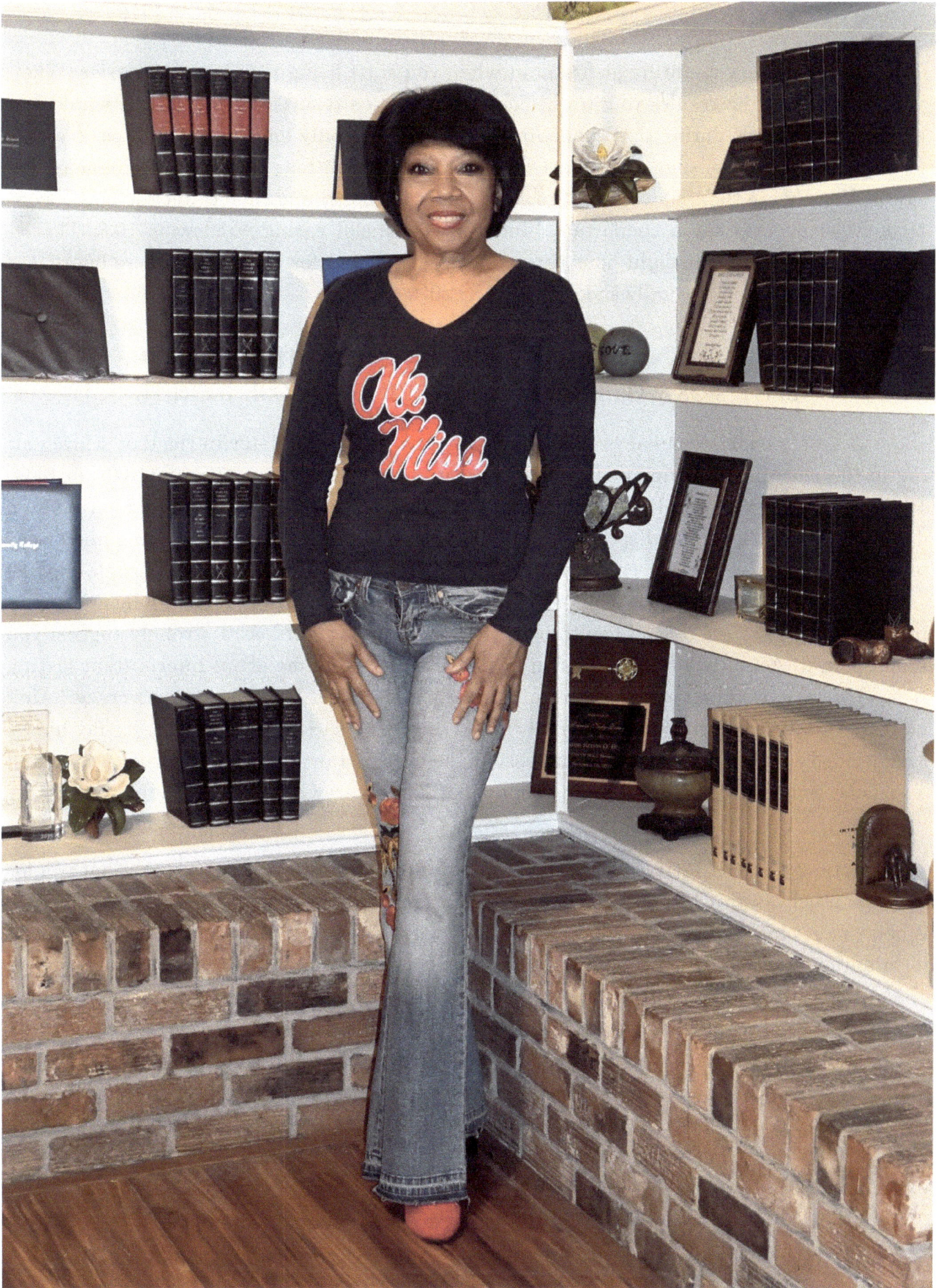

INTERMITTENT FASTING IS REALLY QUITE MAGICAL

It seems very daunting at first, but when you start doing it, it becomes easier. When you start to see the results you are hooked. You will see results. You choose a window of eating and only eat during that time. For best results you only have water and tea or coffee or both Many experts suggest at least drinking some green tea. No sugar or creamer . No juices. You choose the time you want to start eating each day and then count the hours from that. Most experts say a comfortable and very beneficial eating window is 16:8. This is where you eat during an eight hour period and you don't eat for 16 hrs. The more hours you don't eat , the better. I usually shoot for 18:6 or 20:4.

ONE PERSON WHOSE VIDEOS I FOLLOW, SAYS THAT THE 20:4 IS THE "SWEET SPOT" FOR WOMEN WHO ARE TRYING TO LOSE WEIGHT.

A lot of people don't eat breakfast anyway and like eating later in the day. I love eating in the morning. My window is usually   6am-2pm (16/8) or 6am 12noon (18/6) or 6am-10am (20/4). But you can always switch up the times that you start and end your eating window to fit your schedule and special events. Some people do alternate day fasting and swear by it. That is where you eat one day and you don't eat the next day. You alternate days of eating. There are tons of Facebook pages and You Tube videos that you can follow for more information. There are tons of health benefits far beyond weight loss! I strongly suggest you read up on it! Actually a friend/sister in Christ at church told me about intermittent fasting several years ago when I asked her about her weight loss. But, I told her "That's crazy!" Ain't no way. "I'll just be fat!" When I started REALLY getting serious about changing my habits and decided that I wanted to get in my best shape ever, I started looking up information and You Tube videos. Intermittent fasting kept popping up everywhere! I decided to give it a try.

I started with a 12:12 eating window where I gave myself 12 hours to eat. That is a lot. Way too much! But, it helped to ease me in to the routine. Soon, going to 16:8 was a breeze. When you get into the 18 hours and above that's when you really have to dig in with your determination and dedication. You can really eat almost anything during your eating window and still lose weight. But, eating healthier choices is by far much better. A plant based (minimal meat/no red meat) diet is best. This year, when that friend at church started seeing a dramatic difference in my weight, she came up to me and asked, "What in the world are you doing?" I laughed and told her intermittent fasting. I said "Don't you remember YOU were the one who first told me about it? She told me later that a nurse at the hospital had told her about it.

"THE BEST OF ALL MEDICINES ARE RESTING AND FASTING." BENJAMIN FRANKLIN

INTERMITTENT FASTING IS SOMETHING I WANT TO TELL EVERYONE ABOUT

It's really funny , and quite ironic, that my 87 year old mother has been intermittent fasting (16/8) for almost 40 years and really didn't even know it. She eats her breakfast and lunch and usually eats nothing after about 1:00 o'clock until the next morning. She has been a vegetarian that long also. Just recently she decided to go vegan (no eggs, cheese, dairy). Intermittent fasting is something I wish everyone would at least give it a try! Of course, I know, you can lead a horse to water but you can't make him drink . I was certainly a very stubborn horse, at least initially, in most of my fitness journey! We hope that this book might play a part in inspiring others to consider some of the healthier lifestyle choices that we know have benefited us tremendously!

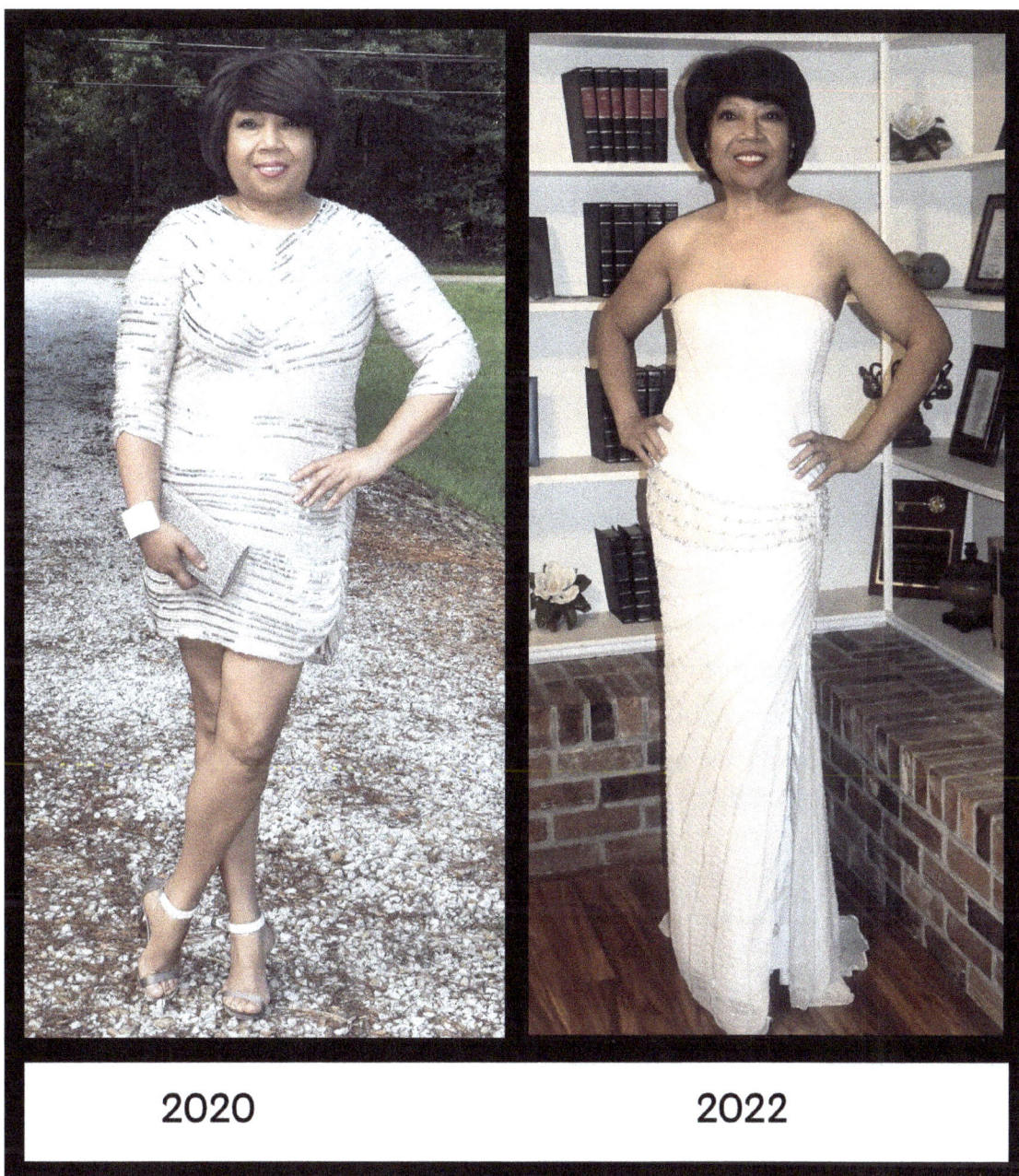

2020   2022

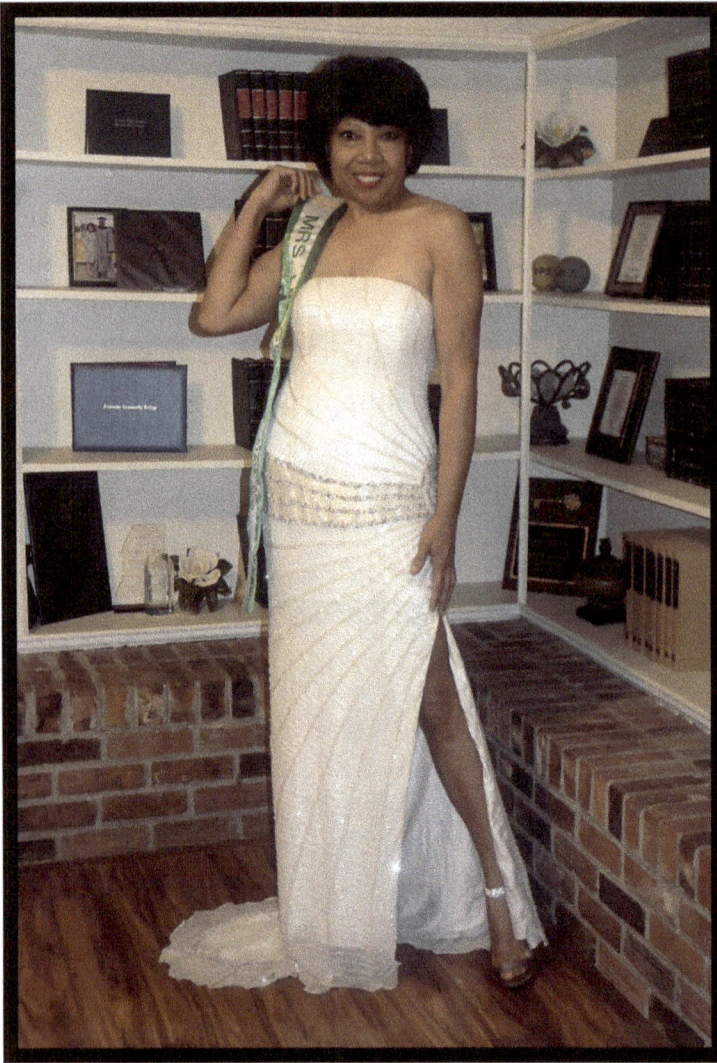

So, you know about my fitness journey and about the post that my fitness trainer posted which included my absolute disdain for exercise! What you might not know is that disdain for exercise and physical exertion goes back a LONG way! My dear lifelong friend, Ronnie Agnew ,who has held many high powered, executive level jobs (including general manager of WOSU Public Media in Ohio and executive director for Mississippi Public Broadcasting (MPB), but is a true journalist at heart. sent me an e-mail with a little "story" of his own about my journey. He has known me forever, so he has some unique insights and observations about it all ! I am sure you will find it amusing :) !

Ronnie Agnew was born in Saltillo, Mississippi. He graduated from Saltillo High School in 1980 and attended the University of Mississippi. He received his B.A. degree in English in 1984 and worked at The Greenwood Commonwealth in Greenwood, Mississippi.

Ronnie moved to Cincinnati, Ohio, where he worked for the Cincinnati Enquirer. In 1993, Agnew became the managing editor for The Hattiesburg American. He worked at The Hattiesburg American until 1997, and was hired as media general and editor at the Dothan Eagle in Dothan, Alabama.

Ronnie served as the managing editor at The Clarion-Ledger in 2001 and was promoted to executive editor in 2002. Ronnie was the first African American to head The Clarion-Ledger. In 2011, Ronnie was hired as the executive director of Mississippi Public Broadcasting, where he worked until 2021.

Ronnie was inducted into the Ole Miss Alumni Hall of Fame .

He Wrote:

You must understand: Pat and sweat never liked each other.
They had a deal that they would never meet. It was ironclad.

Everyday we did the count, 1,2,3,4,5,6,7... Baseball was our game, and we figured that four against four was the best we could do on the open field near our homes. There was an eighth person on the field. Her name is Pat. But when the count got to Pat, well the count was over. Pat wasn't going to play. It was a fact we accepted. You must understand: Pat and sweat never liked each other. They had a deal that they would never meet. It was ironclad. So there was Pat, sitting happily on the ground as we tried to make four against three work. We never held it against Pat. We understood the importance of her vow to leave sweat alone. She was just fine, thank you very much, without it. The years flew by and Pat and her pact with sweat were still very much in agreement. She would get married. She had a baby. She became a successful local author. As life kept churning, as her family unit bonded, nothing changed in the arrangement Pat had with sweat. They had such disdain for each other, something just short of a hate. While others sweated, Pat shopped at local thrift stores. She bought more shoes than Imelda Marcos, more dresses than Elizabeth Taylor. She had a full closet of them that cost no more than about $12 and 35 cents for the whole collection in her stuffed closet.

While others took time to meet sweat, Pat's lifelong agreement to avoid the drippy stuff enjoyed contractual status. She even considered having her brother Brian, an attorney, draft papers. But wait! In the past few weeks and months, something drastic has happened. Superpowers of the Marvel variety have emerged. I've seen my friend Pat shrink to a size I haven't witnessed since we were younger. Against all odds, Pat and sweat finally had a meeting. It must have been in executive session, which keeps it out of the public view. But being a nosy journalist, I had to know how this occurred. So I called Pat the other day and learned of this monumental change in the sweat world. I learned that she's competing in the Miss Magnolia Mississippi pageant this weekend and that she's spent six months getting in shape.

She's lost 35 pounds. Can't be more than a size four. That's a place where the racks in the department store are lonely for lack of visitors. But there's Pat, with pictures to prove that she's met sweat and has a wardrobe that makes her look like that young girl I knew from all those years ago. But there's Pat, with pictures to prove that she's met sweat and has a wardrobe that makes her look like that young girl I knew from all those years ago.   Obviously, I'm rooting for my friend Patricia Neely-Dorsey to be victorious this weekend. And I have this feeling that Pat and sweat will no longer be strangers. Best friends they will be. While I'm sure she may not enjoy the work behind the sweat that has her in such incredible shape, she surely will enjoy its rewards. We've gotten a little older now, but that makeshift baseball field is still outside her house. Wonder if she's ready to be that eighth player we always lacked on the baseball field. She might be in shape for it, but the other members in the count certainly are not. And it's all because Pat rearranged her contract with sweat and lord have mercy, it shows.

A FITNESS JOURNEY

At 50, I made a decision to take charge of my health and fitness again . I starting doing what I used to do, pre-kids! I was a former ballerina & exercised. But, with the hustle & bustle of kids, work & then hospice caregiving of my mother, I definitely LOST my way and totally forgot about me! After my mother's transition, I knew it was time to find myself again. I don't discuss anyone else's weight or lifestyle. And, I applaud those who are fabulous & loving their size. But for me, gaining weight wasn't "me.!" I wasn't happy being a bigger size. Plus, I've always wanted to not only age…quantity of life….but to age well…quality! I want to be here as long as possible & be at my optimal self , not only for my kids, but, more importantly for MYSELF!

So, I made myself a priority again. I roughly walk 5 miles at least 4 of 7 days. I'm a HUGE water drinker, always have been. The biggest thing I cut, was drinking cokes. I love a good ice cold coke, but I had to stop drinking them, although, not entirely. Now, when I have a coke, I treat it like a treat, like having a dessert, only every now and then . My eating isn't about restricting myself. It's more about moderation and actually increasing what I eat. As a mother, I got into running the kids everywhere and sometimes only eating once a day, which was usually a huge meal at night or too much fast food. Now, I force myself to eat several meals a day. It makes me   intentional about sitting down and eating during the day. I only have fast food, every now & then. I have increased my vegetables & fruits. I also strength train with resistance bands AND weights.

As we age, it's crucial that we lift weights. You don't have to be a gym rat or overdo it . Simple low hand weights or kettlebells will do. And, don't forget about the power of stretching the body. My system involves very simple changes that have made a huge difference in my overall health and wellness. I definitely intend to be Fit and Fabulous For Life!

-Kimberly L. Campbell, Esq.
Kimberly joined AARP Mississippi in May 2016 as the AARP Mississippi State Director.
Kimberly is the former Mississippi State Representative for District 72, which encompasses Hinds and Madison counties. She served in the Mississippi legislature for nearly nine years. Additionally ,Kimberly practiced law for 15 years. Kimberly received a Bachelor of Arts Degree in English from Mississippi State University, a Masters Degree in Organizational Communications from Auburn University and a Juris Doctor from the University of Mississippi School of Law. Kimberly lives in Madison, Mississippi.

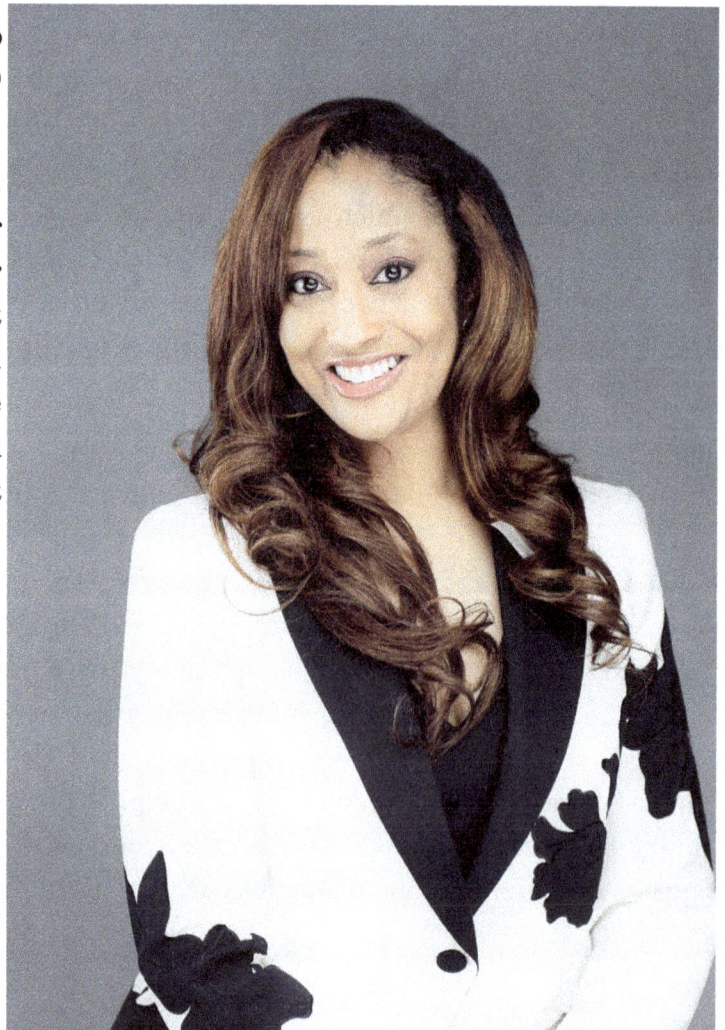

Facebook Friend Cathy Hutchison, Carrollton, TX
Facebook Messages Starting October 2022

Cathy: Do you have time for a call? I want to hear what you did to get in shape.

Patricia: Yes, always. You can call me now.

Patricia: The 14day Keto Cleanse diet will give you step by step instructions to get on track. I think you should start with this. It is not strict keto and it is not all plant based, but a great jump off place.

Cathy: Thank you!! John is on board in doing this. I'm watching videos this weekend and taking the advice you gave on the phone to write out a plan. My hope is to start on Monday.

Patricia: Wonderful! Get the book JJ Smith New Keto Cleanse to give you a really great guideline for a really strong start! Happy Anniversary! Have a great day and weekend!

Cathy: I feel hopeful.

Patricia: You Should!

Patricia: Another great book for deeper insight into fasting is "Fast, Feast, Repeat" by Gin Stephens

Cathy: I'm ready!

Patricia: WooHoo! You/we're off... on an amazing journey!!! Wonderful!

Patricia: Today is the day ! I am so excited for the start of the journey for you (and John)! It will be transformational ! I will be here to cheer you on ! What will be your eating window for your 16:8 fasting? A lot of people choose something like 10am-6pm It's a good comfortable schedule for all the meals. I love eating early so I start my eating window at 6am with a smoothie . So on the 16:8 schedule I would stop eating after 2pm. But, lately, getting ready for the pageant, I most often try to do 20:4 with a four our eating window So after 10am, I am usually not eating. If I extend my window I try to make a rule to stop eating after noon. Months ago, when I started, my journey, I couldn't imagine that ! I am such a grazer and love eating all day ! (or at least I did...until I realized what it does to your body/insulin/fat storage!) For best results I would definitely suggest closing your eating window by 7pm. (That would be 11-7)

Today on the menu is the Vanilla /Avocado smoothie. I love avocados and I love them in my smoothies. It makes them so creamy! I look forward to my smoothies every day ! Everyone says the Pumpkin Chili is delicious! I haven't tried it yet But, I plan on doing so in the future. Let me know what you (and John) think! Make sure to keep in your journal what you eat and what time you eat . Weigh yourself every morning as soon as you get up and put the number at the top of your journal /food chart page each day. At the end of the day, at the bottom of the page write a little note about how you feel . Best Wishes ! Much Love!

Cathy: Yay! You are so awesome and encouraging I'm eating 7-3. Yoga class at 5:30am. Walk in the evening And I have all the turkey pumpkin chili ingredients ready for lunch. I'm having to adjust the smoothies a bit because I'm allergic to tree nuts (also shellfish) but the ratios will be the same. I'll use water instead of almond milk I ate clean keto all weekend and aside from waking very thirsty with a mild headache I'm good! (I wanted to get going!)

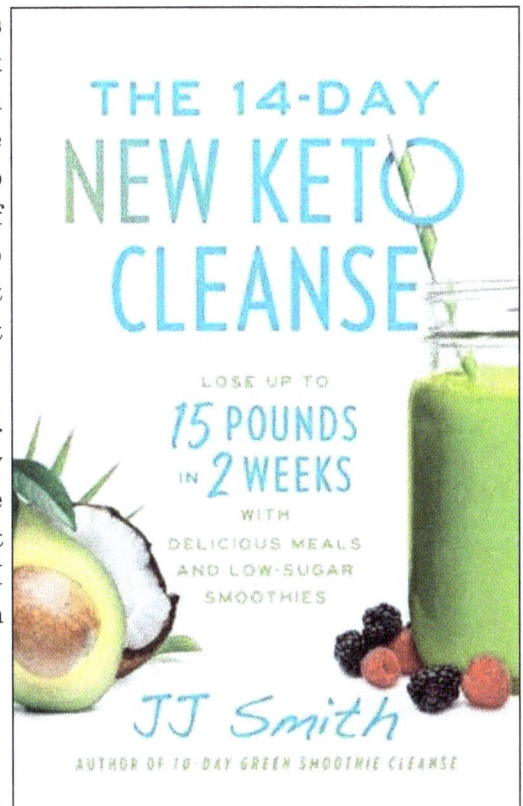

Patricia: Wonderful ! Wonderful ! This is going to be great! The wonderful thing about the smoothies and the intermittent fasting is that it is all adjustable ! After the 14 days you will be ready to basically know the kinds of things that appeal to you, you want to eat and that work for you !

Patricia: That was good to be thirsty waking up Because it will remind you to start drinking your water as soon as you get up

Cathy: Everything went great and the pumpkin chili was delicious tonight I have a fancy client dinner so I'll have to navigate "in the wild ". My strategy is to stay keto and eat only enough to be polite. Herbal tea when dessert comes. Now off to yoga!

Patricia: Going great! Workout good on yesterday ! I have 5 more sessions with trainer and I am going to take a break from trainer during holidays season and probably go to gym now and then . Eating 6am-10am today

Patricia: I can hardly believe that there are only 3 more weeks (a little less) till pageant day ! I feel good about where I am as far as preparation ! P.S. have decided to go with my first choice in dresses. It is more me and I feel more comfortable in it .

Patricia: Just checking in to see how your week went with your new lifestyle changes with lumps and bumps and ups and downs. Remember it is a wellness journey! (A journey of a thousand miles begins with one step...and then another...and another) It is not a quick fix or fad diet. It is a distance run/race and not a sprint. What went well? What went not so well? How did you feel ? How was the weight loss?

Cathy: First, this is very doable. It's my new life It's an identity shift." I'm a person who doesn't eat things that aren't aligned with my goals " Navigating some circumstances is hard. I'm going to the Cowboy game today and packed things I can eat. There's a no food rule and they search bags. Pray they let me take in my boiled eggs and celery sticks otherwise it could be a long day I feel great I lost 6.6 pounds this week. My body likes this way of eating. Thanks for being the best mentor

Patricia: That is more than wonderful !!! Great job !!! It is sooo doable ! You've got this ! Love being your Best Shape/Best Life Ever Buddy !

Cathy: John is doing this too with some adjustments. I can't wait to hear what he lost but I can see it in his face.

Patricia: wonderful!!

Cathy: John lost 9 pounds

Patricia: Wonderful !!!

Patricia: Good Morning ! Happy Halloween ! How did the game go? Did they let your eggs and celery pass through the gates ? What's your plan for today ?

Cathy: They did let it in! Just got back from yoga and am having my smoothie. Salmon and Brussels sprouts on the menu today. How are you doing?

Patricia: Sounds great! Doing good ! Feeling good ! My Sundays lately have been fast days . I am 5 lbs from my goal weight . I should be right on point by pageant day .

Cathy: I lost 2lbs last week. Motivation is high. Was able to stay on plan in social situations. I'm staying on the cleanse this week. It fits nicely into my lifestyle.

Cathy: They did let it in! Just got back from yoga and am having my smoothie. Salmon and Brussels sprouts on the menu today. How are you doing?

Cathy: How is your week going?

Patricia: Sounds great ! 1-2 lbs each week is a good sustainable goal on the road to your goal weight . I am doing good ! I have reached my goal with my trainer and she is very pleased . She will be printing my weight loss journey story next week , The pageant is next weekend ! I am excited ! I am ready ! Please ask friends and family to vote for me for People's Choice ! I want to win that People's Choice crown !

Patricia: Just checking in to see how the week has gone ... Diet, exercise, challenges, triumphs

Cathy: I lost another pound and am very committed to staying on plan. I'm going to yoga 3-4 days a week and have been lifting weights (just 3 reps of 10) in the evenings. How will you navigate Thanksgiving weekend?

Patricia: Wonderful! Sounds great ! Thanksgiving won't be hard for me because we won't be having any type of large family gathering . It will just be me , James , Henry and Mom ...so really we will be eating like we usually eat and Mom has been doing the heathy eating /vegetarian thing for over 35 years !

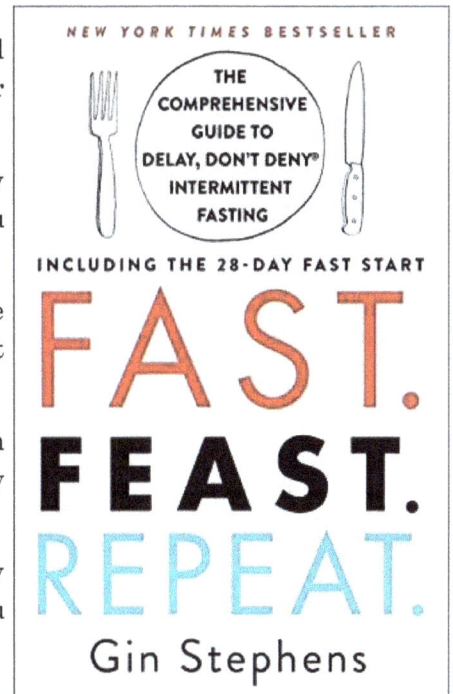

NEW YORK TIMES BESTSELLER

THE COMPREHENSIVE GUIDE TO DELAY, DON'T DENY® INTERMITTENT FASTING

INCLUDING THE 28-DAY FAST START

FAST.
FEAST.
REPEAT.

Gin Stephens

Photo taken the weekend I called Patricia to ask what she was doing to improve her health.

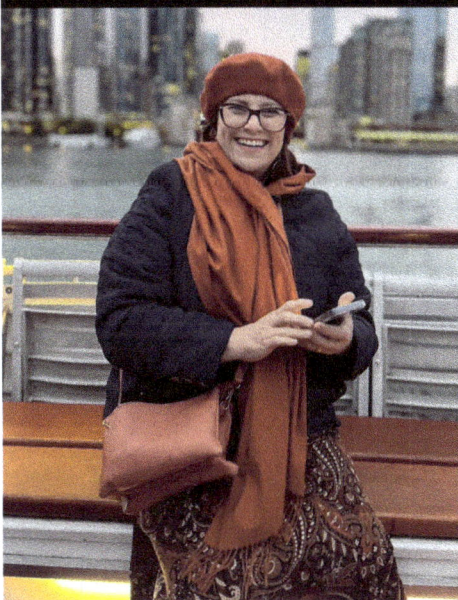

Photo taken four months later after following Patricia's advice.

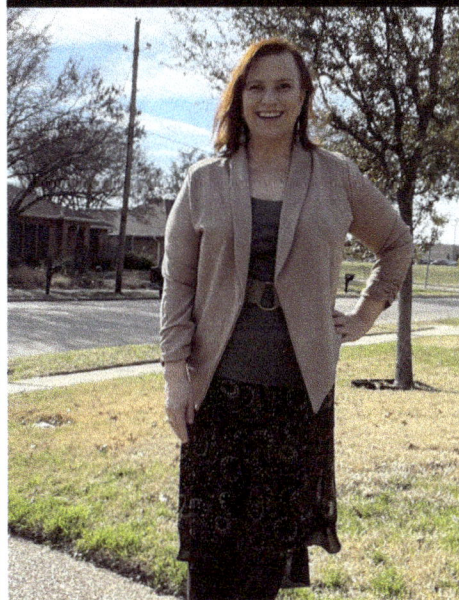

Message : January 14, 2023

Hi Patricia! I have some exciting news this morning! I am down 20 lbs from when I first called you back in October sitting at the airport. And while this isn't my final destination, it is a REALLY IMPORTANT MILESTONE. So I 100% had to reach out to celebrate. Thank you for being so inspiring and sharing your knowledge with me and others.

You shine so beautifully and teach the rest of us to do that too. Thanks for mentoring me.

BEING INSPIRED

Throughout the year 2022, I watched in awe & admiration as Patricia Neely-Dorsey embarked upon a journey of getting into the best shape of her life. She openly shared with the world the things that she was doing to hit milestones & achieve her fitness goals. One of the things that she shared that really stood out to me was that she was changing her diet to mimic more the diet of her mother Mrs. Elaine Neely.

Mrs. Neely had been a long term vegetarian and in recent years has become a vegan. And though she is a woman of a certain age; Patricia stated that Mrs. Neely is on NO medication!! This fact was remarkable to me because I was/am aware that nearly 70% of all Americans are on at least 1 prescription drug. Yet, Mrs. Neely, as a senior citizen, is not. Amazing!

Patricia also shared that she was also combining intermittent fasting along with modest exercise throughout the week to help her reach her goals. And boy could we see the results! Not only that, I knew for myself that each of the things that she mentioned really did work because I had incorporated them into my own lifestyle for many years to great results but in the last few years had given in to the SAD (Standard American Diet) lifestyle.

It saddens me to now admit that though I watched and applauded Patricia's progress throughout 2022; at that time I made no personal changes myself. That is, until the end of 2022. At that time, I determined that starting in January 2023; if things were going to change; I had to change them. And I DID! Now I haven't done things perfectly and I give myself plenty of grace when I don't quite meet the mark; but I DO keep showing up for myself. And, just 4 months after beginning; my blood pressure is consistently great for the first time in years, I sleep wonderfully, I have little to no inflammation or joint pain and I am over 20+ pounds lighter. So I must sincerely thank Mrs. Neely and Patricia for being a source of inspiration for not only me but countless others. Our health is truly our wealth.

-ChristyRenee' Williams

I want to be healthy more than anything. I want to be free from meds, bad feeling day, no energy and lots of things. Diabetes is hereditary in my family and I've gone from size 12-20 over the years. On February 1/23 I began a healthier life changing journey. Inspired by Mrs. Elaine Neely and my lifelong friend and classmate ,Patricia Neely Dorsey I decided to eat a plant based diet. Patricia has shared on Facebook that her mother had been a vegetarian for years and was 80+ and was not on any meds or had any health issues. I knew that was my goal in life, to get off meds, and live a long healthy life.

So far I've been dedicated to my choice and have lost 15 lbs. I'm determined to stay on this journey for myself, my grandchildren, and to enjoy the freedom from medicine. I want to personally want to thank Mrs. Neely and Patricia for sharing their journeys and inspiring me to want to eat healthier so I can live longer and be around for many more years to come. I have cut out a lot of bread. I eat fruit and veggies, lots of greens, cabbage, sweet potato and blackeye peas (which I never ate before) that's the honest truth... never liked them . But, Mrs. Neely eats them, now so do I. I am drinking more water (which I hate drinking) Again, I'm following my Inspiration. Also, I have cut out eating sweets on a regular basis .

Jewel (Mabry) Bumphis

MICHAELA: A FITNESS JOURNEY

Losing someone close to you unexpectedly will have you rethink your lifestyle and way of living. For me, that is what led me to my decision to get back on track on becoming a healthier me. I made a choice back in 2020 during the pandemic ,that I was going to start working on becoming a healthier me. Before I started , I did my research on different types of diets, including diet pills, supplements ect. that I thought might help start my weight loss journey. After doing the research, I finally choose what I felt would work best for me and my body type. I chose to go with intermittent fasting. Intermittent fasting is where you have different time frames where you eat and fast. I chose to do the 16:8 intermittent fasting where I would fast for 16 hours and only eat 8 hours throughout each day. My time frames lately are from 12noon-6PM (6hrs0 or some days I do 1-7PM (6hrs) it just depends on my schedule on that day. During the times that I eat , I incorporate the Keto diet along with doing low carb and eating smaller portions. The keto diet consists of less carbs and all the healthy foods and fats with no sugar or bread. I also drink tons of water. Water is your friend even if you are not trying to lose weight. We all need water on a daily basis. Keto is good for you but you have to be careful with staying on this kind of diet for a long period of time.

I also knew I had to begin to get active. I started by going to the track and taking slow brisk walks for 30-45 minutes. I started with a mile and worked my way up to 3 miles and started doing that 5-6 days a week. At the gym, I started going to different work out classes along with lifting weight, leaving myself a day during the week to rest which is usually on Sundays. Throughout my weight loss journey I have struggled and sometimes I find myself wanting to stop. I always remind myself the journey won't be easy but it will be worth it. Becoming a healthier version of yourself is a commitment. If you are serious about it then once your mind changes, then your body will automatically follow. My motto that I live by is "ONE DAY AT TIME", because it won't happen overnight. I can honestly say throughout my weight loss journey I have grown spiritually, emotionally, physically, and mentally within all the areas in my life. I am definitely becoming a better version of myself not only for me but for my family as well. My confidence and self worth is through the roof, now! I chose to love myself first this time around and it feels amazing! Self love is mandatory so whatever you have to do to get to a healthier you then do just that no matter how long it may take. Just stick with it, because the results are worth it.

PND: Slow and steady wins the race! Michaela says that she has lost a total of 55 lbs since starting her journey and says that she averages 2-4 lbs a month. Michaela is the absolutely gorgeous daughter of my classmate, Evangeline Burks Hayden, who passed away at the age of 49 from a heart attack. #GoneTooSoon She is also is my sister in Christ and a member of The North Green Street Church of Christ.

Michaela Fitzpatrick

Work in progress

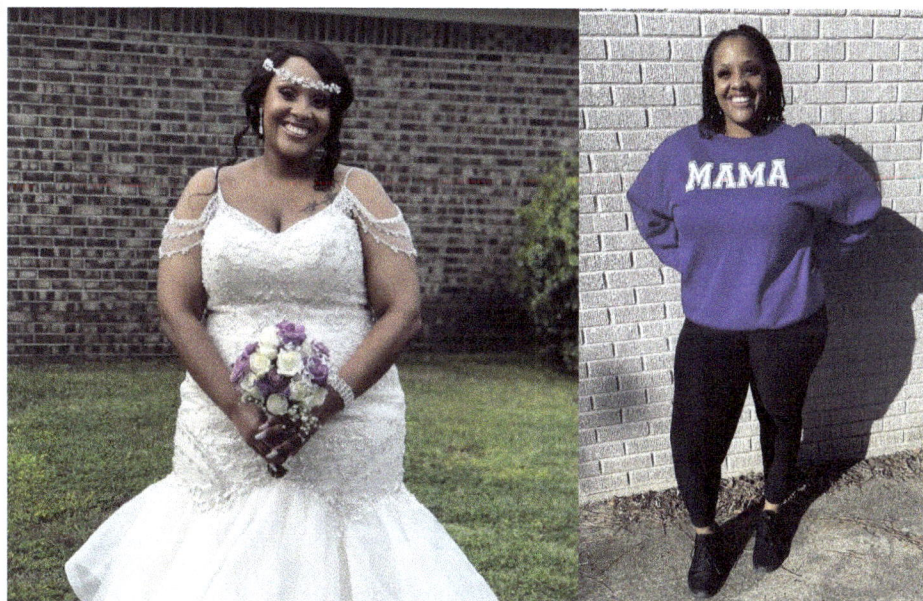

Thirty-eight years ago I became a vegetarian. One Sunday I cooked a pot roast with potatoes, carrots, and onions. I ate two servings of vegetables and no meat. From that day forward I ate no meat. I continued to prepare the regular meals for the family with emphasis on healthy foods. I ate all foods except meat. We ate our share of mangoes, strawberries, kiwi, bananas, grapes, asparagus, broccoli, carrots, collard, mustard, and turnip greens, green peas, green beans, squash, and tomatoes. Prior to becoming a vegetarian I was always health conscious.

Every month I purchased Woman's Day and Family Circle magazines. Those magazines introduced me to healthy ways of eating. Wheat germ was a grain that gained a lot of attention. Berries and cinnamon were mentioned frequently. I kept berries and wheat germ in the refrigerator. One-half teaspoon of cinnamon sprinkled over cereal was a daily breakfast for thirty-eight years. One magazine recommended cinnamon to help prevent high blood pressure. At one point during those years I began to eat two meals daily. The magazines also suggested eating no food after a specified time. I had no idea I had begun to practice intermittent fasting. I was aware that my weight during those years never went five pounds above or below my normal weight. Walking was my exercise routine. The local mall was a favorite place for many walkers. I chose the mall for safety reasons. As a vegetarian I was fortunate to have access to vegetarian meals. As an active member of Alpha Kappa Alpha sorority I attended numerous conferences. Vegetarian meals were available. As an elementary school teacher the midday meal would be my last one for the day. The school cafeteria always had an array of delicious vegetarian options.

I was aware that my weight during those years never went five pounds above or below my normal weight.

Becoming a Vegan

I have been aware of the vegan diet for many years. I never paid attention to it. I felt the vegetarian diet was healthy enough for me. During the month of July 2022 I read the book Healthy at Last by Eric Adams, the current mayor of New York City. He was not mayor when he wrote the book. His recommendation of eliminating dairy and eggs from your diet made me take note. I had been pouring dairy on my cereal for thirty-eight years. After reading the entire book I decided to try the vegan diet. After eliminating dairy and eggs and eating the recommended in the book I noticed some amazing things happening in my body.

The first thing I noticed was the bloat I had experienced for years suddenly disappeared. I became aware that I was lactose intolerant. Secondly, I noticed a glow my skin that I had not seen before. Thirdly, my gray hair had at the roots its original hair color. After taking note of the impact I knew that I would become a true vegan. I eliminated all the foods that the book recommended.

The next step was to make a list of foods that were crucial to the diet. Once the cabinets and refrigerator were clear of the unhealthy foods I went shopping with the recommended list.

After cooking and eating a variety of foods I have selected those that I eat on a regular basis: bananas, kiwi, strawberries, peaches, tomatoes, steel-cut oatmeal, brown rice, sugar-free whole wheat bread, collard greens, turnip greens, sweet potatoes, broccoli, red bell pepper, red onions, black eyed peas, almond, nutritional yeast, unsweetened soy milk (B-12 fortified) pure maple syrup, peanut butter, lentils.

Preparing meals is not a chore for me. I prepare most of my foods in advance. I am aware of the importance of staying hydrated; I drink enough water. Many of the foods I eat have a high water content. I have been drinking distilled bottled water for many years. When the water from the faucet became unfit to drink I resorted to bottled water and continue to drink it daily. This book is a result of my love of healthy eating on a daily basis. It made me want to share the benefits of proper eating with others, mainly the vegan diet.

The foods that I eat daily are among the healthiest fruits, vegetables and grains. They include steel cut oatmeal, 100% whole wheat bread, bananas, wild blueberries, strawberries, pears, collard greens, sweet potatoes, red bell peppers , red onions, and black eyed peas. I keep Vitamin B12 fortified soy milk and nutritional yeast in the refrigerator to have a daily supply of Vitamin B12.

Note: One serving of Braggs nutritional yeast has five grams of protein and two grams of dietary fiber. One serving also has 6% of your daily required iron. It is also fortified with (vitaminb1), riboflavin (vitamin b2), niacin (vitamin b3), vitamin b6 and vitamin b12. I learned about the benefits of nutritional yeast from reading one of many books that I have healthy eating.

I reserve desserts for the holidays. My favorites are pumpkin pie, pecan pie and ambrosia.

I have acquired a taste for peanut butter. I love the taste. As a result, my midday meal is not complete without a peanut butter sandwich on 100% whole wheat bread. After eating my midday meal, I have no desire for any food until 6am the following day.

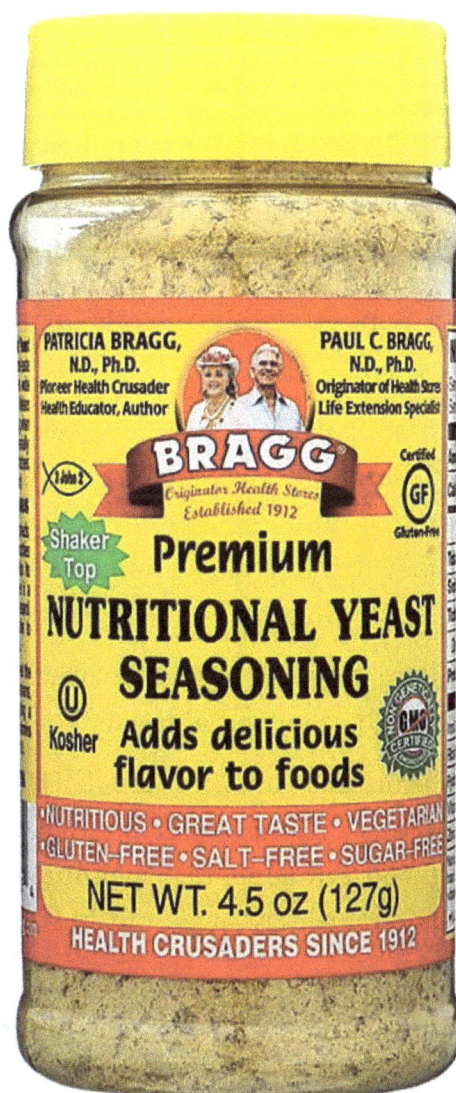

Breakfast: 6 a.m.

One banana

1/2 cup blueberries

One cup steel cut oatmeal

One cup unsweetened soy milk

One slice 100% whole wheat toast

Midday meal: 12:00 noon

One cup collard greens

1 cup mashed sweet potatoes

1/2 cup black eye pea salad

(This is my last meal for the day.)

I drink four to six glasses of water during the day. I cannot drink eight glasses. The reason is probably due to some foods I eat having high water content namely bananas, red bell peppers, celery, and tomatoes.

I have included some healthy alternative recipes to some traditional favorites .

Foods to Eat Daily

1. Upon awakening drink an 8oz glass of water.

2. 5am Eat breakfast each morning. 2)kiwi 1)banana 1 cup steel cut oats with 1/2 tsp cinnamon. While preparing breakfast drink 1) 8oz glass of water with 1/2 tsp of ginger.

3. 9am drink 1) 8oz glass of water and eat 1/2 tbs chopped almonds

4. 1pm eat midday meal. 1)cup collard greens, 1)cup sweet potatoes, 1/2 cup of diced red peppers, 1-peanut butter sandwich with 2tbsp peanut butter.

5. Do not eat any food after the midday meal until 5am the following morning

Steel Cut Oats with blueberries
Sliced bananas

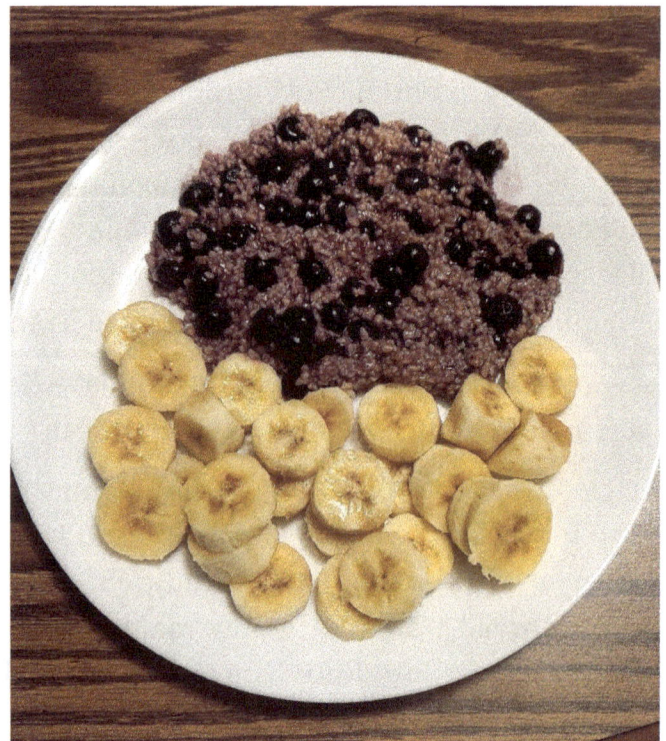

Breakfast

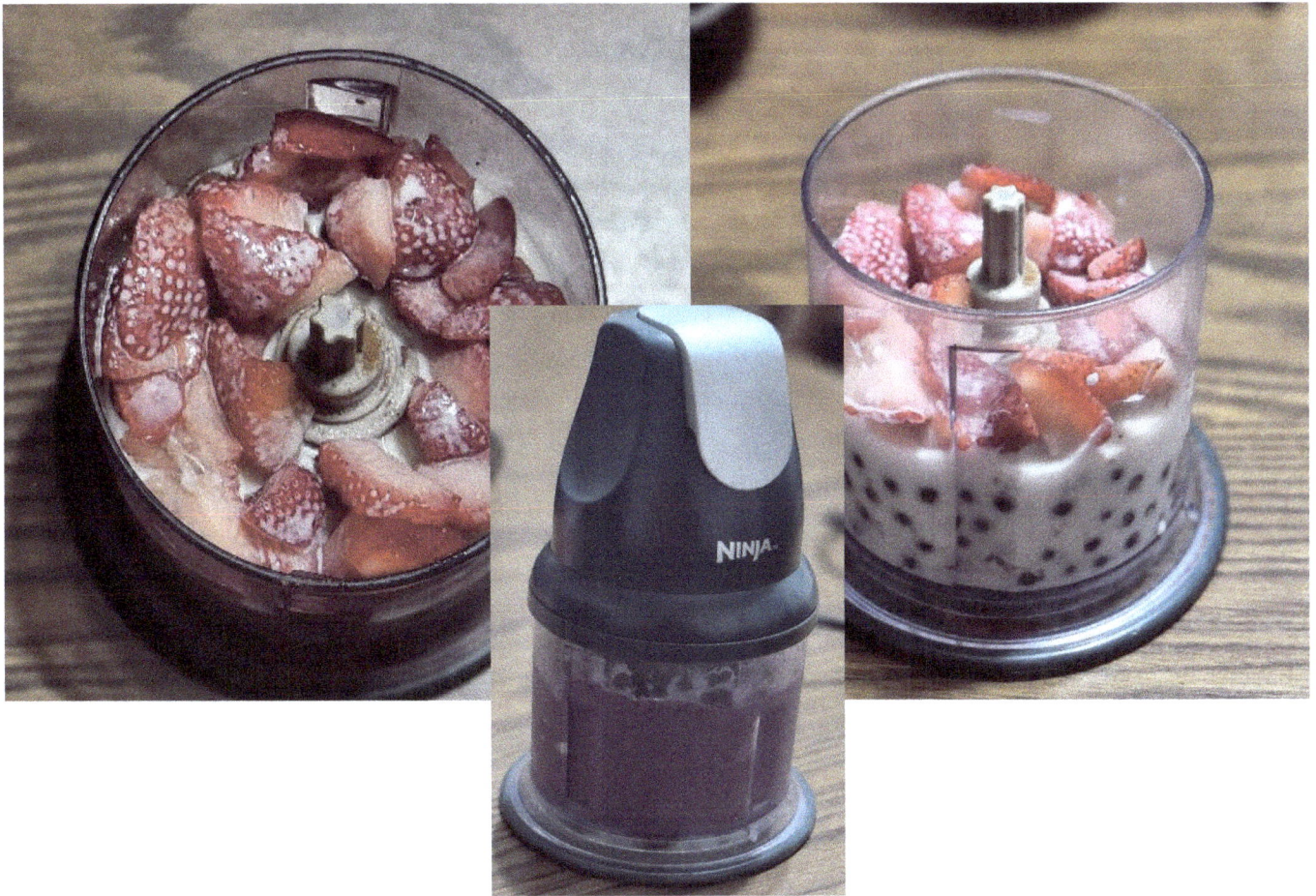

After reading numerous books about the plant-based diet, I changed my breakfast routine. One book stated that we do not necessarily need to eat grains daily, but should make sure to eat fruits and vegetables daily. I began to substitute a green smoothie for my breakfast of choice, instead of the oatmeal that I had been eating.

The green smoothies have been such a refreshing way to start the day. I have noticed a difference in the way that my body feels. My body certainly seems to like the Change !

I have never felt such a "clean" feeling! One book mentioned how a single father used smoothies as a way to ensure that his five year old daughter ate fruits and vegetables daily. Putting them in smoothies does the job and the daughter loves them.

Green Smoothie

1Cup frozen collard greens

1/2 cup frozen wild blueberries

1/2 cup fresh strawberries

1/2 tsp parsley

1/2 tsp powdered basil

1 cup unsweet soy milk B12 fortified

In a blender combine the ingredients. Blend for two minutes or until contents reach a smooth creamy consistency.
Serves 1

Breads

Vegan Cornbread

1 cup yellow cornmeal

1/2 teaspoon baking powder

One cup unsweetened soy milk

1 tablespoon maple syrup

Preheat the oven to 425 degrees. Pour two teaspoons of extra virgin olive oil into a loaf pan. Set aside. Mix cornmeal, baking powder and milk until blended. Add the maple syrup. Pour mixture into the oiled pan. Baked for thirty minutes. Remove from oven. Let sit for five minutes. Transfer to a plate and slice.
Variation: you can also add 1 cup frozen broccoli florets (microwaved for two minutes) in the batter.

Gingerbread

1/2 cup extra virgin olive oil

1/2 cup pure maple syrup

One cup whole wheat flour

One teaspoon cinnamon

1 tsp ginger

One teaspoon nutmeg

3/4 teaspoon baking soda

1/2 cup hot water

Preheat oven to 350 degrees. Mix olive oil and maple syrup. Set aside. Mix dry ingredients. Add 2 tablespoons of oil and two tablespoons to dry ingredients. Stir in 1/4 cup of hot water. Add remaining oil, syrup, and dry ingredients. Stir in 1/4 cup of hot water. Oil a loaf pan and pour mixture into the pan. Baked for thirty minutes. Let cool for five minutes. Transfer to a plate and slice.

Minestrone Soup

2 tablespoons olive oil

1 clove garlic, minced

3/4 cup chopped celery

3/4 cup chopped onion

3/4 cup green beans

One half cup frozen sliced carrots

1/2 cup kidney beans

3/4 cup frozen green peas

1/2 can salt-free chopped tomatoes

5 cups water

One cup whole-wheat macaroni

Heat oil in a large pot. Add garlic, celery, and onion. Sautee for five minutes. Add remaining ingredients except macaroni. Bring to boil, reduce heat, simmer for forty-five minutes. Add uncooked macaroni and cook for 15 minutes. Yields eight cups.

Salads

Layered Salad

Lettuce
1/2 cup chopped celery
1/2 cup chopped bell pepper
1/2 cup chopped red onion
1/2 cup frozen green peas, thawed
Vegan mayonnaise
One teaspoon pure maple syrup

Tear lettuce into fine pieces. Place in the bottom of a dish. Layer remaining ingredients except mayonnaise and syrup in the order listed. Mix mayonnaise and syrup. Spread over salad covering it completely. Chill for eight hours or overnight. When ready to serve toss salad.

Green Leaf Salad

6 leaves of lettuce, washed
2 stalks of celery, chopped
One apple, cored
One fourth cup walnuts, chopped
1 tablespoon pure maple syrup

Tear lettuce leaves into bite-size pieces and place in a bowl. Add chopped celery, apple, and walnuts. Stir in maple syrup. Serves four.

Broccoli Salad

One cup frozen broccoli florets
1/2 cup finely chopped red onion
One teaspoon pure maple syrup
1/2 cup sliced almonds

Thaw broccoli. Toss together with chopped onion. Drizzle maple syrup broccoli mixture; toss gently to coat. Before serving, add sliced almonds. Serves two.

Green Pea Salad

One cup frozen green peas, thawed
1/2 cup finely chopped red bell pepper
1/2 cup finely chopped onion
One teaspoon red wine vinegar
1 tablespoon maple syrup, optional

Mix peas, bell pepper, onion, red wine vinegar, and syrup. Stir well. Chill until ready to serve.

Black Eyed Pea Salad

One half cup black eyed peas,
    (rinsed and drained)
1/2 cup finely chopped red bell pepper
1/2 cup finely chopped red onion

Mix ingredients in a bowl. Cover and chill until ready to serve.

Vegetables

Mashed Sweet Potatoes

6 large sweet potatoes
One half cup soy milk
1 tbsp pure maple syrup

Wash potatoes. place in a large pot and cover with water. Bring to boil. Cover pot, lower heat, and cook for thirty minutes or until potatoes are soft. Remove from water and place on a baking sheet. Remove skins from potatoes and place in a large pan a few at a time. Mash with a hand masher. Do not use a food processor. Add the soy milk and maple syrup. Mix well. Potatoes may be prepared a day ahead and placed in the refrigerator. When ready to serve, microwave for two minutes. They also freeze well.

Green Bean Casserole

One package frozen green beans
1/2 cup chopped mushrooms
1/4 cup chopped red onion
2 tablespoon extra virgin olive oil
2 tablespoon whole wheat flour
1/2 cup unsweetened soy milk
1/2 teaspoon soy sauce
1/4 teaspoon black pepper
Chopped almonds

Cook beans and drain well. Sautee mushrooms for five minutes in olive oil. Add flour, mix well. Add milk and let thicken. Add soy sauce and black pepper. Mix beans into the other ingredients. Place in an oiled baking dish. Sprinkle with chopped almonds. Bake at 400 degrees in the oven.

Collards

1 tablespoon extra-virgin olive oil
1 teaspoon garlic powder
1–10-ounce package frozen collard greens
1/4 cup water

Place oil, garlic powder, and greens in a pot. Cover pot and steam over medium heat for ten minutes stirring occasionally. Remove cover, add water, and steam for ten minutes. Makes three cups.

Spinach and Brown Rice

1 tablespoon virgin olive oil
1/4 cup chopped red onion
1/2 cup frozen chopped spinach
1/2 cup cooked brown rice

Sautee onion in oil. Add spinach and steam until heated. Add cooked rice and turn heat off. Let steam.

Brown Rice

1/2 cup brown rice
1 cup water

Place rice and water in a pan. Bring to boil. Stir with a fork. Cover pan. Cook for 15 minutes. Lift top immediately and then replace. Turn off heat and let stand for 45 minutes

Grains

Barley

2 cups water
One cup barley

Bring water to boil. Stir barley into water. Cover and reduce heat. Simmer for ten to twelve minutes. Remove from heat and let stand for 5 minutes. Use immediately or store in the refrigerator up to one week.

Red Rice

2 tablespoons olive oil
1/2 cup chopped onion
1/4 teaspoon garlic powder
One cup cooked brown rice
One can salt-free diced tomatoes
One teaspoon vinegar

Heat oil in a saucepan. Add onion and garlic powder. Sauteed until onion is tender. Add cooked rice, tomatoes, and vinegar. Stir well. Cover pan and simmer for ten minutes.

Seitan

1 8 Oz package of seitan, thinly sliced
1 1/2 teaspoon extra-virgin olive oil
1/2 tsp garlic powder
1/2 tsp onion powder
1/4 tsp paprika
1/8 teaspoon black pepper
1 tbsp whole wheat flour
1 cup water

Heat seitan, olive oil, and spices over medium heat for 5 minutes, stirring occasionally. Add flour and water. Heat for 2 minutes. Served hot. Serves two.

Basic Quinoa

One cup quinoa
2 cups water
One bay leaf

In a small saucepan bring all the ingredients to boil. Reduce heat and cover pan. Cook until quinoa is tender and the water is absorbed (about 15 minutes). Make 3 cups.

Desserts

Ambrosia

Three oranges
14 ounce can of crushed pineapple in juice, drained and reserved
2/3 cup unsweetened grated coconut

Peel and section oranges. Place 1 1/2 of the oranges in a bowl. Top with 2 ounces of crushed pineapple. Sprinkle one third cup of coconut. Repeat with 1-1/2 of oranges, 2 ounces of crushed pineapple, and one third cup coconut. Pour reserved juice over ingredients. Cover bowl with plastic wrap. Refrigerate until ready to serve.

Pecan Pie

1 cup pecan halves
1 cup chopped pecans
3/4 cup maple syrup
One half teaspoon cinnamon
One teaspoon vanilla
One fourth cup unsweetened soy milk
2 tablespoon extra virgin olive oil
2 tablespoon whole wheat flour
One whole wheat pie crust

In a food processor add 1 cup pecan halves and process until a coarse meal is formed. Place the meal in a bowl and add the chopped pecans. Stir until just combined. In another bowl combine the maple syrup, vanilla, milk, and oil. Add the pecan mixture to the wet mixture. Stir in the flour. Pour the batter into the pie crust. Bake in a preheated 350-degree oven for forty-five minutes. Remove from the oven; let the pie cool completely so it can set.

Vanilla Pudding

1/2 cup pure maple syrup
2 cups soy milk
3 tablespoon cornstarch
One teaspoon pure vanilla extract

Combine the syrup, milk, and cornstarch together in a saucepan. Whisk until combined. Add vanilla extract. Place the saucepan over medium heat and stir until mixture to begin to thicken. Stir constantly until mixture is thick. Pour into individual dessert bowls. Wrap each bowl with plastic wrap and refrigerate ready to serve. Serves two.

Pumpkin Pie

2 tablespoon maple syrup
1 tablespoon whole wheat flour
1 teaspoon ground cinnamon
1/4 teaspoon ground nutmeg
1/4 teaspoon ground allspice
One 1/2 cups canned pumpkin
One 1/2 cups unsweetened soy milk
1 unbaked whole wheat pie crust

Preheat oven to 375 degrees. Combine maple syrup, flour, and spices. Stir pumpkin and soy milk. Mix until smooth. Pour into an unbaked pie crust. Bake for forty-five minutes. Allow it to cool. Refrigerate for at least 4 hours to allow the filling to set.

Herbs and Spices

Allspice
Basil
Black pepper
Cayenne pepper
Celery seed
Chili powder
Cinnamon
Cloves
Cumin
Garlic powder
Ginger
Mace
Nutmeg
Onion powder
Oregano
Paprika
Parsley
Rosemary
Sage
Turmeric

Vocabulary

Agave (ah GAH vay) nectar: a natural sweetener often provided from the sap of blue agaves that grow in Mexico.

Herbs: a leaf

Intermittent fasting: letting at least 12 hours elapse between your last meal one day the first meal the next day.

Lactose intolerant: inability to digest milk products.

Legume: any plant that carries fruit inside a pod

Lentil: a legume that is healthy and can be used as a substitute for meat

Nutritional yeast: yeast that is different from brewer's and baker's yeast.

Quinoa (keen wa): gluten free plant-based food

Spice: dried seeds, roots, and barks

Steel-cut oatmeal: less processed than rolled oats. It is 100%.

Seitan (say-tan): made from wheat. It is known as wheat meat.

Vegetarian: someone who abstains from meat, fish, and fowl as food.

Vegan: someone who does not eat meat, fish, or dairy

I do understand the sentiments of people who say that they have tried many diets or fitness plans before. Most of us are not as strong willed and strong minded as my dear mother. She decided on what she wanted to do for her health and has stuck with it almost four decades! I on the other hand have yoyo-ed with my diet and size over and over again. I would never stay committed to the changes that I had made to achieve the long term weight losses. The thing about the basic plan: PLANT -BASED WHOLE FOODS DI-ET, WATER, WALKING INTERMITTENT FASTING. (NO FRIED FOODS) (NO FAST FOODS) It's a very SIMPLE plan. It does not cost boatloads of money. Besides buying food, which you are going to do anyway, it's TOTALLY FREE! It can be a very hard plan to maintain if you don't stay FOCUSED, COMMITTED, DEDICATED and DETERMINED. If you work the plan the plan will ABSOLUTELY work for you. JUST DO IT!

I plan to stick to this plan this time because I have a different reason. My reason is HEALTH! Believe me HEALTH IS WEALTH! As I am nearing 60, and have seen so many friends and relatives suffer and battle with poor health, it has jolted me into a different mindset and reality. I saw high-blood pressure wreak havoc on my father's life. I have seen so many (too many) of my classmates not make it to the 55 year mark and many more not made it to where most of us are now, at 59. The memorial ceremony at our 40th year class reunion (2022) was a real eye-opener and sobering moment.

I want to follow in the example that my mother has set in how to be re-sponsible for the FABULOUS gift of life that we have been given. I want to take care of my body as a temple. It is the only one that we have. I want to ex-perience optimal health for the rest of my days. I want to stay FIT and FABU-LOUS FOR LIFE! FIND YOUR WHY and STICK WITH IT.

I want you to understand that I do TOTALLY understand how you might be feeling or thinking about making any drastic   lifestyle change(s). Two of my favorite sayings/quotes that I lean on with tackling any "project" are:

1. Question How Do you Eat An Elephant?

   Answer: One Bite At A Time.

Take It One Bite/One Little Bit at a Time of whatever you or trying to accomplish or tackle) Of course we aren't going to be eating elephants because we are gonna be vegans, Right?

2. **The Journey of a thousand miles begins with one step**.

Translation: Just start somewhere. Just get started . Take one small step/piece and then another and another. You don't have to take the attitude that you have to conquer this whole thing all at one. It can seem too overwhelming, in our minds , to even start. That is what keeps many people from even trying at all. It seems too daunting of a task. Whatever it is , It is NOT TOO HARD to accomplish . YOU CAN DO IT! Another Nelson Mandela quote that I love is:

> "IT ALWAYS SEEM IMPOSSIBLE, UNTIL IT'S DONE."

It's never too late. You are not too old. You are not too out of shape. You are not TOO anything. Your situation is not too bad, for you to start a plan to make it better. START WHERE YOU ARE. START TODAY .

NOTE:

You have to be on a PERSONAL mission to live your best life, REGARDLESS or what other people are doing or not doing around you. I have a friend who moved to Tupelo several years ago from a more northern city. We were having a conversation about the town and the overall environment Then, we got on food, diet, exercise etc. I knew that   before she moved here she had a really stringent exercise routine and did a lot of walking and was very interested in keeping a certain look and size. I told her that one pitfall she would encounter if she was not very careful would be gaining weight. I told her that for the most part, she would not be around people who are putting a great deal of emphasis on exercise and fitness or healthy eating habits. Her husband is a minister, so the sources of food temptations would be multiplied tremendously! I explained that people would be cooking and bringing them all kinds of cakes and pies, fried foods, barbecue and other southern delicacies They would be constantly inviting them to their homes to eat and inviting them to birthday parties reunions, cookouts, etc. We all have these things going on. But, when you have a whole congregation of people bringing you food and asking you to all of these food-filled events it's a whole different story! The impact is multiplied. In the south we center almost EVERYTHING around food. And, in the South we FRY almost everything, not to mention putting loads of sugar in everything, especially TEA. People add sugar to things you might not even suspect , like spaghetti. We have some AMAZING cooks, both male and female. Southern food is like non other and really cannot be compared. We all know that the food is absolutely AMAZING!

It is always amazing ,but not always necessarily healthy! Most times it is very unhealthy. We all know about the astronomical and steadily skyrocketing numbers of obesity high blood pressure, heart disease and diabetes, especially in the South. You have to stick by your own PERSONAL commitment to healthier lifestyle choices. I told her that I was a size 5/6 when I moved home. She immediately asked; "What happened?" That was a very valid question considering my size at the time. My response: "Life" I told her about my experience with some lifestyle choices and changes I made , but did not follow through on., when I moved back home to Tupelo from Memphis, in 2007. I had lived in Memphis since 1988. Of course, Memphis is very Southern and is especially known for amazing barbecue and soul food. Over the years, I gained a lot of weight eating that food with friends and co-workers.

My co-workers would come into work eating totally unhealthy fast food breakfasts and immediately start planning what we were going to eat for lunch. We seemed to want to make it our goal to try out EVERY SINGLE   eating place in Memphis. We probably came very close.

As the years go by, it is unfortunately, much more difficult to lose the weight without significant effort. We all remember those days , when in our teens and early twenties we could skip a meal or two or cut back a little and lose 5 lbs in a few days. It takes much more effort as we age. During this time, I had gotten up to one of my high weights , like around 185. I began a fitness journey to lose the excess weight in my early forties (43). I started working out at a Curves facility EVERY DAY. (I love the Curves Circuit routine!) I would have a Smoothie King smoothie for breakfast and a Smoothie King Smooth for lunch (not the sugar laden ones) and a low carb dinner (meat and vegetables).

My friends at work called me the Smoothie Queen. They knew my order at Smoothie King would be a Strawberry Gladiator Smoothie with Acai I still love them! I even got several of my co workers to start drinking healthy smoothies for breakfast and lunch. A couple of them accompanied me to Curves a few times. One placed membership. I lost a significant amount of weight and was down to about 140 lbs. when I moved back home in August 2007. I was wearing a size 6. IT'S A SMALL WORLD!!! After going to the Smoothie King that was near my job, every day, for months. I found out that the owner was the son of a longtime family friend from Tupelo, Malcolm Jackson. A few years later, I found out that the owner's wife and I are cousins, when we showed up at the same Townsend family reunion, in Tupelo!

I was super excited when I returned home that they had a Curves which I immediately joined and faithfully continued to work out. I hated that we did not have a Smoothie King (although we did get one later on, for a time ,and we have another come coming) Unfortunately, the Curves closed several months after I returned home. I did not like going to gyms, so I basically stopped doing any kind of consistent exercising. From my pictures, you can absolutely see that I did not remain at that 5/6. It takes personal CONSISTENCY and COMMITTMENT to maintain the desired results. You must take CONTROL of your life CHOICES to MAINTAIN the results that you desire.

FIND WHAT WORKS FOR YOU! JUST DO IT ! KEEP GOING!

REMEMBER WHY YOU STARTED. DON'T QUIT!

BE COMMITTED TO BEING FIT AND FABULOUS FOR LIFE!

PLEASE REMEMBER FOR WEIGHT LOSS, YOU CAN'T OUT EXERXCISE A BAD DIET!!!

Some gurus say It's 80% diet and 20% exercise.

Daniel 1: 8-16

8 But Daniel resolved not to defile himself with the royal food and wine, and he asked the chief official for permission not to defile himself this way.

9 Now God had caused the official to show favor and compassion to Daniel,

10 but the official told Daniel, "I am afraid of my lord the king, who has   assigned your [food and drink.

Why should he see you looking worse than the other young men your age? The king would then have my head because of you."

11 Daniel then said to the guard whom the chief official had appointed over Daniel, Hananiah, Mishael and Azariah,

12 "Please test your servants for ten days: Give us nothing but vegetables to eat and water to drink.

13 Then compare our appearance with that of the young men who eat the royal food, and treat your servants in accordance with what you see."

14 So he agreed to this and tested them for ten days.

15 At the end of the ten days they looked healthier and better nourished than any of the young men who ate the royal food.

16 So the guard took away their choice food and the wine they were to drink and gave them vegetables instead.

COMMERCIAL BREAK:

I signed up in February for the Prevention Heart Screening that is done by The Cardiology Associates in Tupelo. The screening consists of: CT calcium score ·EKG (electrocardiogram)· Lipid Profile. They usually offer the screening for $99 . In February, for Heart Health Month ,they had a special of $50 . My results were great! The main test was the calcium score. Interpretation Summary :Your Cardiac Calcium Score : 0. No evidence of calcified plaque, which means that there is less than 5 percent chance you have coronary artery disease (CAD). Your risk of a heart attack is very low Percentile : 10th (Which means 90% of people have a higher score) You are at low risk for coronary heart disease. General recommendations for heart health on the print out include: RED MEAT ONLY ONCE A MONTH Sweets, Eggs, Poultry, Fish ONLY ONCE A WEEK. Fruits, Legumes, Nuts, Seeds, Vegetables ·DAILY 6 Glasses of Water DAILY , Daily Physical Activity

From the printout: Research has shown that a diet low in simple carbohydrates is beneficial in long term successful weight loss and reduction in premature death related to obesity. Those foods that contain simple carbohydrates include sugar or foods containing sugar, , potatoes (other than sweet potatoes) , white rice, corn or corn meal, and foods made from refined flour such as bread , cake, rolls, pasta, etc.. Additionally , avoiding fatty cholesterol loaded meats such as beef and pork and NOT frying foods is also beneficial.

GO FORTH AND BE FABULOUS ON A SHOESTRING BUDGET

As I mentioned in the previous chapter, to get myself motivated for my fitness journey. I decided to enter the Miss Magnolia State Pageant. (Mrs Division.) I knew that trying on dresses and trying to look my very best on stage, would really kick me into gear. Being the Down South Diva on A Dime that I am, I competed in all yard sale, thrift shop or Poshmark resale site attire. My dress and shoes "below" for opening number were purchased from Poshmark for sooo much less than they cost at retail price. The dress has a very classic style cut. It reminded me of a 50's style cocktail dress (if you take away all the pageant glimmer/glitz /sequins of course). No, I didn't win. But, I held my own for a 58 year old with the young-uns! I also placed first runner up for the Viewers Choice Awards.

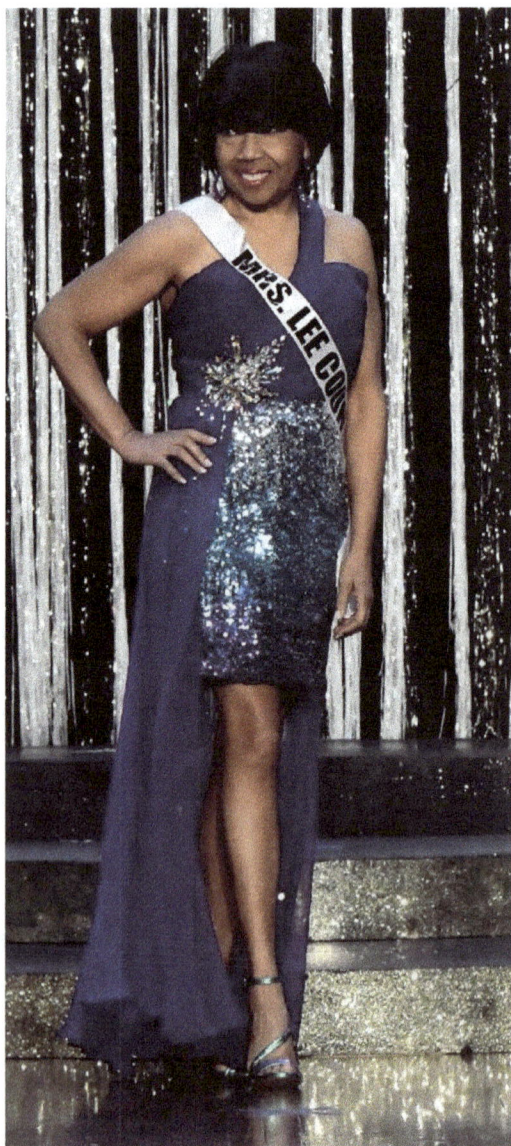

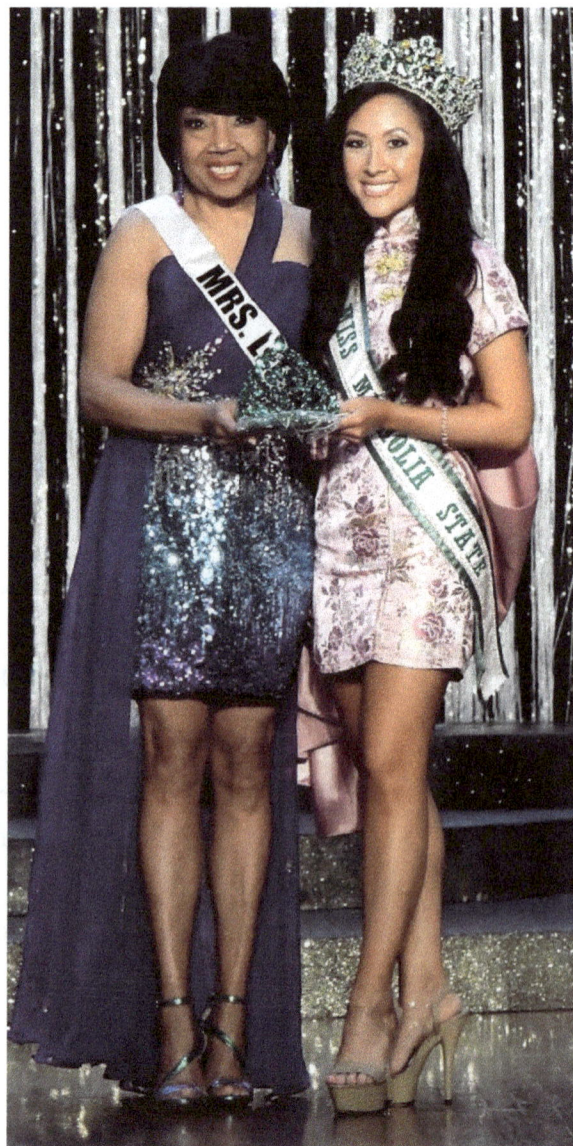

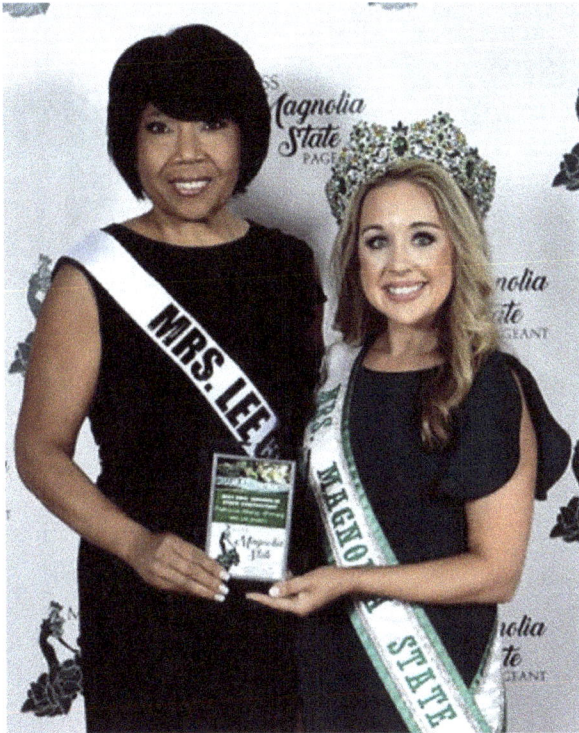

My interview dress was purchased from a thrift shop for Under $10.

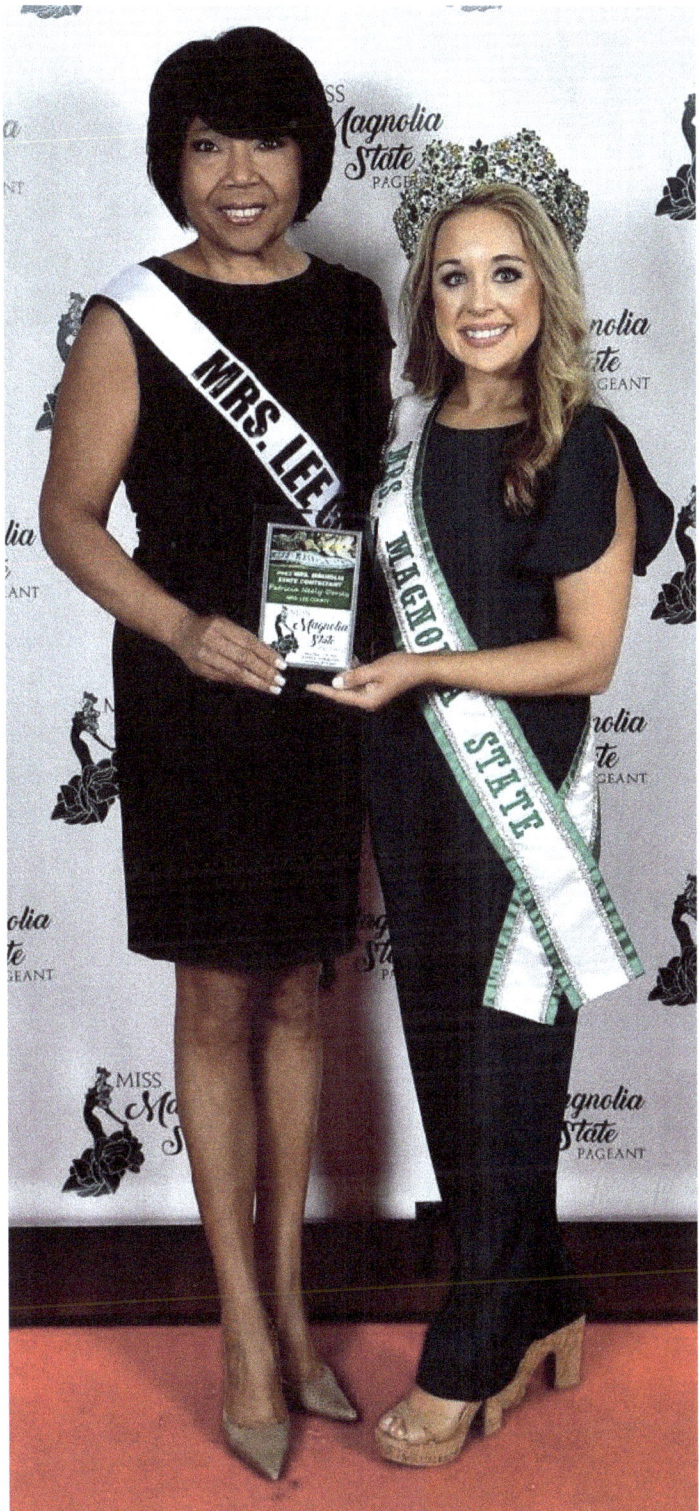

Photogenic
4th Jeanne Elise LaFontaine
3rd Brooke Gilpin
2nd Pat Kelly May
1st Tiara Brown
Winner Brandi Jo Middleton

Fashion
4th Wendy Bullard Smith
3rd Pat Kelly May
2nd Tracy Owens
1st Jennifer Howard
Winner Brandi Jo Middleton

Viewer's Choice
4th Abigail Huffstatler
3rd Tiffany Swinney
2nd Melinda Brown
1st Patricia Neely-Dorsey
Winner Wendy Bullard Smith

Photo taken after interview with previous year's
Mrs. Magnolia State, Kayla McMinn.
She won the title on her 10th try!

The dress that I wore for casual wear was an over ten year old $1 yard sale find that I purchased at a yard sale in Saltillo in 2011.

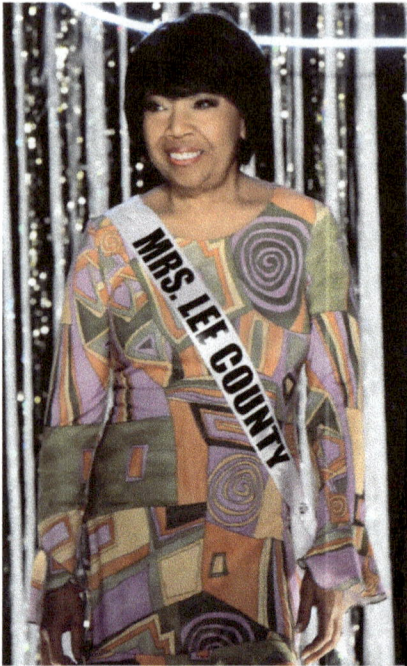

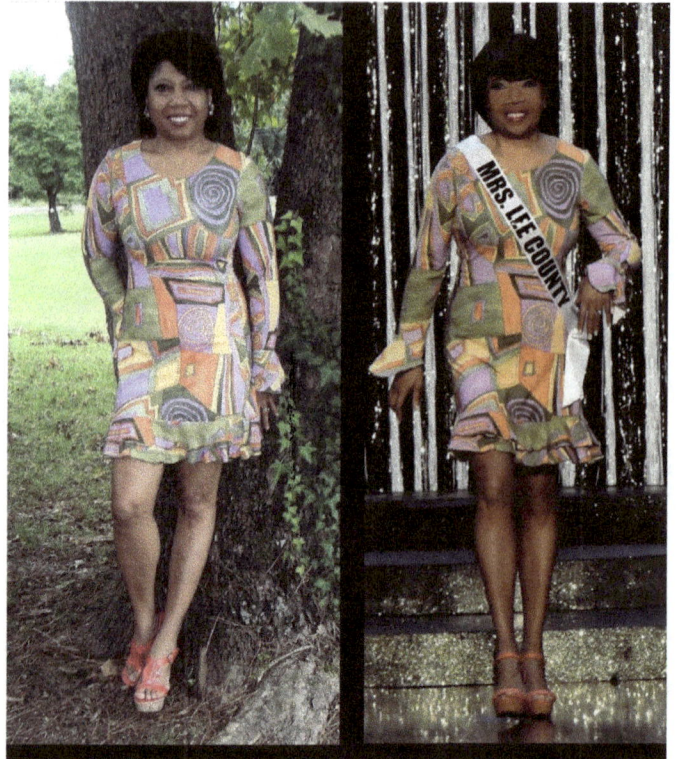

2011   2022

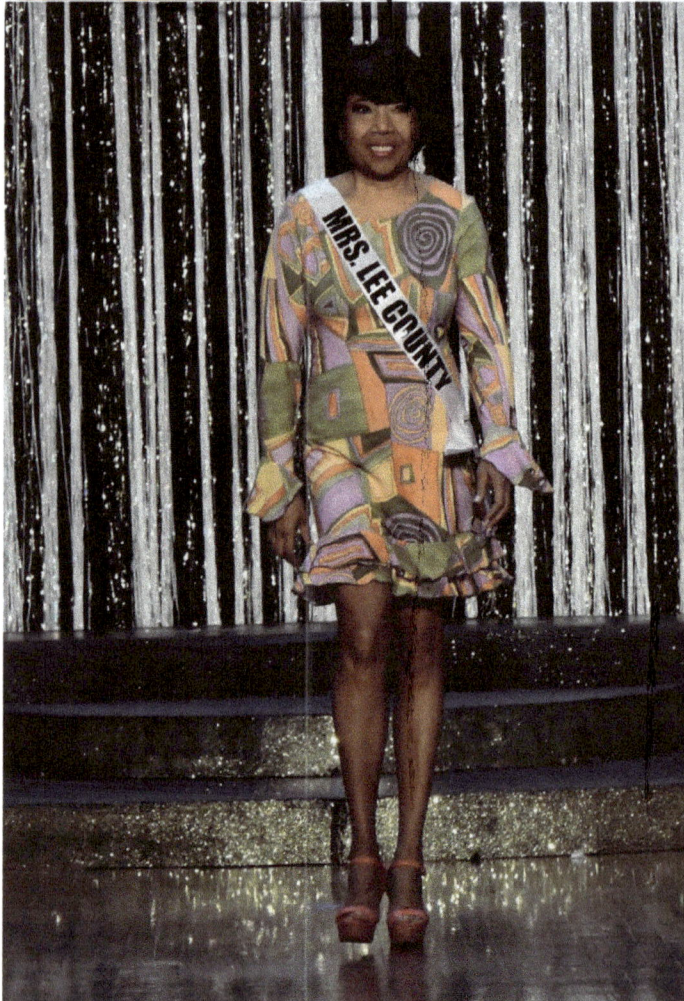

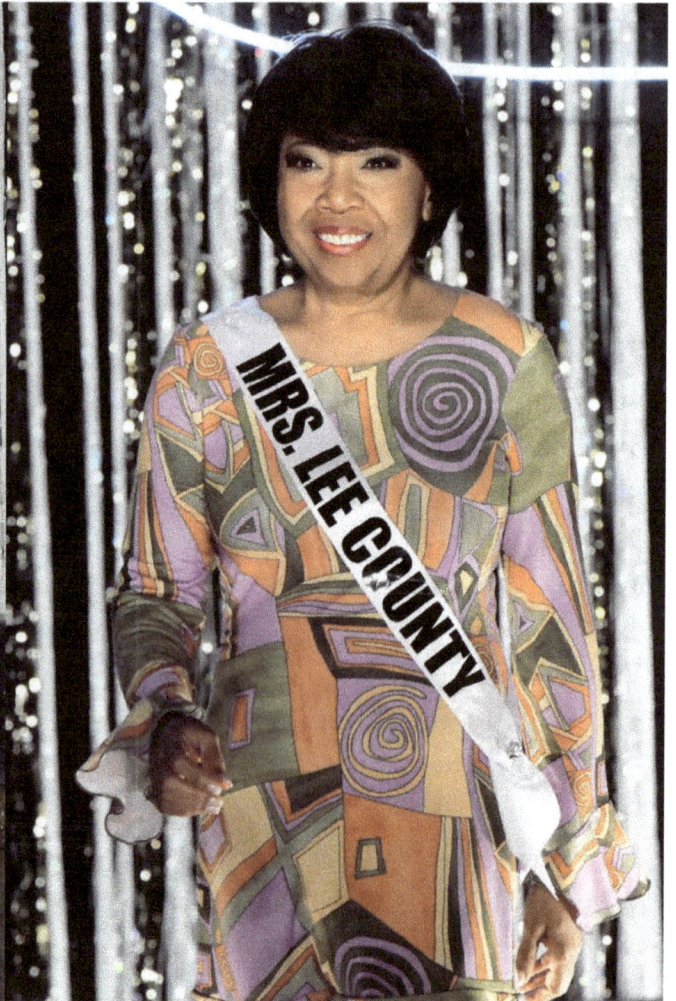

I purchased my evening gown from Poshmark resale site for so much less than retail prices.

Age 58

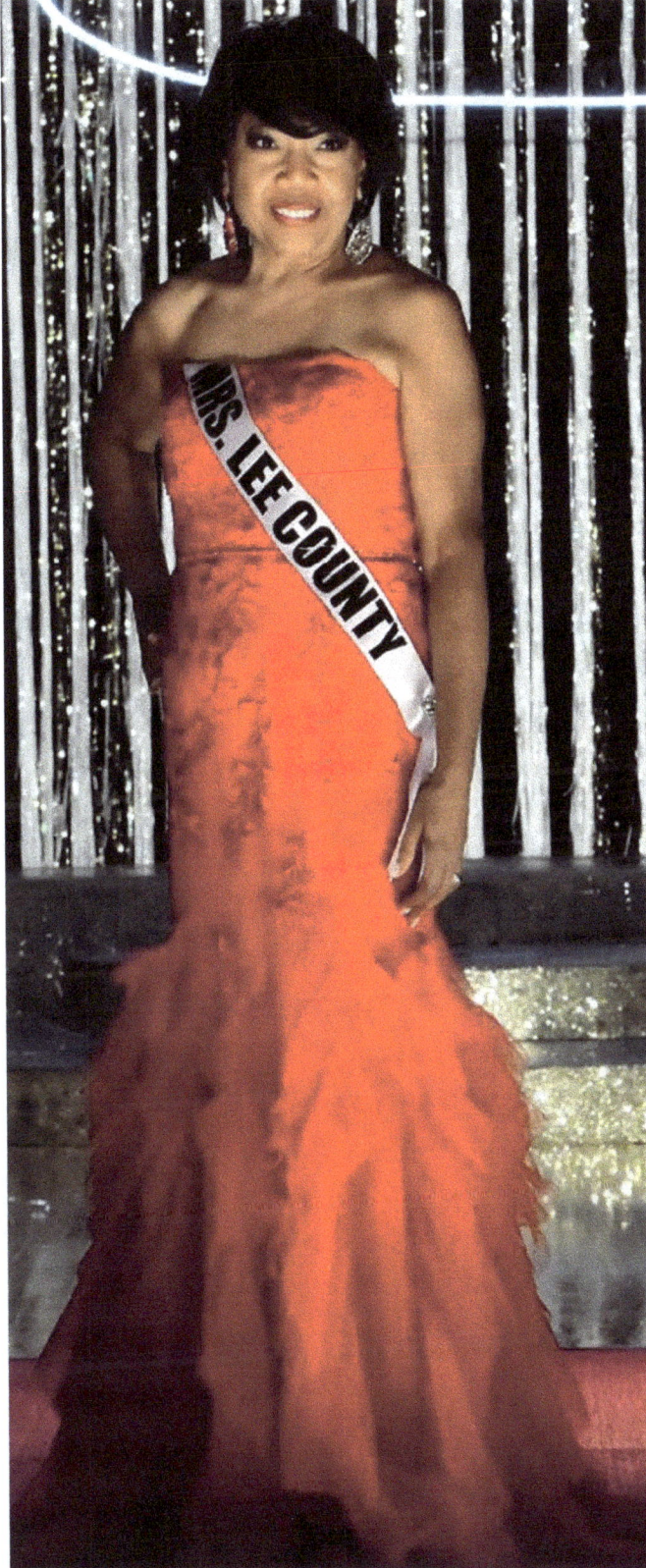

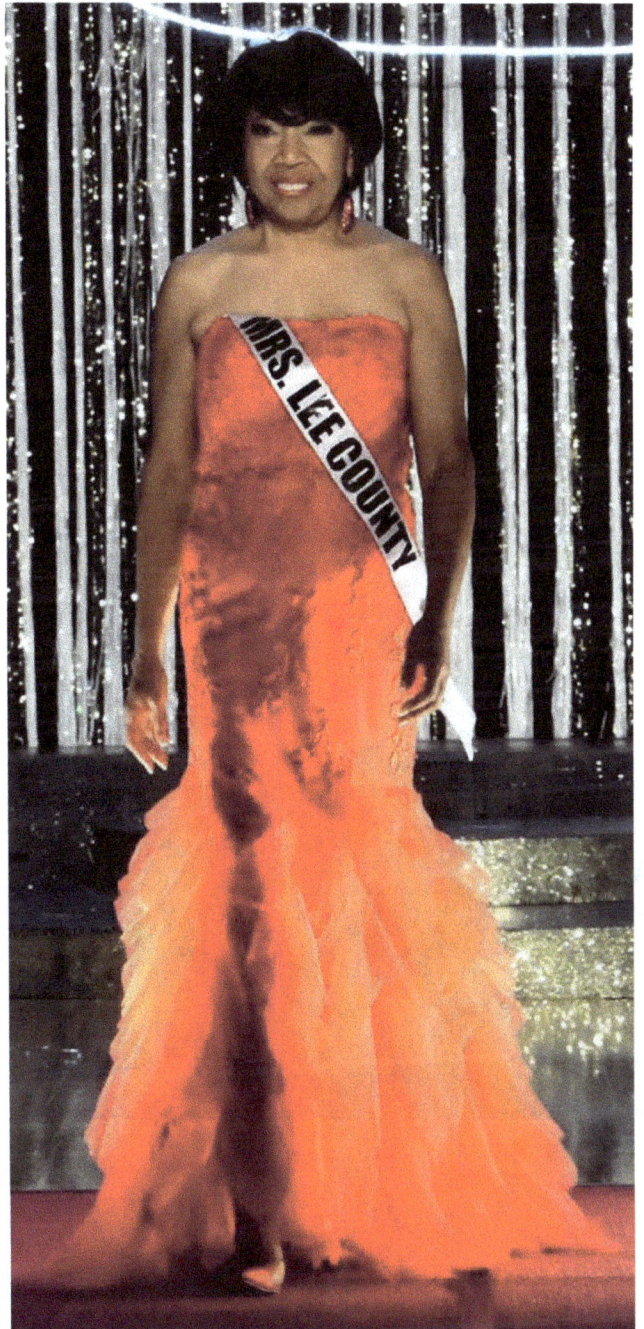

I'm not really a pageant girl. This was only my 3rd pageant. The first one was Miss Northside at age 16. The second was Mrs. Mississippi at age 47. My dresses for headshot, orientation, interview and banquet came from Ross, at prices much less than regular retail.

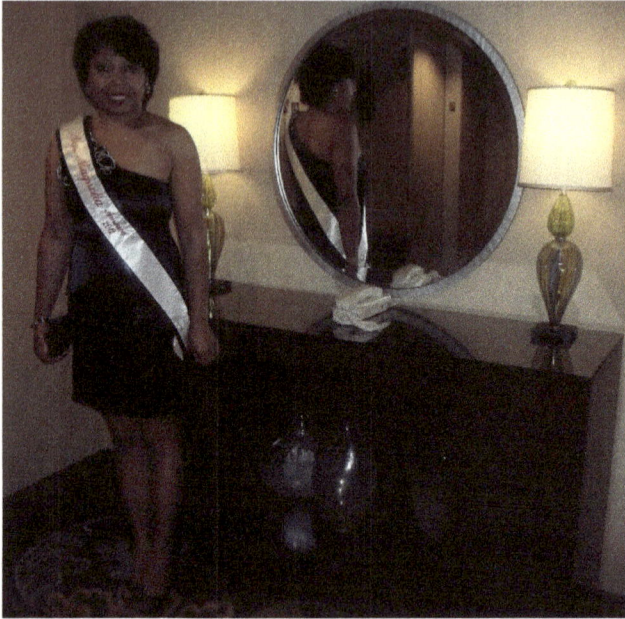

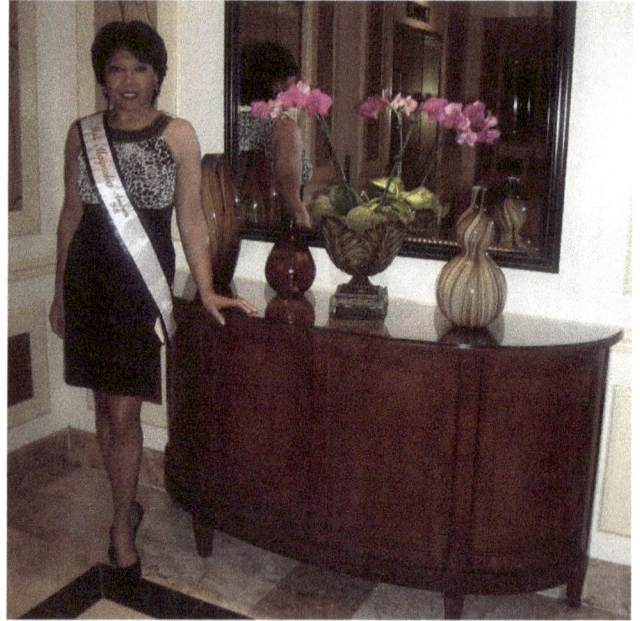

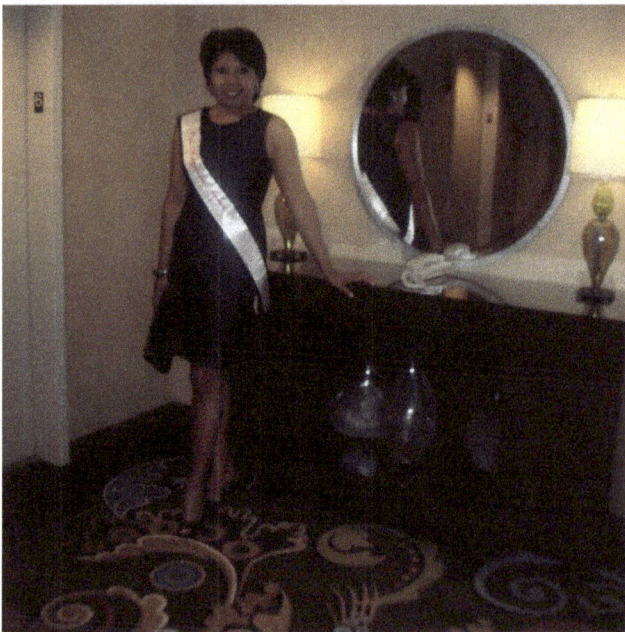

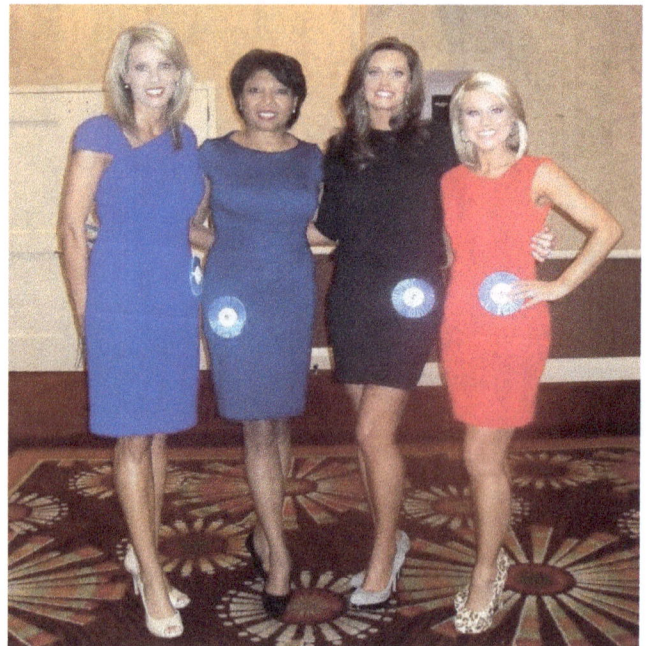

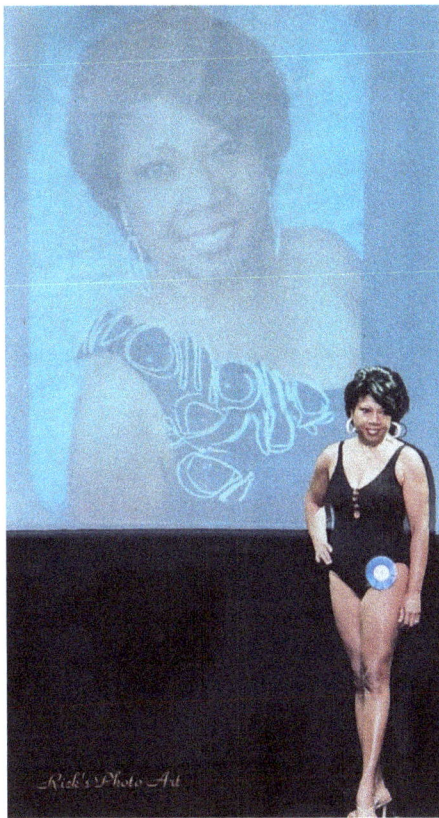

Age 47

My gown was purchased for $5 from
a yardsale in Saltillo

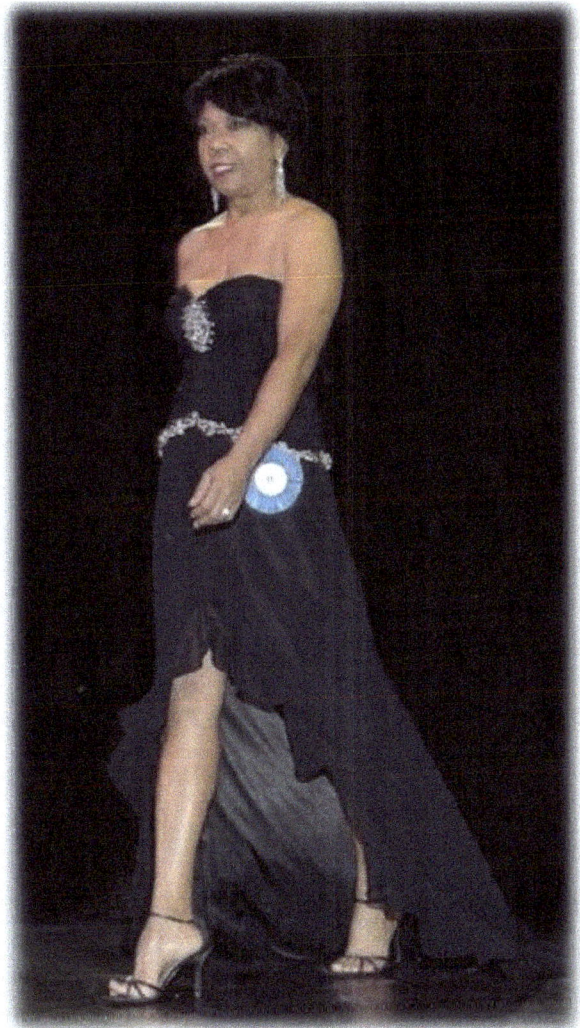

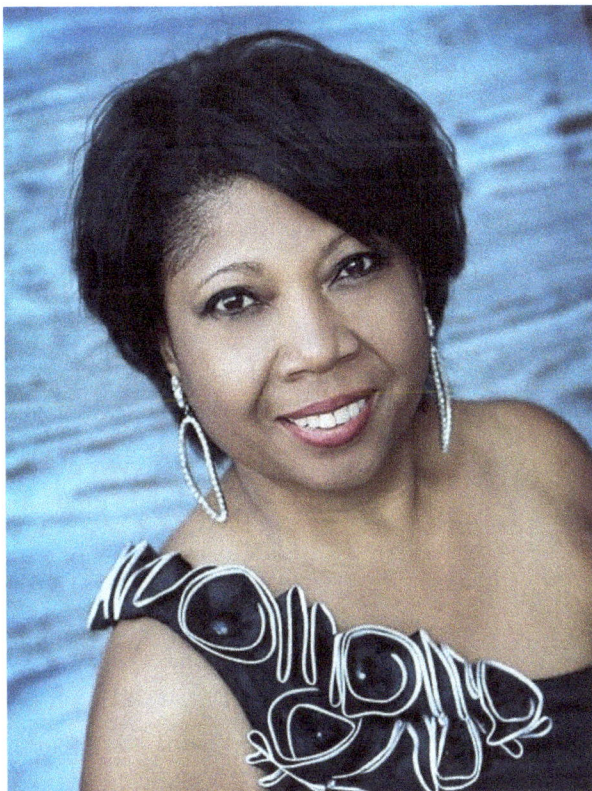

A Facebook friend suggested that I
enter the Mrs Mississippi Pageant to
highlight my platform of Promoting a
Positive Mississippi. I thought it was
a good idea.

November 2011

NEVER PAY FULL PRICE FOR FABULOUS

The Marshall's chain of discount stores has a advertising campaign slogan:

"Never pay full price for fabulous!"

I have adopted this as my own personal mantra. I am always encouraging & prompting my friends to "Go Forth and Be Fabulous." I am, however, not one that advocates fabulosity at any cost. I am one who believes in fabulosity at little or almost NO cost at all. I have been thrift shopping and yard saling for my personal wardrobe for many years. I would estimate that for the past 25 years, about 90% of my wardrobe has been acquired this way. Along with saving a tremendous amount of money, it can be SO MUCH FUN. I am always trying to proclaim the joys and benefits of thrift shopping and "Yard Saling" to everyone that I know and anyone who will listen.

POSSIBILITY THINKING: THE MUST HAVE MINDSET FOR THRIFT SHOPPING

In the shopping realm, possibility thinking means evaluating what can be done to make any item exactly what you want or need it to be. Of course, everything won't, ultimately, fit into that category, but the challenge is to mentally give everything a fighting chance and not dismiss it too quickly. Sometimes, just a few small adjustments can be made to make it absolutely perfect for you. But, you must acquire the ability to look beyond what is to what could be.

Sometimes, a person will disregard something and miss an absolutely fabulous find, simply because it is not exactly the right fit, the size that the person usually wears, or has a few minor flaws, at that time. There might be a button or two missing, a slight tear or other small flaw. Not only can these things, usually, be easily and inexpensively fixed, when they are pointed out, you can often get an added discount on an already unbelievable deal. If you came across a wonderful suit that you know normally retails in the $100 - $200 range and is offered for $1 - $5 but has a button or two missing or a small tear under the arm, why in the world would you NOT buy it? The tear can easily be sewn and buttons can very inexpensively be replaced. The worse thing that could happen is that it won't work out exactly as you had hoped and you are out of $5! Boo Hoo! You can always re-donate an item or pass it on to someone who would be glad to have it. Like Me !!! I can hook it up!!! If you pass up an item like this in a thrift shop or at a yard sale, it just means that you will have made someone like me a very happy camper when they come across it!

POSSIBILITY THINKING

Once, I took a friend thrift shopping because she wanted to see how I do my Diva on a Dime style of purchasing. We went to City Thrift on West Main Street in Tupelo on their 99 cents day, which was every Monday back then. (They no longer have the 99 cents day) I was, of course, like a kid in a candy shop grabbing all kinds of things that I thought that she would like. She did like the style of almost everything that I pulled off the racks, but for so many of them, she had some reason that they were not QUITE right. Most of the time, the reason that she gave for not getting an item was that it was too long, because she is petite. An item being too short might sometimes be a problem, but too long should NEVER be a problem! I cannot even fathom turning down a new , very expensive designer dress with tags on it at a price of 99 cents, because it is TOO LONG!! WOW!!!

It is one of the mysteries of the universe. Any item can be hemmed by yourself, a friend, or very inexpensively, by a seamstress. All I can say about that is one of my favorite sayings. You can lead a horse to water, but you can't make him (or her) drink! I still shake my head over that! I came out of the store with several very large bags, as usual and she came out with four or five items. She was absolutely thrilled with all of her finds She later told me about the many compliments that she got on the items that she purchased and wished that she had taken my advise and purchased the other items I had shown her and suggested. Oh! The Possibilities missed!!!

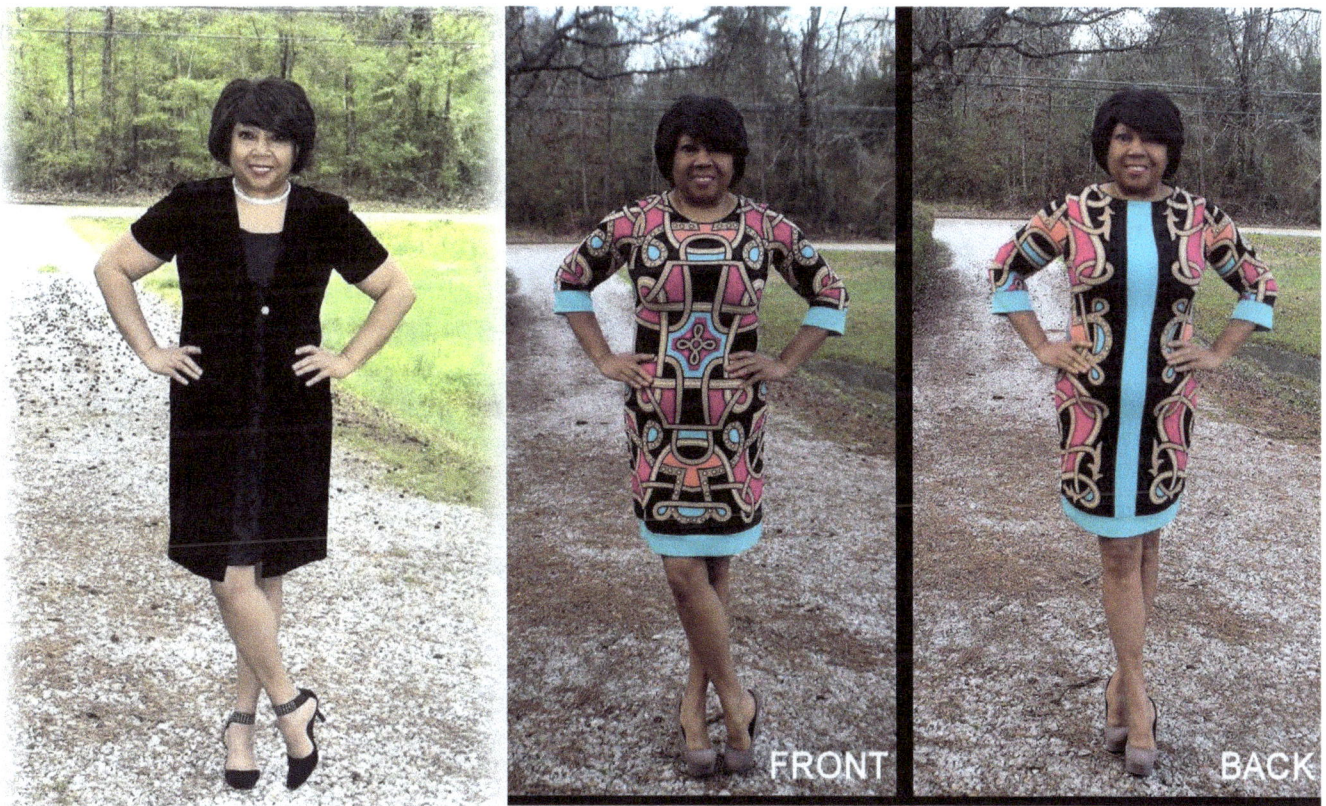

FRONT

BACK

Velvet Dress with attached faux jacket
99 Cents-City Thrift-Tupelo ,Mississippi

Dress 99 Cents - City Thrift

I have a wonderful example of working with the possibilities. Dear Hubby found a beautiful ankle length evening dress with a lace overlay for me at the thrift shop on 99 cent day. I absolutely loved it! It is one that I would have picked, if I had seen it. But, after trying it on a few times, I kept thinking that something wasn't quite right. I felt that it could be more fabulous and more ME! I decided to have the dress shortened to knee length while having the lace overlay remain long. It cost $10 to have altered, but it looked like a million bucks on me with the changes! The dress was perfect and I rocked it! I wore it to a black tie affair and got tons of compliments.

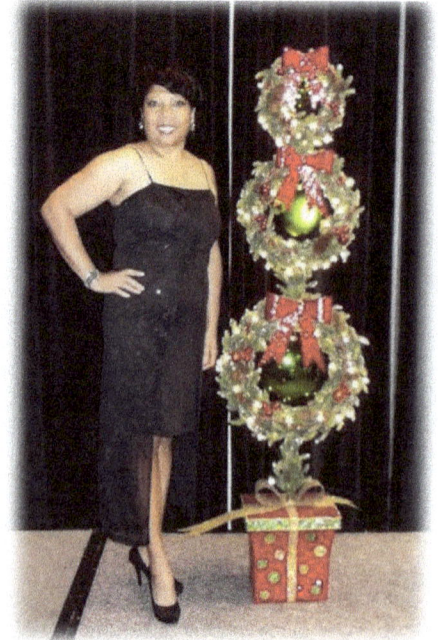

Black dress with lace overlay skirt
99 cents— City Thrift – Tupelo,MS

For all of those special occasions, when people can shell out an outrageous amount of money for that perfect dress, if you are a thrift shopper you have no worries . You can find semi-formal and formal gowns all of the time. There are always dresses that will certainly satisfy your needs for pageants ,banquets, parties and black-tie events for pennies on the dollar. It is not unusual to find exquisite gowns for $20 or less! For any wardrobe requirements, from casual to super fancy, thrift shops have you covered literally!

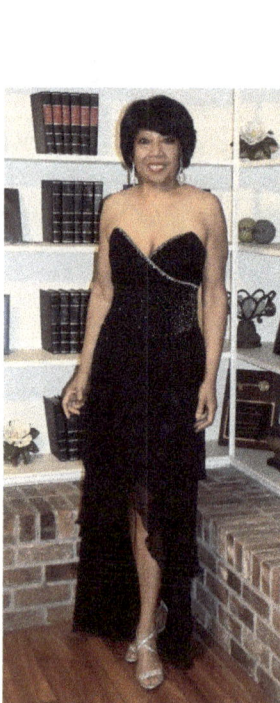

99 Cents
City Thrift-Tupelo, Mississippi

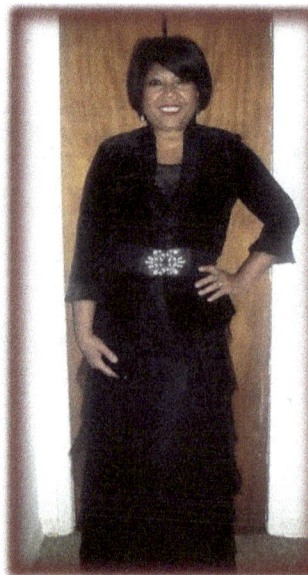

Jessica McClintock evening gown $10
Sanctuary Thrift Shop
Jacket $2

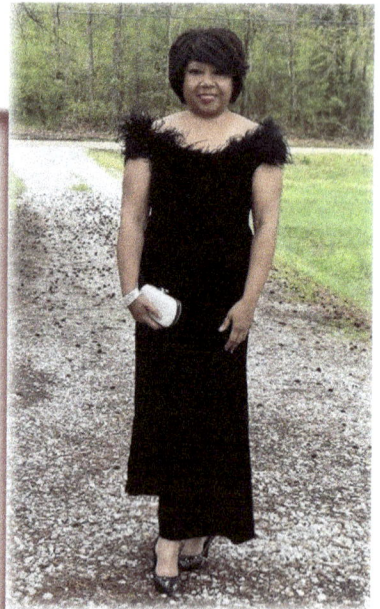

VELVET DRESS
$19.91 City Thrift Tupelo, MS

$20 City Thrift - Tupelo, MS

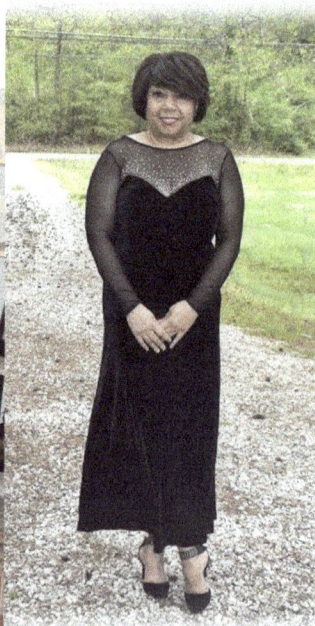

There is a huge misnomer about thrift shops that there are only great fashion treasures/gems to be found in small sizes. This is far from the truth. There are women of all sizes who donate to thrift shops. There are amazing pieces in every size imaginable. I have gone up and down over the years in sizes ranging from 4-16 (you can see that in my pictures). There is an abundance of 18, 20, 22 ,1x 2x and 3x to be found. I have ALWAYS found an ABUNDANCE of fabulous finds in ALL sizes. I have purchased items for friends in sizes 18 and up. There is no shortage of XL and XXL sizes. If you have lost or gained weight, you will have no worries in ever finding something to wear, at whatever size you happen to be, at any given time.

I often buy for other folks besides myself and LOVE IT! The treasure hunt aspect of thrift shopping is exhilarating! One of my friends has a whole , super extensive wardrobe of pure fabulosity ..courtesy of me PND! You are not ready for all the Fabulosity! She loves lots of glitz and lots of glam! When it's a little too much for me, it goes straight the her! She also loves black as much as I do but she takes sparkle and accessorizing to another level! If you ever run across her, you would need to get you some shades! The SHINE will be bright!

She is not 20 something or 50 something. She is 70+ something !!! You cannot give the excuse that you can only find great bargain stuff for young folks. She is not a size 6 or a size 10..She is a size 16 /18. You cannot give the excuse that you can only find great bargains in small sizes. There is absolutely no excuse not to just give it a try! You will not regret it!

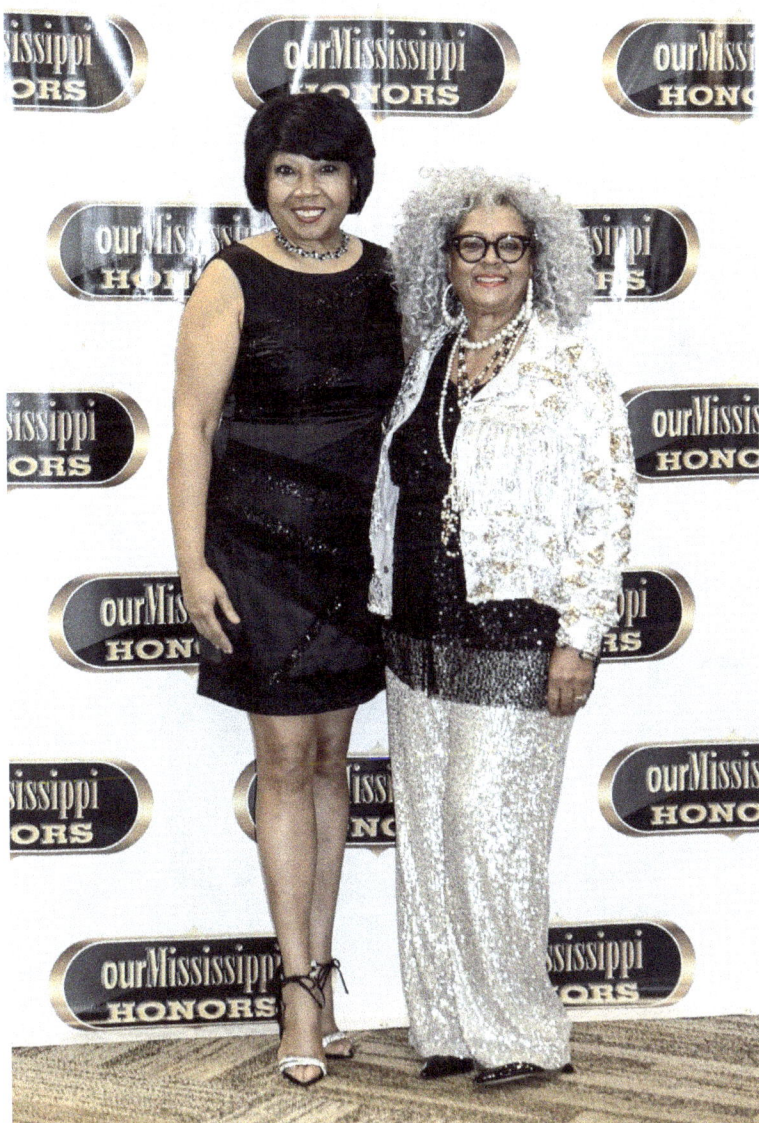

Note: My friend is so vibrant and FULL OF LIFE. She is the epitome of FABULOUS! She always says " I'm gonna LIVE 'til I die!" I always give a big amen to that sentiment . We have a running joke between us, which is not really a joke at all for her . She always tells me "When I die you make sure they put me on something shiny and some bright red lipstick." I have agreed to that .

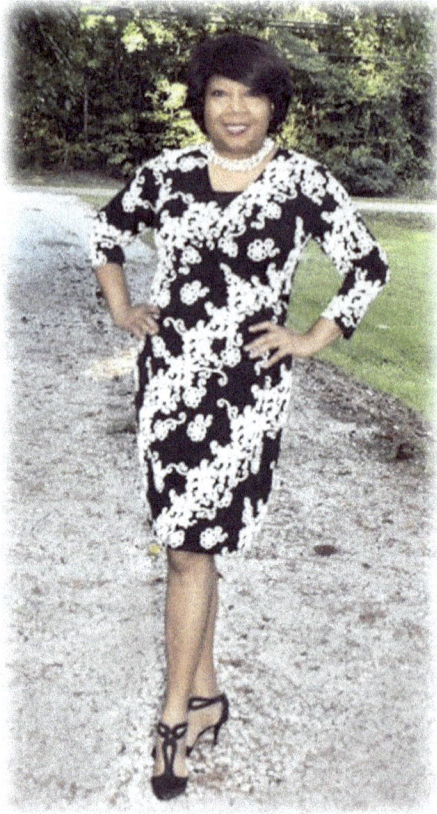

DRESS $5.99 - Nine West SHOES: $5.99
Goodwill -TUPELO

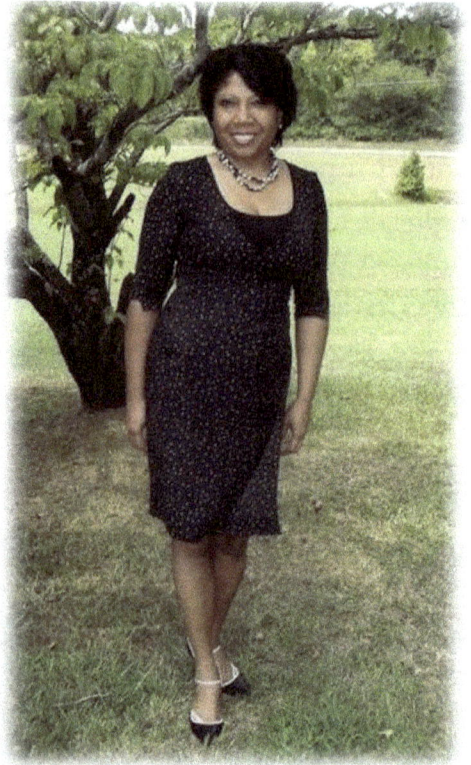

Dress 99 Cents – City Thrift
Shoes $1 Salvation Army
Necklace $1 Yardsale – Saltillo

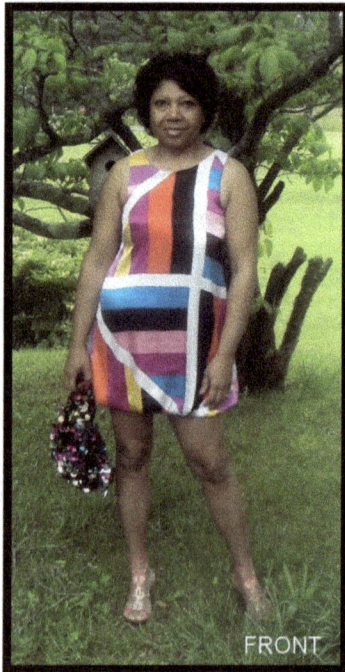

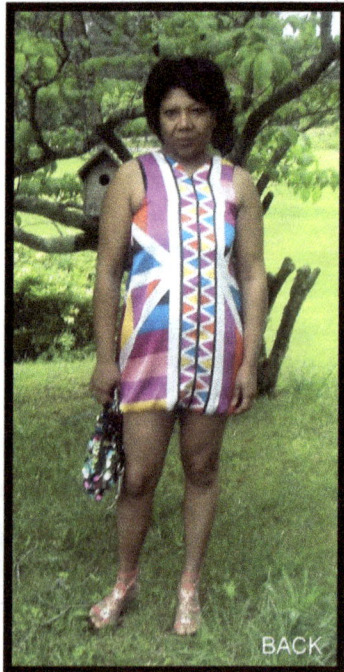

FRONT

BACK

Dress $2   Purse $1

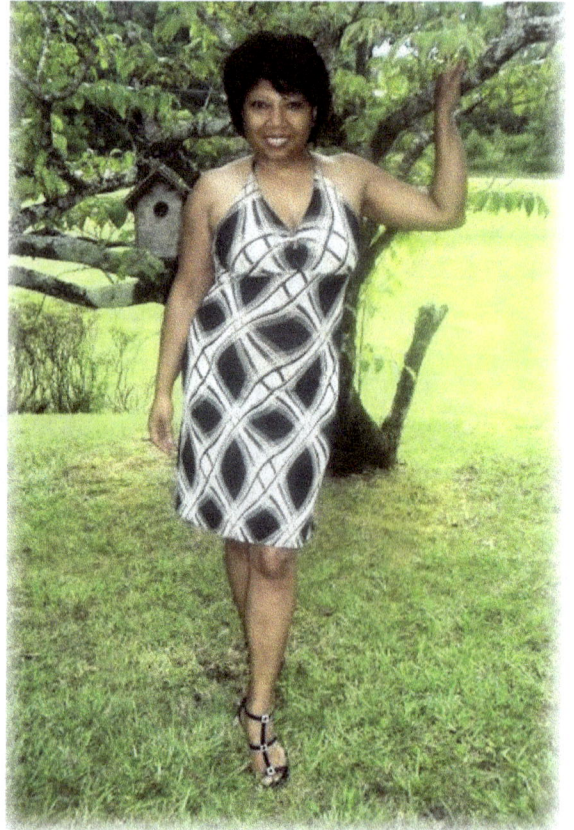

Sundress $2 - Salvation Army

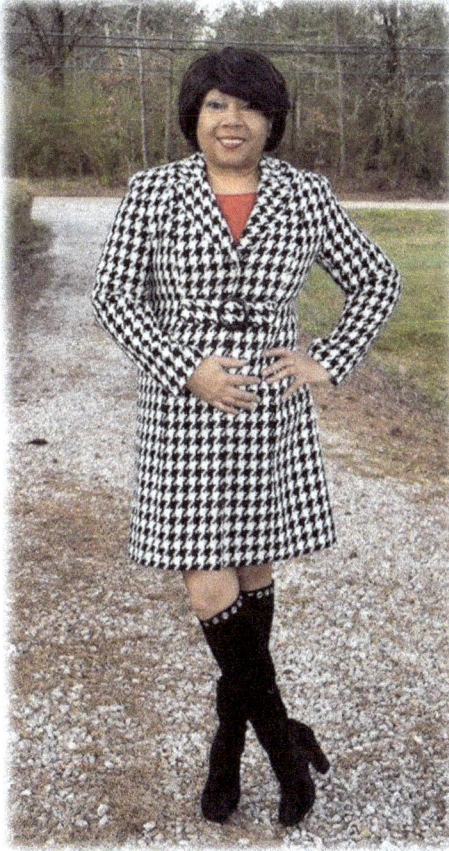

Coat Under $5 Salvation Army
Boots $8

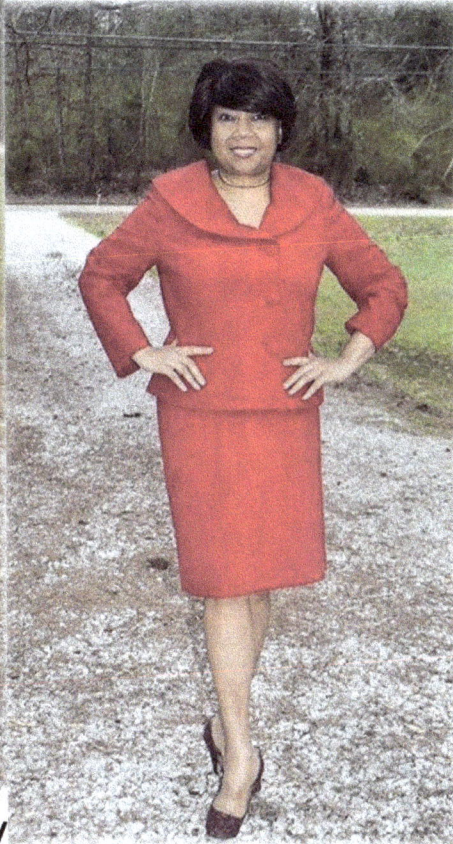

TAHARI SUIT $7.99 ~ Goodwill -Tupelo

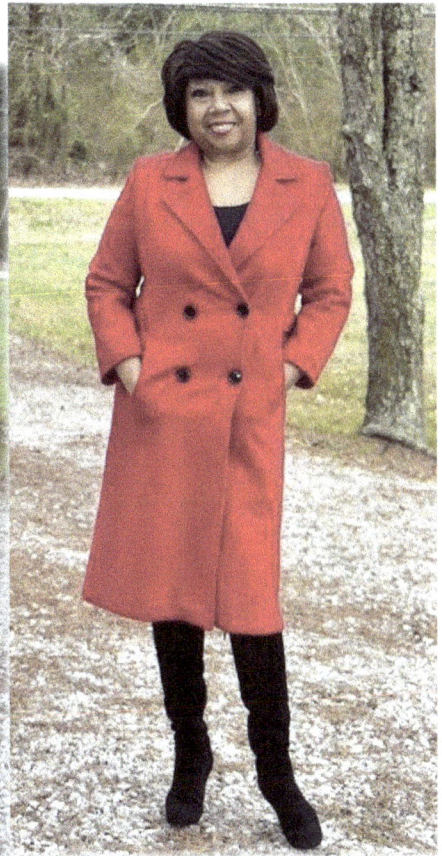

Coat $5 ~ Boots $8

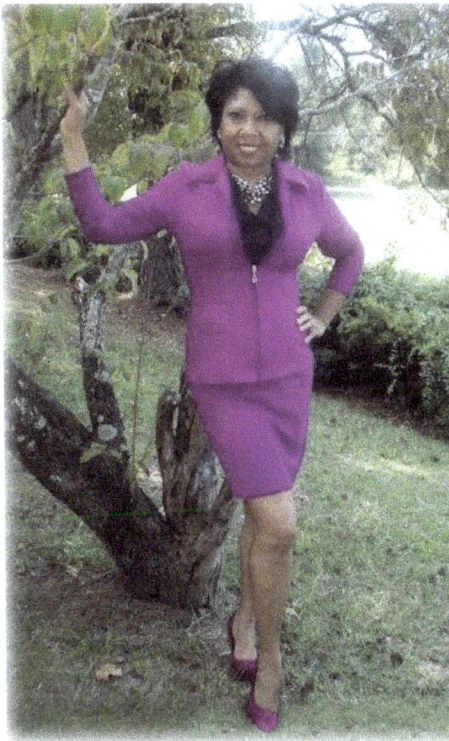

Magenta Suit - Under $10
City Thrift- Tupelo, MS

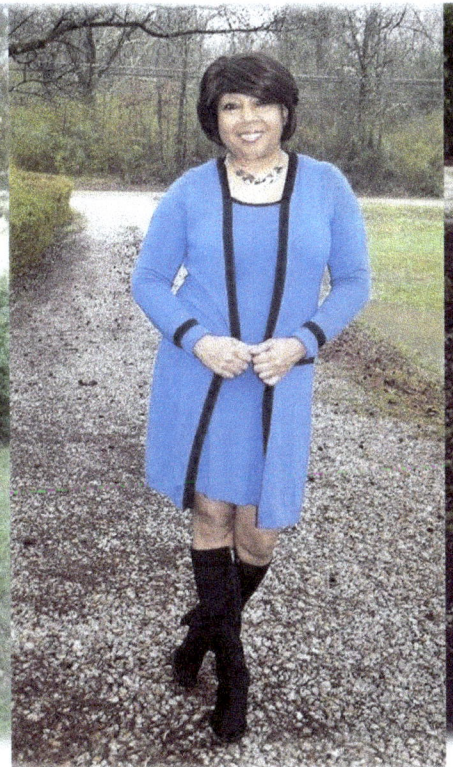

Dress with faux jacket $5.99
Goodwill - Tupelo

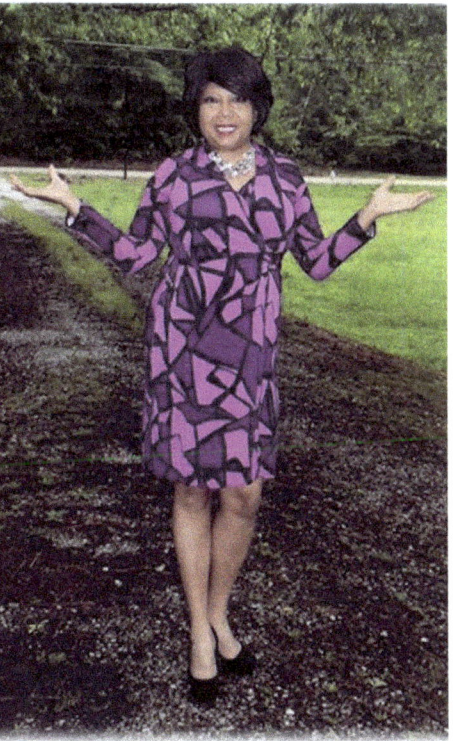

Nine West Dress-$5.99
Goodwill -Tupelo

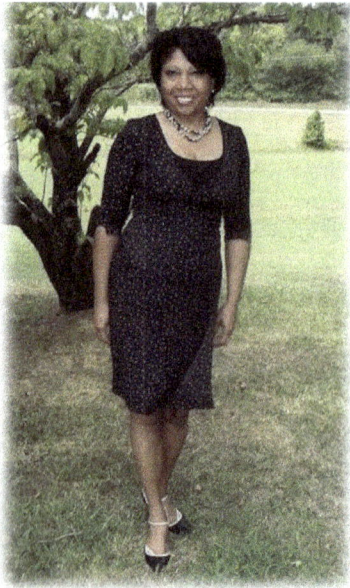

Dress 99 Cents – City Thrift
Shoes $1 Salvation Army
Necklace $1 Yardsale – Saltillo

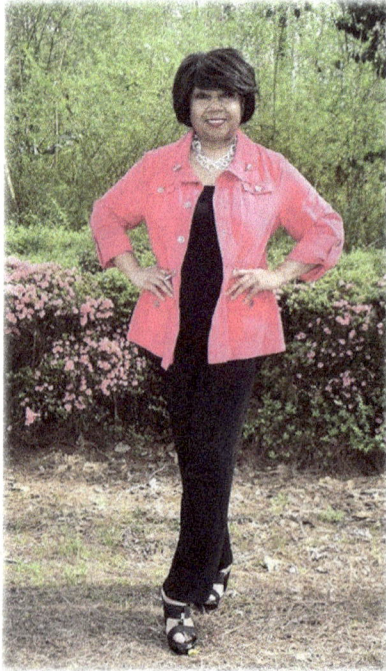

Jacket 75 cents -Salvation Army

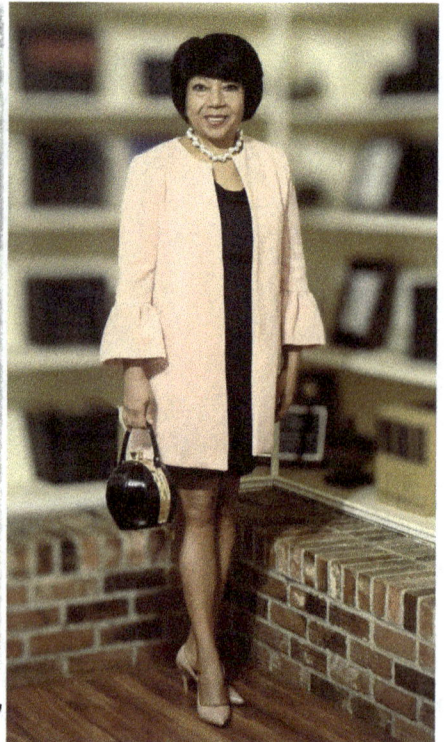

Jacket $5.99 Goodwill
Black Slip Dress $1 Yard Sale
Shoes $3 Salvation Army

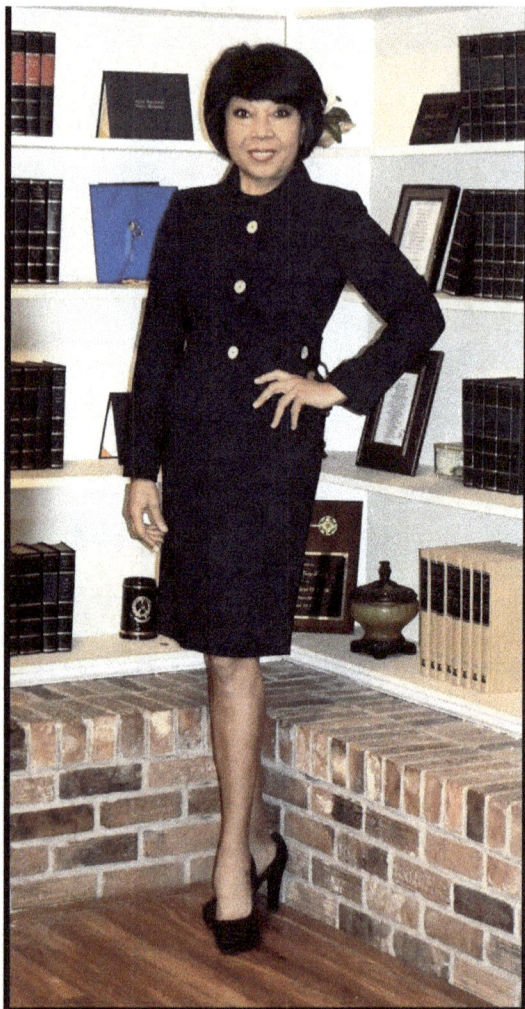

Liz Claiborne Navy Suit
$5-Thrift Shop

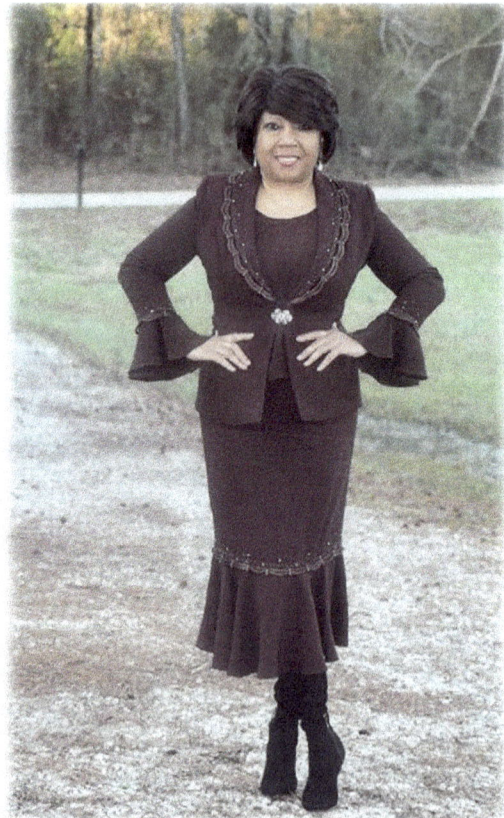

Chocolate Brown
3 -Piece Outfit $9.99 Goodwill -Tupelo
Boots $3.50 Salvation Army-Tupelo

This suit was $5 dollars from a thrift shop. It was three pieces and came with the camisole. I loved it and wore it often.

OCTOBER 1, 2009
BELOW
Guest Speaker -Rust College Lyceum Series along with friend , barber and fellow author John Campbell
It was the first time I had presented my book/poems in front of such a HUGE crowd.

JANUARY 2011
RIGHT
Guest Speaker-Itawamba Development Council
Annual Awards Banquet
FULTON

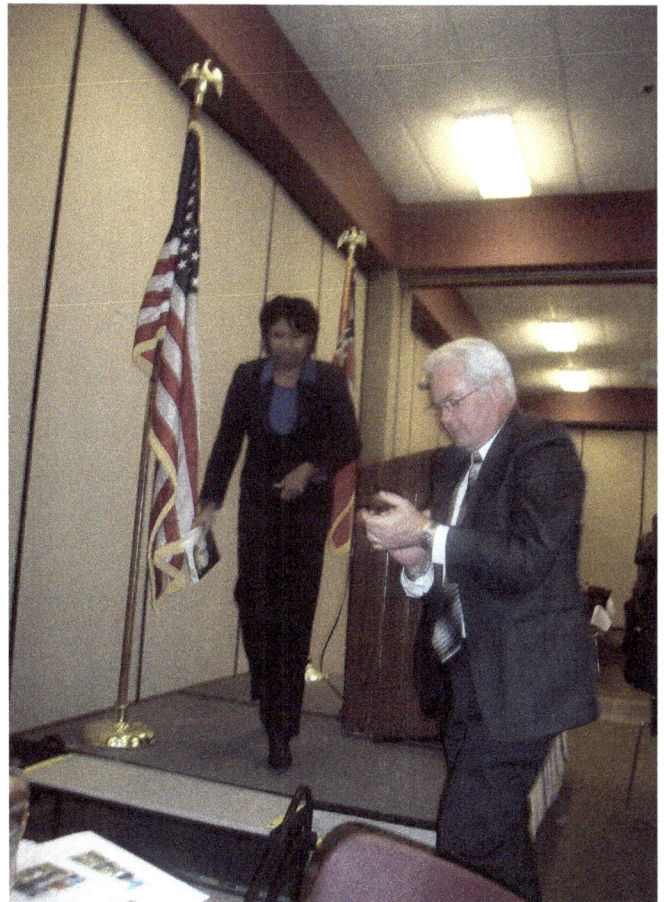

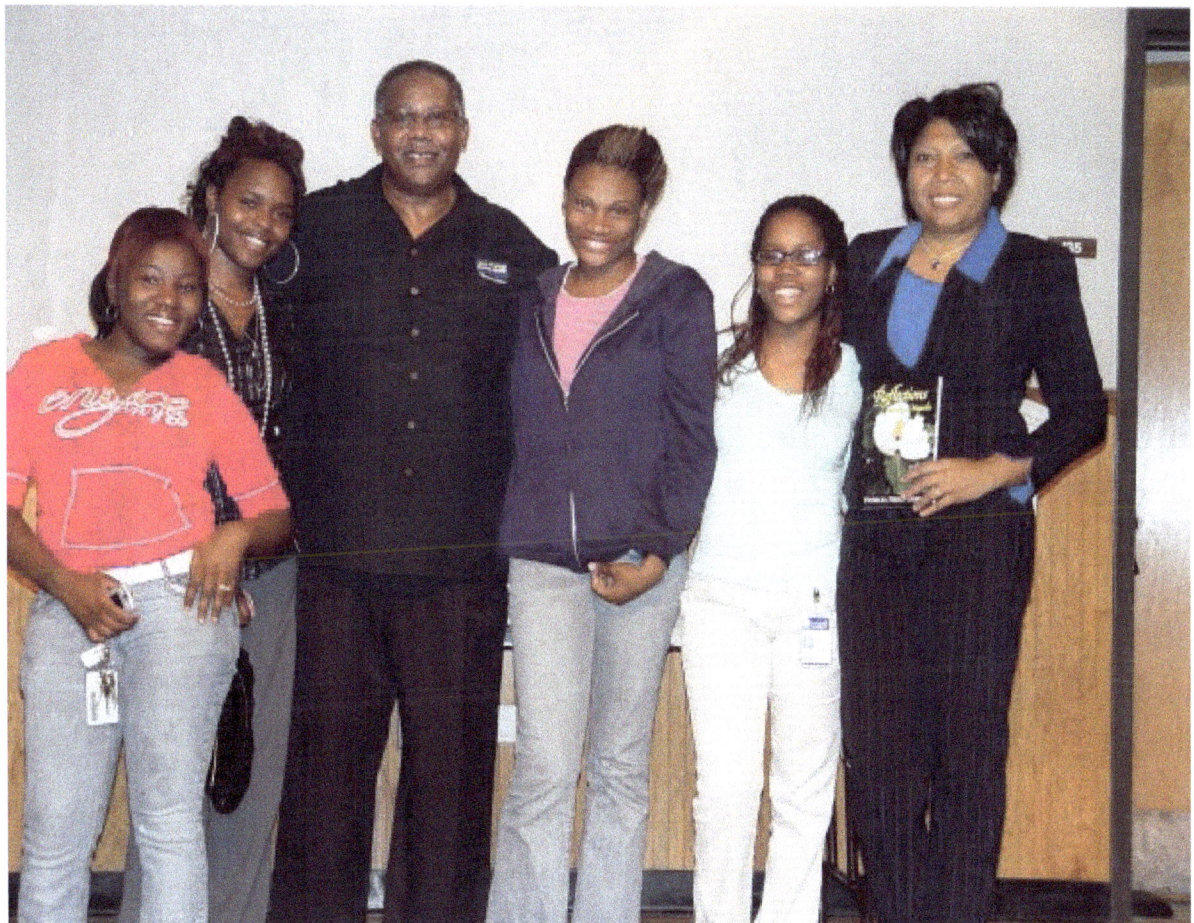

Many people will say that they do not like wearing used clothes. What most people don't know is that you can often find new clothes that have never been worn. There are clothes that have come straight out of a retail store and have landed in your local thrift shop. The only difference is you will be paying pennies on the dollar. In retail stores you are paying for the bright lights, organization and fancy merchandising. What I love about thrift shopping is that you can try out/ explore/ experiment with all types of styles and "play dress up" as much as you want without breaking the bank and purchase pieces that you would not even consider purchasing at regular retail because of the price and/ or impracticality. Trina Turk cocktail dress (NWT) New With Tags. Under $10 from thrift shop Salvation Army Tupelo, Mississippi. retail price on tag $398. Oct.2022

As I have mentioned before, you can find MANY items in thrift stores that are brand new with the tags still on them. Retail stores often donate out of season or last season's fashions. Some people buy clothes and just don't decide to wear them. PND: Whatever the reason is that anyone donates, I want to thank you personally! (smile) #MoreForMe

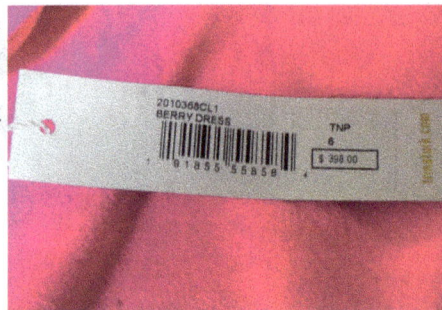

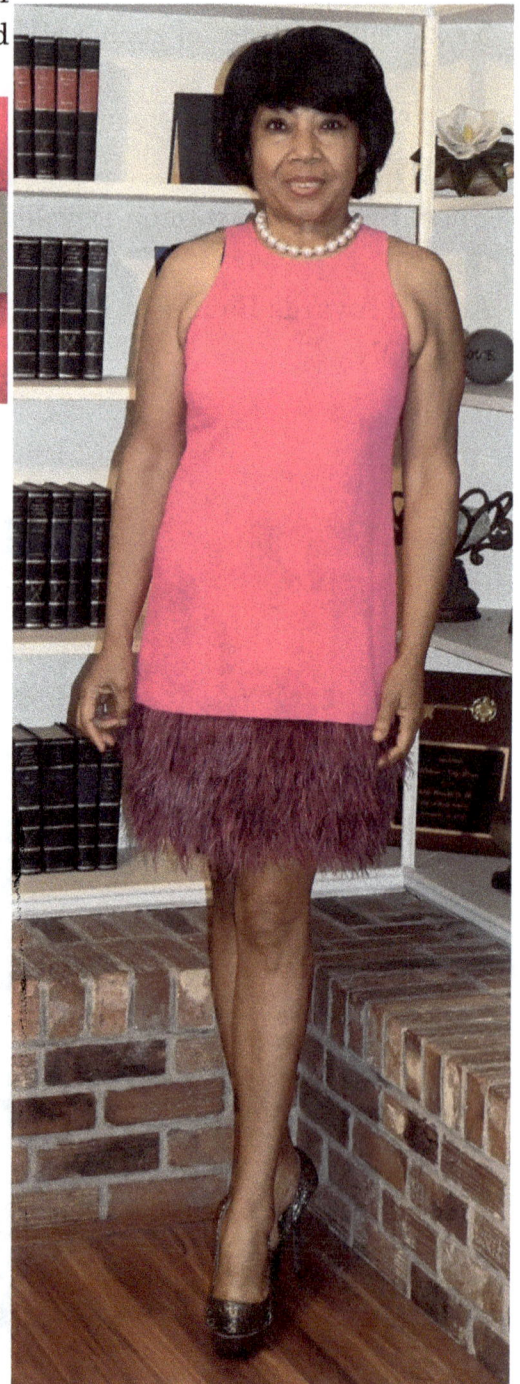

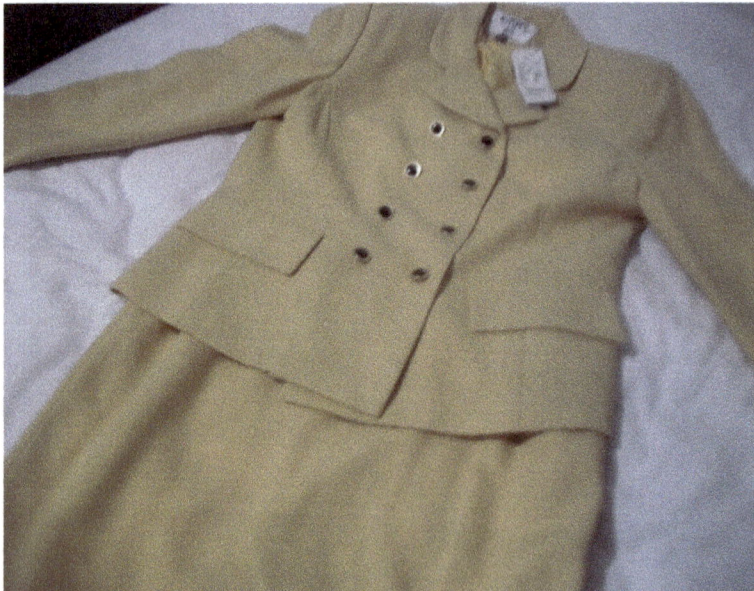

Several years ago , I purchased several BRAND NEW suits from Salvation   Army for $4 each ($2 for each piece)

They were most probably donated from a local retail store.

Here is a bright mustard yellow KASPER suit with all of the tags and a $199. 00 price still on it

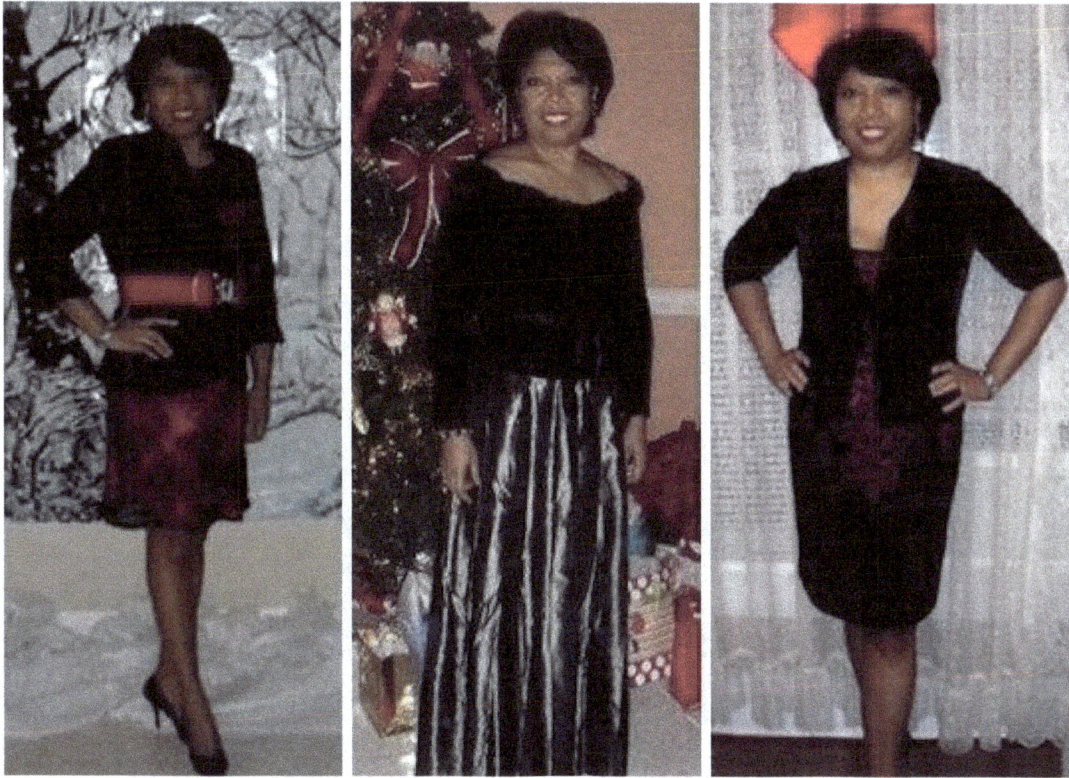

ALL of these outfits COMBINED cost LESS THAN $50

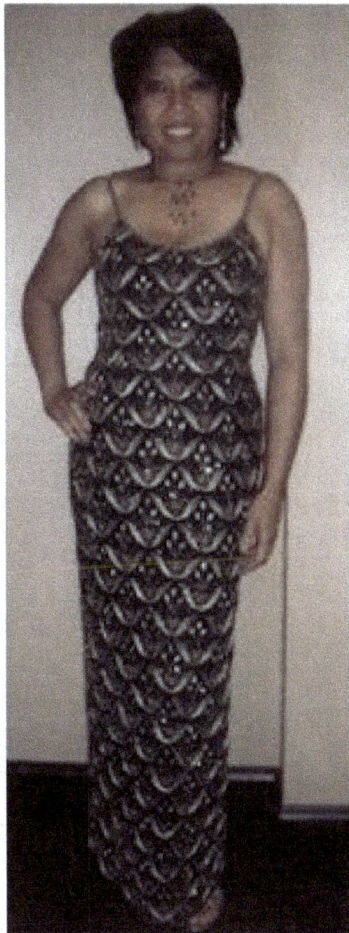

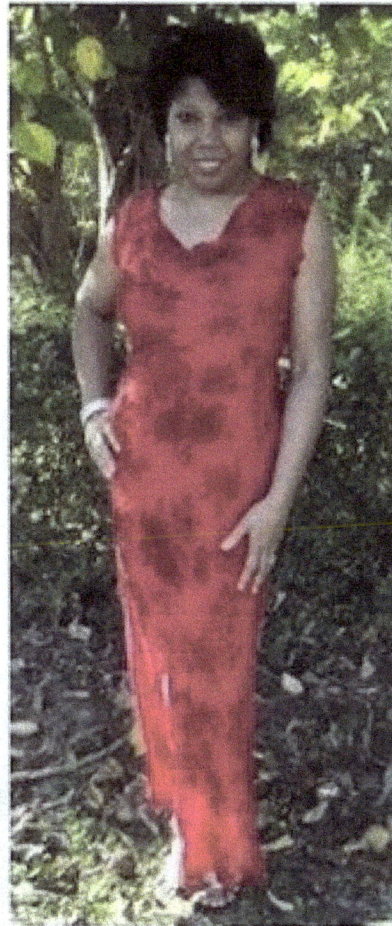

Wonderful time sharing my favorite yard sale /thrift shop tips as the Guest Speaker- NEWMS Escape Lunch
November 13, 2014
My wonderful model (friend Yvonne Jackson Roberts) helped show off some of my finds!
The ladies even got to take home lots of yard sale goodies!

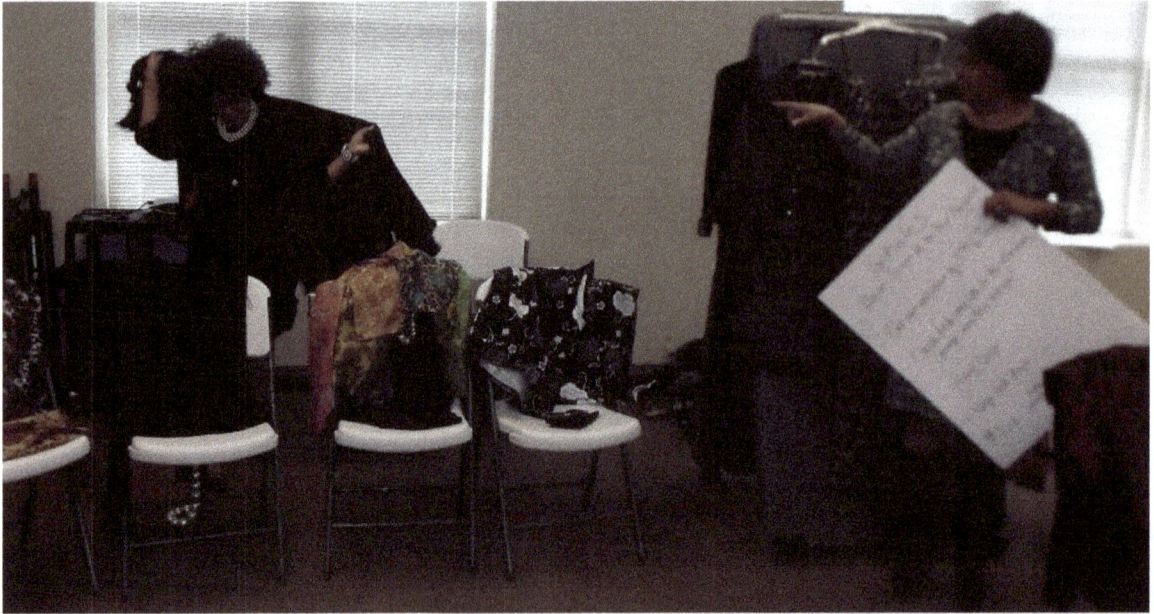

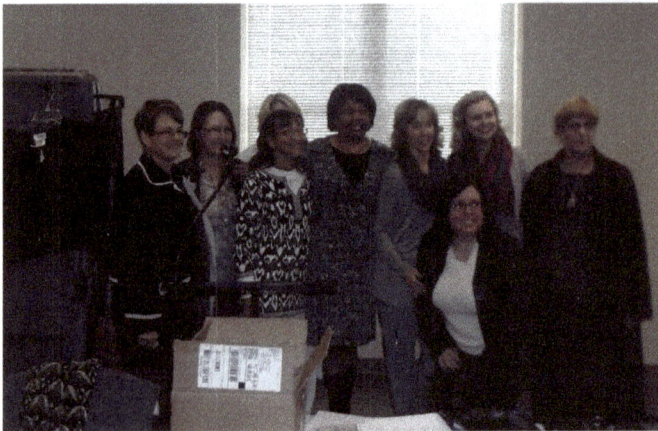

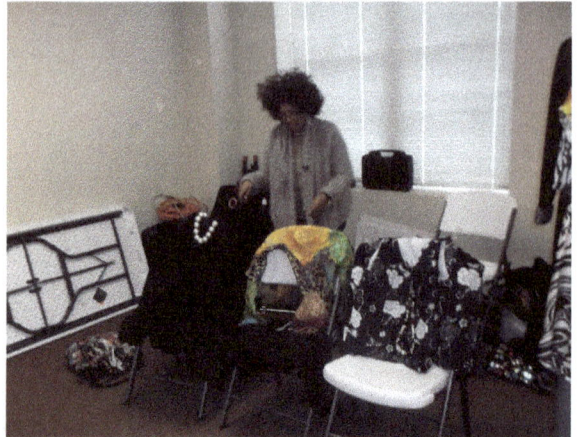

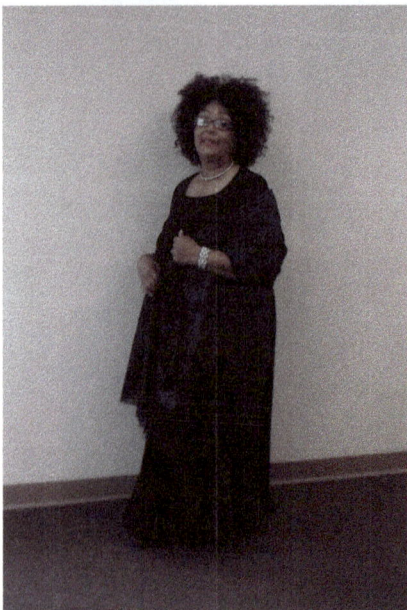

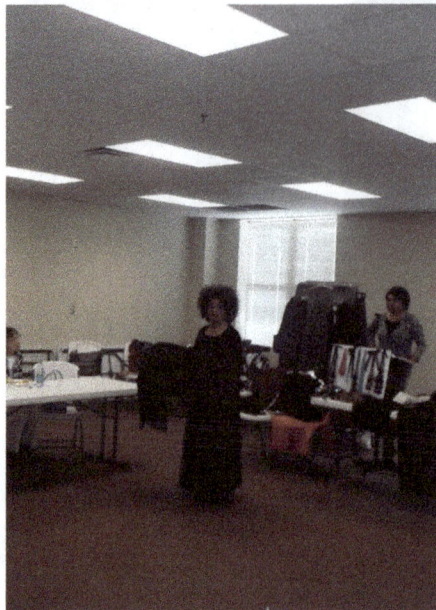

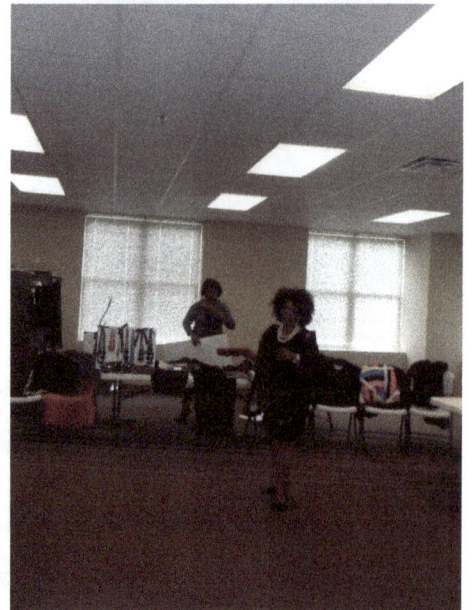

GOODWILL BARBIE

The day I met "Goodwill Barbie". (April 22, 2019)

I was doing my usual Goodwill rounds of shopping, planning to run in and run out I went directly to the dress wall and started "filing" through the dresses. I usually kind of quickly flip through them like turning pages in a book . If it's not my color or style, it does not even get a blip on the radar. I am a "spotter when it comes to shopping .My eyes have become trained to hone in on my favorite styles and colors immediately. As I was going down the aisle, there was a lady standing right in front of a black and white dress that I instantly spotted. I was a little annoyed because she was just standing there staring. She wasn't taking anything off of the rack or anything ..just standing and staring. I didn't want to be rude and reach in front of her. So, I went past her and kept looking through other dresses, thinking that I would get my black and white dress as soon as she moved. She didn't move. Finally I said, "excuse me" and got the dress. She was still just standing there staring. I thought to myself that she must be having some type of melt down or going through something. It was very strange. Later, a few aisles over with my basket full and checking out the shoes, we met up again. She said that she was looking for an outfit for an interview and was just totally overwhelmed. She said that she didn't know what she should get or how to decide.

She said that she had been watching me and wondered how I could go through and pick things so fast. She said that she had noticed that black and white dress and was thinking about getting it. I said, "What? This dress?" as I pulled it out of the pile of things in my cart. I told her that the dress would be perfect for an interview I told her it would look really good on her and fit her perfectly. ...I could tell. I had her try it on ...and it did! (It was actually banging on me too, because I had tried it on...I don't even know why, because I rarely try on anything) I have to admit it was a lot tighter and lumpier because of my size at that time. But, you know, that's another story ! LOL!

Long story short...I told her how I do what I do She came out of the store that day with "my dress" and a big bag or clothes that I helped her pick and a big smile. I dubbed her Goodwill Barbie (she loved that) because she is a perfect size to dress! She confided that she had been over 250 pounds and she went on the Keto diet and got to her current size. She showed me a picture on her phone. The transformation was amazing! Yep, we had to take a selfie to document the beginning of a wonderful friendship and epic crisis management shopping spree. I had to talk her out of wearing this blouse and PANTS for her dream job interview! The blouse is really cute and the pants were nice, but wasn't THE LOOK! PND Personal Diva on a Dime Shopper Extraordinaire to the rescue. P.S And we still think we're cute with the no make up all about the shopping , trying not to be seen mode

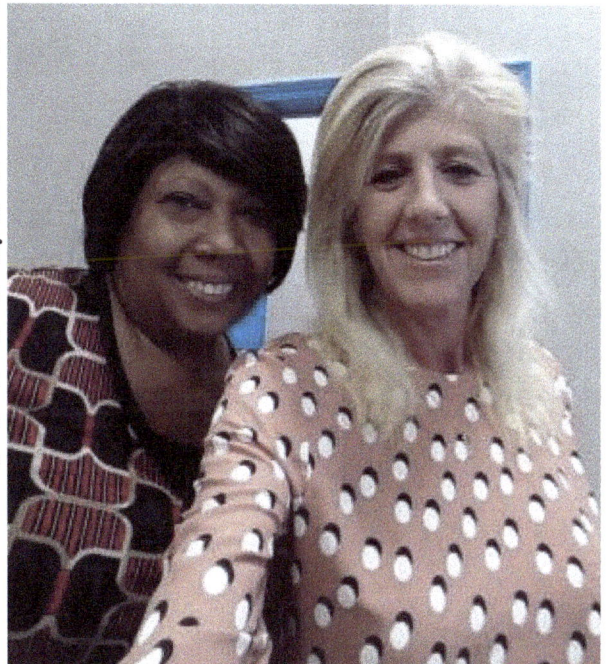

I made this Facebook post the next day April 23, 2023

This is the beautiful new friend that I met in Goodwill on Monday! (April 22) This is the dress and shoes that I insisted she wear. Trust me, the picture doesn't even do it justice! (She wanted to wear pants! Not on my watch !) I received this message from her today: You were RIGHT! I felt so pretty this morning! After this interview, will you go with me to get jewelry and accessories and more clothing? My hubby was impressed! So am I! Thank you so much for the help! You're amazing! Diva on a Dime in the House! Mission accomplished! I'm on the case. The dress was $5.99 .

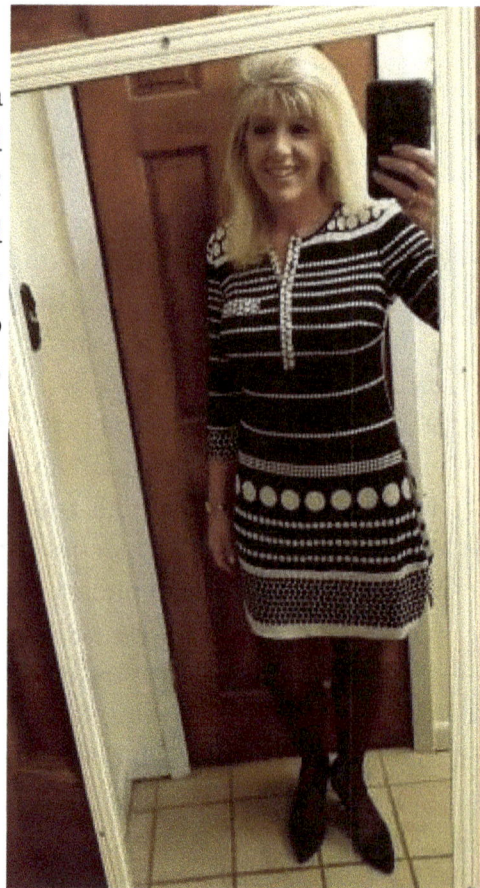

We met for round two of shopping and she was wearing the dress.

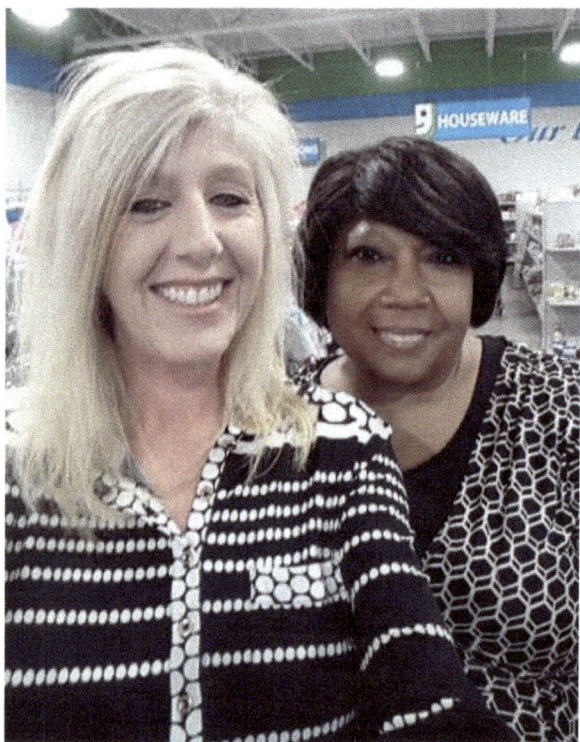

May 2, 2019 Look at that pair that was loose, again, in Goodwill. PND and "Barbie" ! This is the kind of smile you have when you walk into Goodwill. there is already a basket of clothes custom selected just for you. You try them on. You LOVE them all. You buy them all. Checkout lady says, "Wow you made some great finds!" You point at your friend PND and say I didn't find anything. She did.

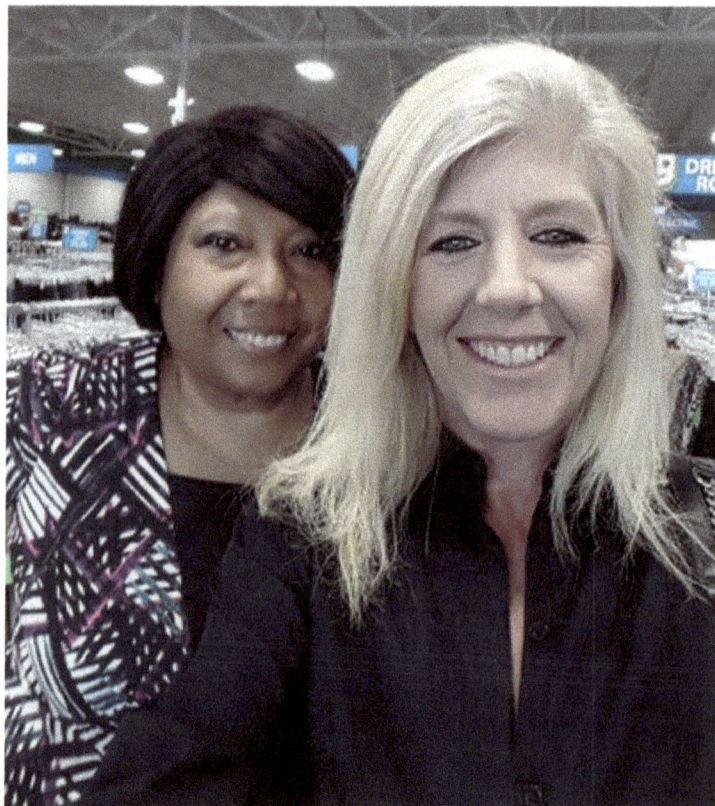

GOODWILL BARBIE FOLLOWUP

This story shows that shopping can be fun and not a chore and there is a science to it. The key is to Know Thyself! It is an example of women helping women ...people helping people ..We all should ..in any small way possible. (Even if it's just giving fashion tips or shopping assistance) It is an example of a Maya Angelou quote that I try to live by ..." Be a rainbow in someone's cloud"

#RandomActsofKindness

The night after our meeting and shopping excursion She sent me this message after going to her interview in the dress that I knew would be a hit : She wrote: You were RIGHT! I felt so pretty this morning! After this interview. Will you go with me to get jewelry and accessories and more clothing? My hubby was impressed! So am I! Thank you so much for the help! You're amazing! Barbie was offered the job and said she did not have a lot of dresses or professional clothing. She had recently moved from Florida and said she had mostly "beachy" clothes.

(Hmm maybe I should have renamed her Malibu Barbie) We met up after her interview and found more fabulous outfits for her. We met up a couple of more times for accessories and miscellaneous.

Over the next month, I gave her several huge bags of clothes from my closet that I though would look good on her. She looks great in black and in every shade of blue! Navy is wonderful on her ! Red is great on her!

She said that she had never had that many clothes in her LIFE! LOL! P.S. We didn't have to go on anymore shopping trips. I gave her all of the clothes and jewelry that she needed! Here are a few of the items from the bags .

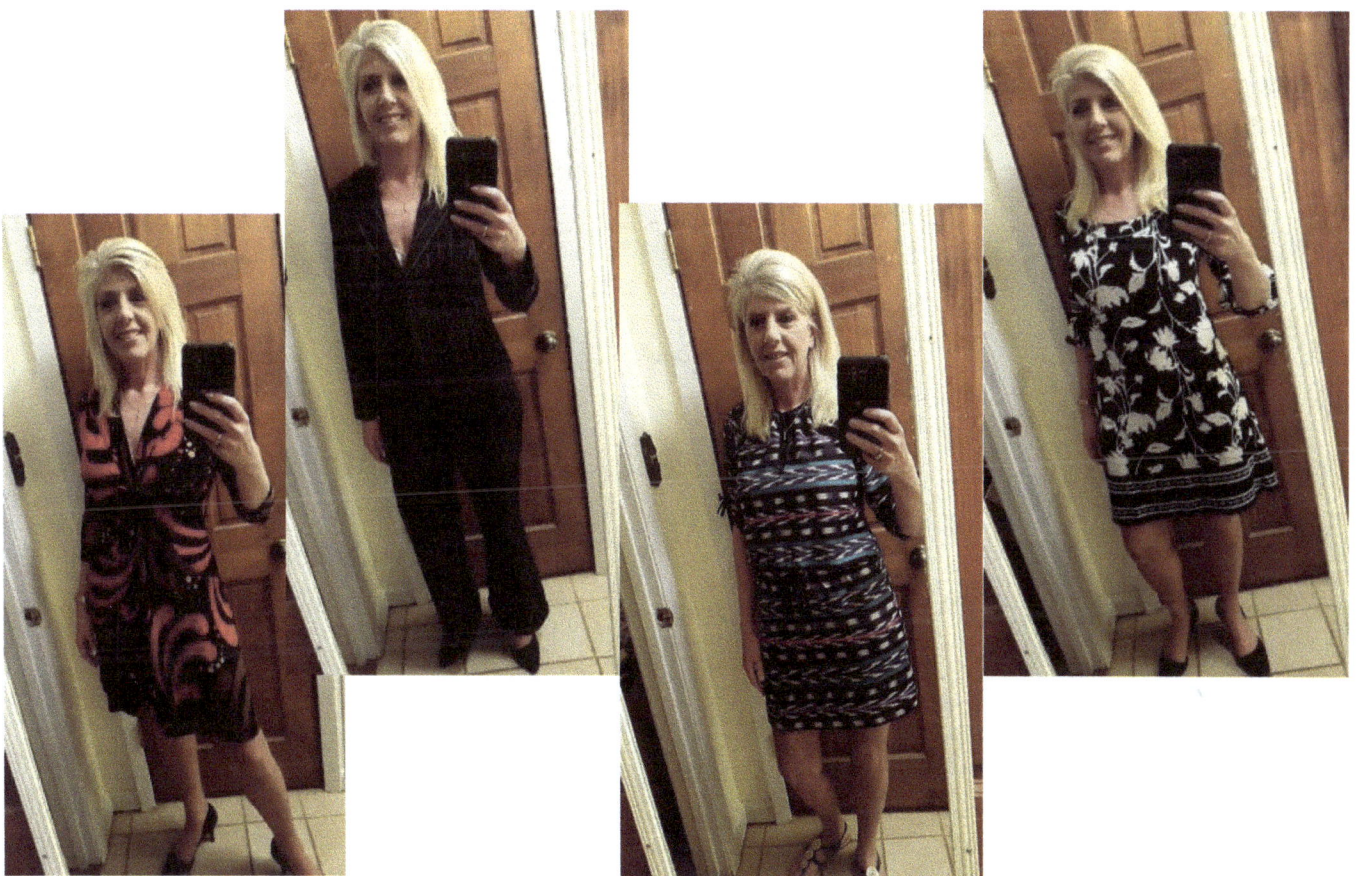

DIVA ON A DIME

I am always and forever doing the Diva on a Dime thing! Do you remember this thrifty shopping article with a familiar poet you might know? I was interviewed about my Diva On A Dime Shopping habits/tips.

Sunday January 23, 2011- Daily Journal

From the article: Tupelo poet Patricia Neely-Dorsey advises friends to be "Divas on a Dime" by shopping at thrift stores, consignment shops and garage sales.

"When I was younger, I spent crazy mounts of money on clothes," said the former mental health worker. "In my 20s, it was nothing for me to spend $100 on a blouse or $150 on a sweater."

Neely-Dorsey, author of "Reflections of a Mississippi Magnolia," said now her upper limit for even an evening gown is $10, but she aims to buy most items for 50 cents to $2. "Most times I'll be clothed from head to toe – dress, jacket, shoes and all – for less than $10," she said. Neely-Dorsey said it was years after she'd furnished her college apartment at garage sales that thrift clothing finally got her attention.

"I didn't think of the clothing thing until I was in my church in Memphis. My friend would have clothes that were phenomenal, that she got at yard sales, and she'd paid something like 50 cents or a dollar," she said. "Once you start, you really feel sorry for people who shop regular stores."

The Tupelo native regularly features her finds on Facebook and has been urged to offer her "Diva on a Dime" insights as a book or a seminar. "Thrift shopping is totally guilt-free shopping," she said. "If you decide you don't really like something after all, you can give it away; at 50 cents a shirt, you can afford to buy for your friends. And you're usually supporting a good cause."

READ FULL ARTICLE HERE:
http://djournal.com/news/pinching-pennies-the-new-austerity-savings-can-mean-sacrifice-or-serendipity/

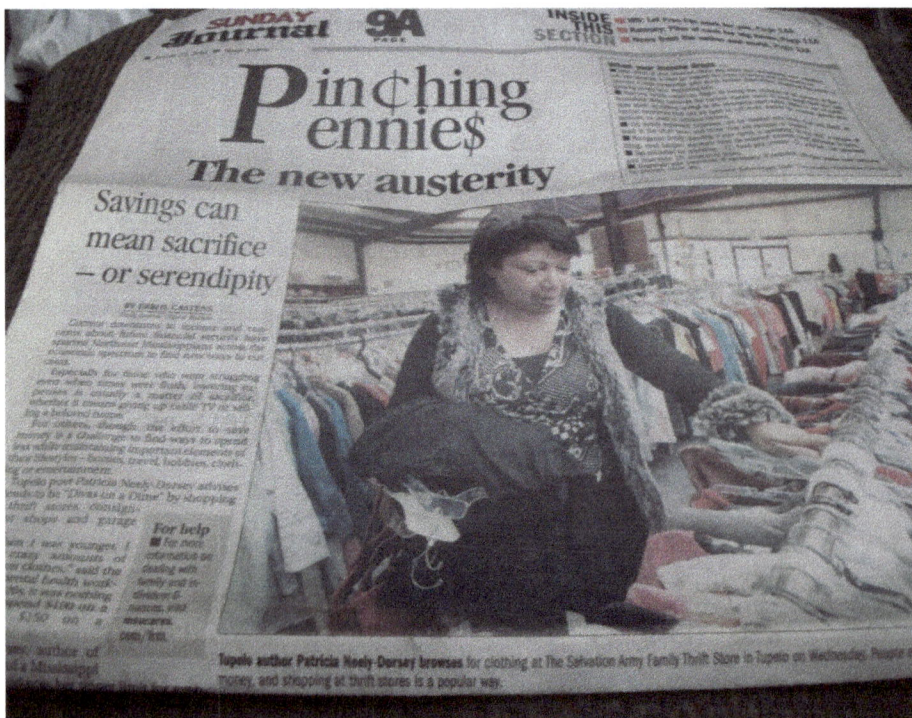

Pinching Pennies: The new austerity. Savings can mean sacrifice – or serendipity

Posted on **January 23, 2011** by **Errol Castens** in News

By Errol Castens / NEMS Daily Journal Oxford Bureau

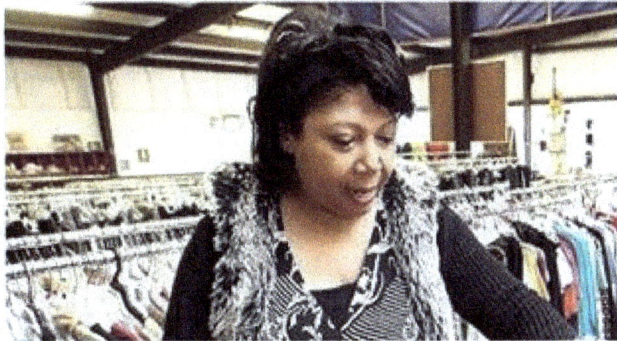

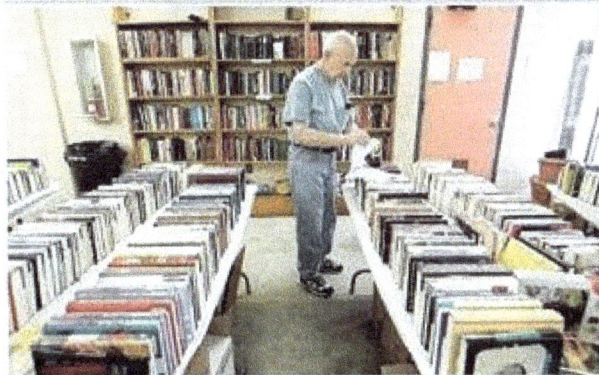

Current downturns in income and concerns about future financial security have spurred Northeast Mississippians across the economic spectrum to find new ways to cut costs.

Especially for those who were struggling even when times were flush, lowering expenses is usually a matter of sacrifice, whether it means giving up cable TV or selling a beloved home.

For others, though, the effort to save money is a challenge to find ways to spend less while maintaining important elements of their lifestyles – homes, travel, hobbies, clothing or entertainment.

Tupelo poet Patricia Neely-Dorsey advises friends to be "Divas on a Dime" by shopping at thrift stores, consignment shops and garage sales.

"When I was younger, I spent crazy amounts of money on clothes," said the former mental health worker. "In my 20s, it was nothing for me to spend $100 on a blouse or $150 on a sweater."

Neely-Dorsey, author of "Reflections of a Mississippi Magnolia," said now her upper limit for even an evening gown is $10, but she aims to buy most items for 50 cents to $2.

"Most times I'll be clothed from head to toe – dress, jacket, shoes and all – for less than $10," she said.

Neely-Dorsey said it was years after she'd furnished her college apartment at garage sales that thrift clothing finally got her attention.

"I didn't think of the clothing thing until I was in my church in Memphis. My friend would have clothes that were phenomenal, that she got at yard sales, and she'd paid something like 50 cents or a dollar," she said. "Once you start, you really feel sorry for people who shop regular stores."

The Tupelo native regularly features her finds on Facebook and has been urged to offer her "Diva on a Dime" insights as a book or a seminar.

"Thrift shopping is totally guilt-free shopping," she said. "If you decide you don't really like something after all, you can give it away; at 50 cents a shirt, you can afford to buy for your friends. And you're usually supporting a good cause."

February 2012

Book Signing /Poetry Reading Coldwater Books Tuscumbia, Alabama

Can you believe they had me speaking on being a Diva on a Dime, too? LOL!!! I brought some fab finds with me for show and tell! During almost every speaking engagement that I have been to over the years, except for the schools, I have been asked to talk about my thrift shopping. I have been asked over and over to write a book about it, showing my thrift shop finds and sharing tips. It's amazing how the universe has answered. Through my mother, the wishes have been granted. If it were not for her, everyone would just have to follow on Facebook for any gems.

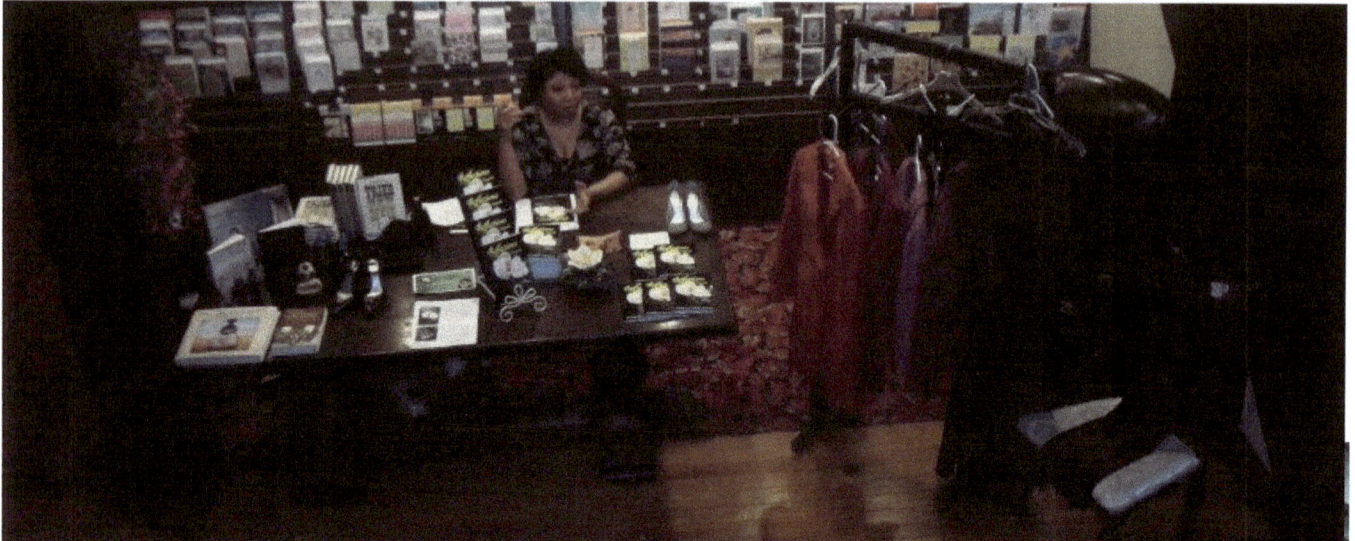

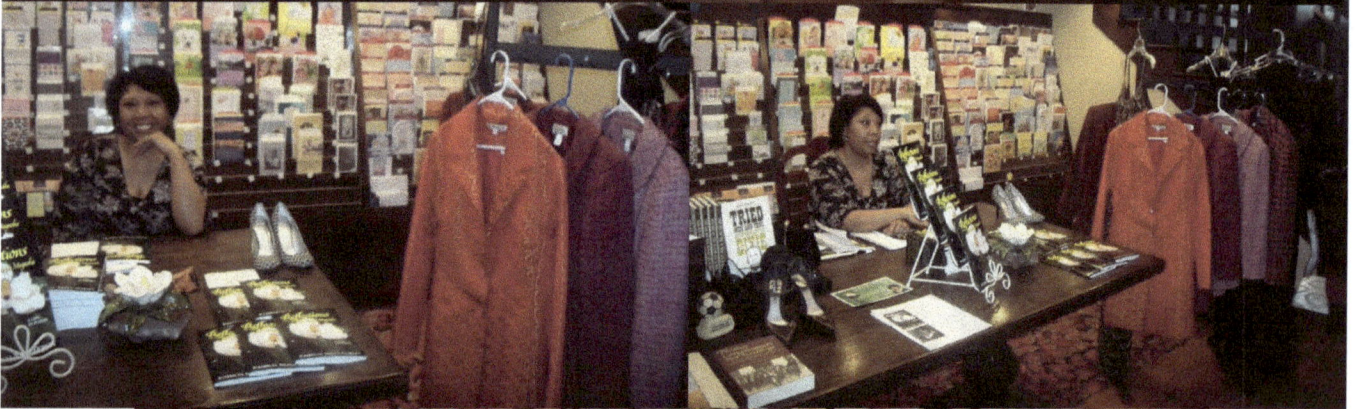

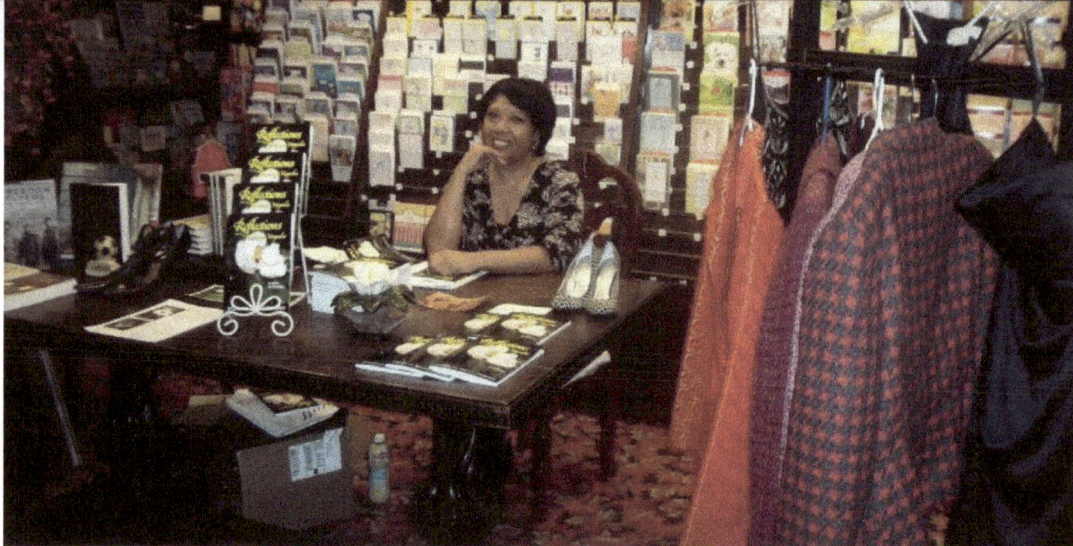

THE ART OF THE DEAL IN YARD SALES

If you are thinking about getting into the game, it would be good to know one of the major rules of engagement. In the yard sale game, everyone is looking for a BETTER deal. Even if an item already seems to you to be an absolute steal, it NEVER hurts to try to negotiate for a lower price. Sometimes, you will find sellers who are firm and stubborn about their prices and say no to your efforts. But, more often than not, sellers will say yes to reductions. So, it never hurts to ask. Always keep in mind: Sellers want to SELL! Slight flaws or defects in any item that you are thinking of buying can give you leverage in negotiating for lower prices. If you point out a tear or clip in an item, to the seller, he or she is often more willing to discount that item. Of course, you don't want something that is irreparable and you never want to buy junk. But, an item with some small imperfections can turn out be a tremendous bargain! In any transaction be sure to ask the seller if they will take any less for an item. Sellers are very accustomed to hearing: "Will you take anything less for this?" or "What is the lowest you are willing to go on this ?" So don't be shy! You can offer your own lower price suggestion and the seller will usually meet you somewhere in between. Also, the more items that you buy, the more the seller is likely to go down on individual prices or give you a fantastic deal on the total purchase. If you are thinking about buying three dresses and the price is $5 on each dress, ask if they will take $2 per dress.

You will more than likely get the $2 a dress price that you offered or a slightly higher $3 counter price by the seller. Either way, you have come out ahead. Furthermore, you can often get unbelievable deals near the end of the yardsaling day. Yard sales usually start winding down after the noon hour, with sellers eager to get rid of their wares and end the day without having to drag items back inside. If a seller was stubborn about the price of an item earlier in the day, and you were not willing to pay that price, it might be beneficial to you to stop back by that sale later in the day. The seller will probably be more than happy to give you that lower price that you were seeking. I have been to sales later in the day where the sellers were practically giving things away. So, make your rounds and then maybe backtrack a bit. You might hit the jackpot! Now you have a few cards in your hand to play in winning at the yardsale game.

1. Yard sales usually start around 6:00am (sometimes earlier). So be prepared to be UP, DRESSED and OUT OF THE HOUSE before 6:00am. The early bird really does get the worm, in this case. You will get the pick of the litter, when you are one of the first ones to arrive.

2. Scout out the locations where you plan to go. Many yard sales are listed in the newspaper on Friday and Saturday . But, these are not all of the sales that are out there, by any means. There are too many to count. You cannot possibly make it to all of the sales, so, decide on some of the locations that you want to try from the descriptions in the paper or decide on a certain part of town. Over time, you will start to discover where you find your favorite things and where the best sales are for the things that you like.

My husband goes all over Tupelo and surrounding areas because he loves to drive. My favorite areas, and where I purchase most of my Diva Finds, are in North Tupelo (Barnes Crossing Mall area, Northridge Subdivision) and Saltillo. I have taught Hubby very well! He knows my style , my sizes and my favorite brands. These days I hardly have to shop for myself at all! He finds amazing bargains! One day several years ago, he brought home about ten formal dresses that he had purchased for $1 a piece! I loved them all!

3. Take lots of small bills ($1 and $5) and lots of change. It is much easier to make your purchases when you have the exact amount. You can get in and out with no hassle. Also, you really don't want to take all of the sellers change because they need it for the day. They will appreciate your small bills.

4. As soon as you approach a yard sale, give the whole yard sale a once over glance to see if there is anything that catches your eye. If you start in one area and just focus on it, thinking that you have time to leisurely browse, you might miss something that you really wanted. .You will be amazed at how many shoppers are at the sales . Everyone is out to get that great find ,Try not to let them get to it before you do!

5. Have Fun !

6. You can often find great bargains on rainy days. Because so many would-be shoppers think that the sales might have been canceled, they decide not to go out. Sellers often decide to have their sales in their garages, anyway. Because there are fewer shoppers out looking for the goods, you will be able to have first choice of the merchandise without much competition. And, because there are fewer shoppers, the sellers are more likely to let items go at lower prices, just do get rid of them. Sellers want to sell their merchandise and not have to take all of the things back in. This will work to your advantage.

You will meet some great people while yardsaling and even learn a lot of things! It's amazing the things you can learn at a yard sale. You might get to know some of your neighbors that you didn't know before. You can find out where some of the best sales are that day. You can even find out about future sales and other activities going on it the city. Any way that you slice it, Yard Sales ROCKS !!!!

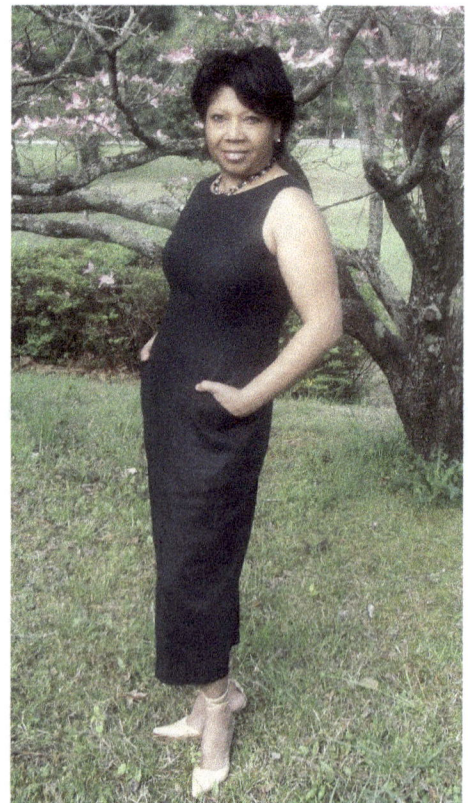

Black Linen SANTE FE Dress
from Yard Sale under $5
Shoes Yard Sale $1

~ YARDSALING ~

Yardsaling is a southern art,
And to some it's a way of life;
It's a way of getting almost anything,
Without the stress and strife.
You meet all kinds of people,
And you see how others live;
And while the kids sell lemonade,
You negotiate what you'll give.
There's always a faithful crew,
That gets up before the dawn;
To see what treasures they might find,
On some neighbor's lawn.
There's much anticipation ,
Of the next bargain 'round the bend;
And everyone knows in yardsaling,
The possibilities never end.
There's always something
You've been searching for,
Suddenly , staring you in the face;
And when your eyes lock on to it ,
Your heart begins to race.
There's nothing like the yard sale game,
Or should I say, the sport;
It quite easily becomes an addiction,
If you're of that sort.

Patricia Neely-Dorsey @2008
from Reflections of a
Mississippi Magnolia-A Life in Poems

83

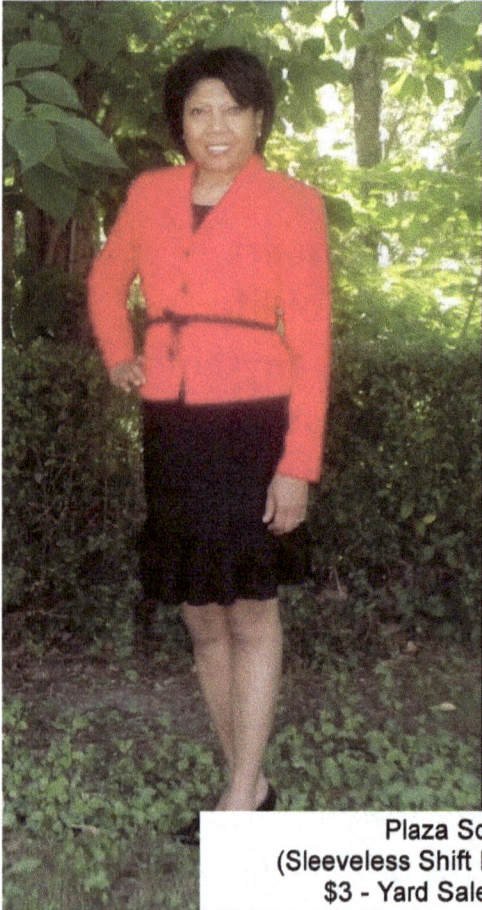

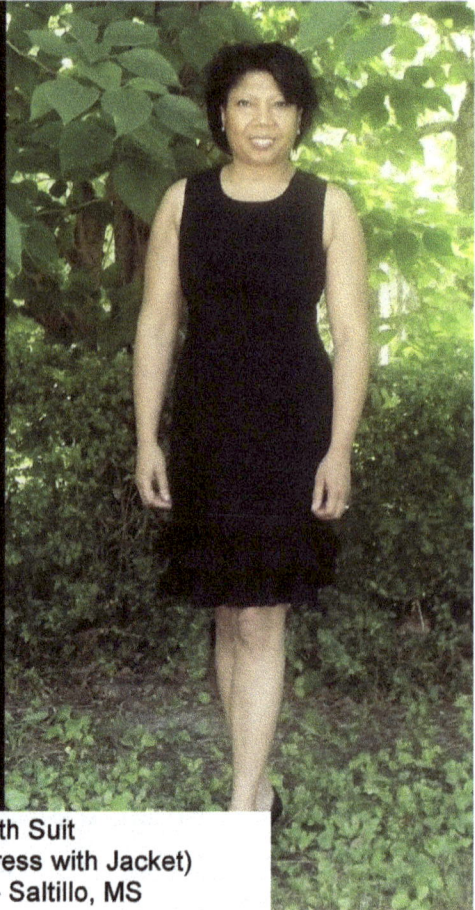

Plaza South Suit
(Sleeveless Shift Dress with Jacket)
$3 - Yard Sale - Saltillo, MS

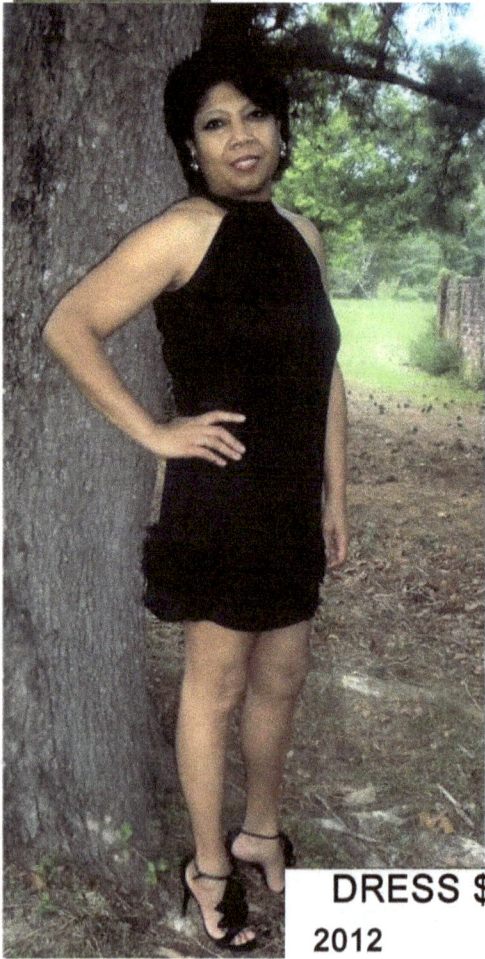

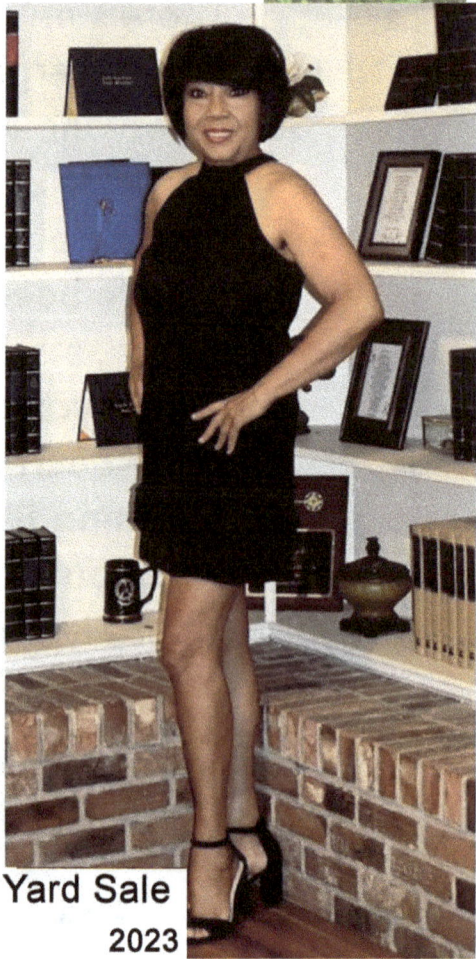

DRESS $1 Yard Sale

2012   2023

Yellow Suit
$2 from Yard Sale

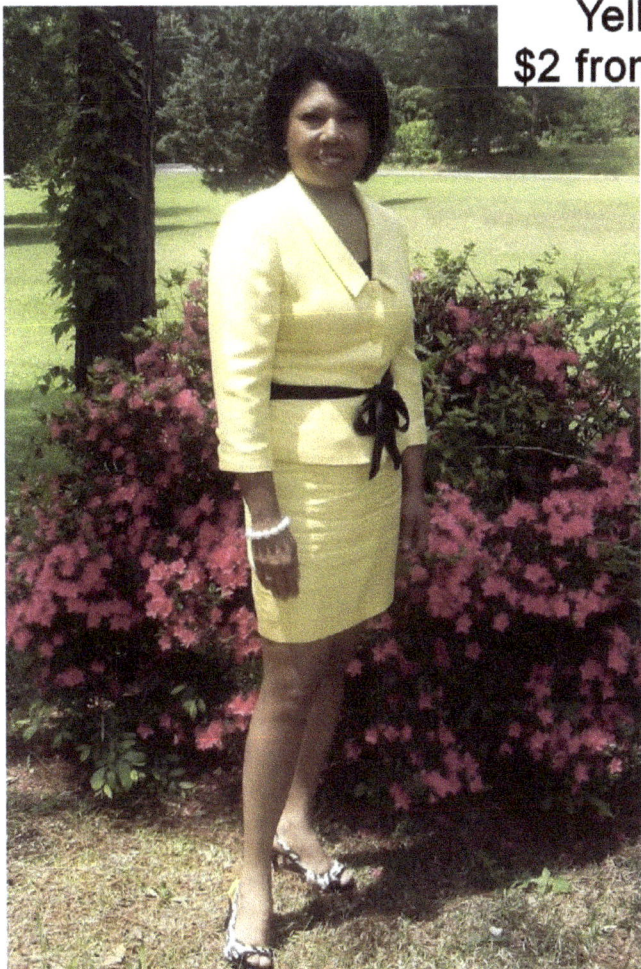

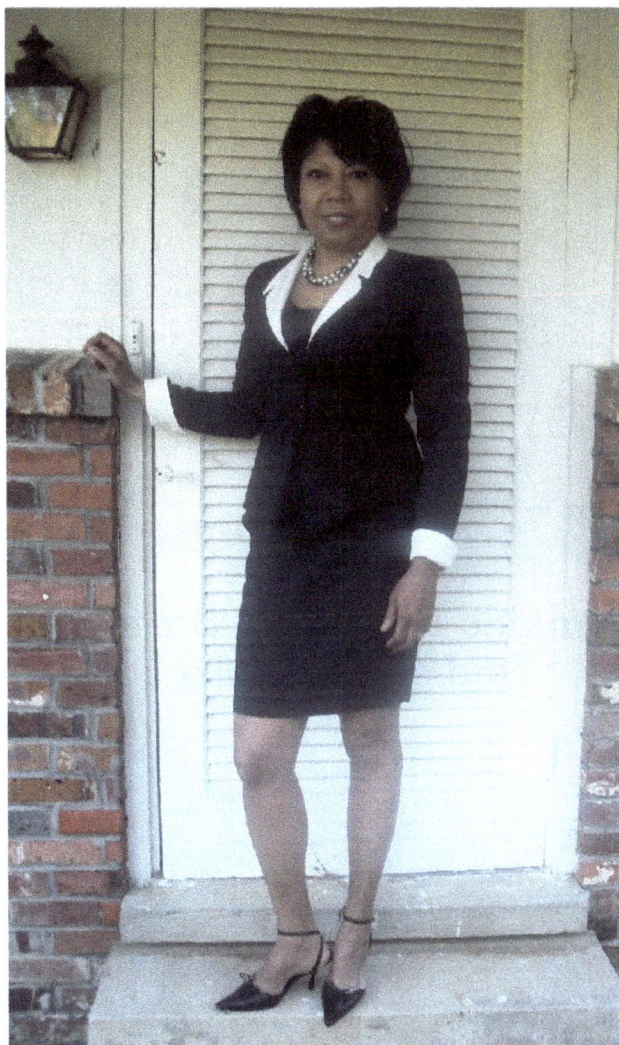

Black and White Suit - $2 Yard Sale

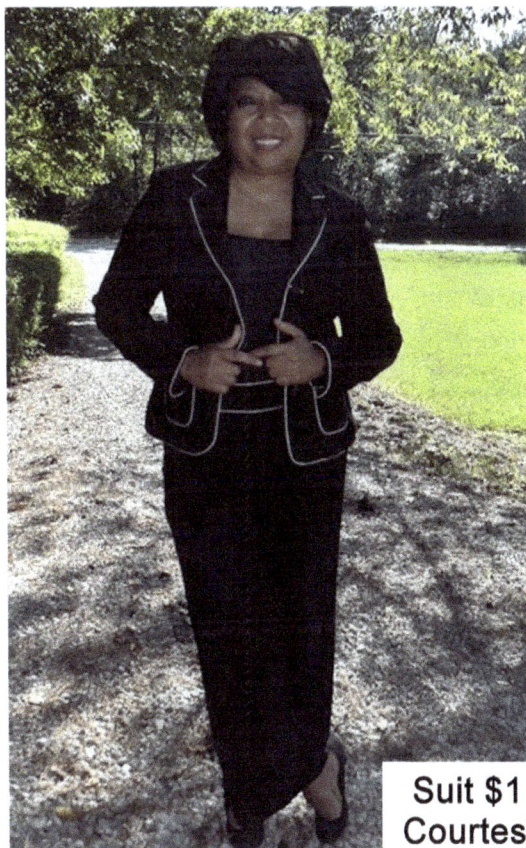

Suit $1 Yard Sale
Courtesy of Hubby

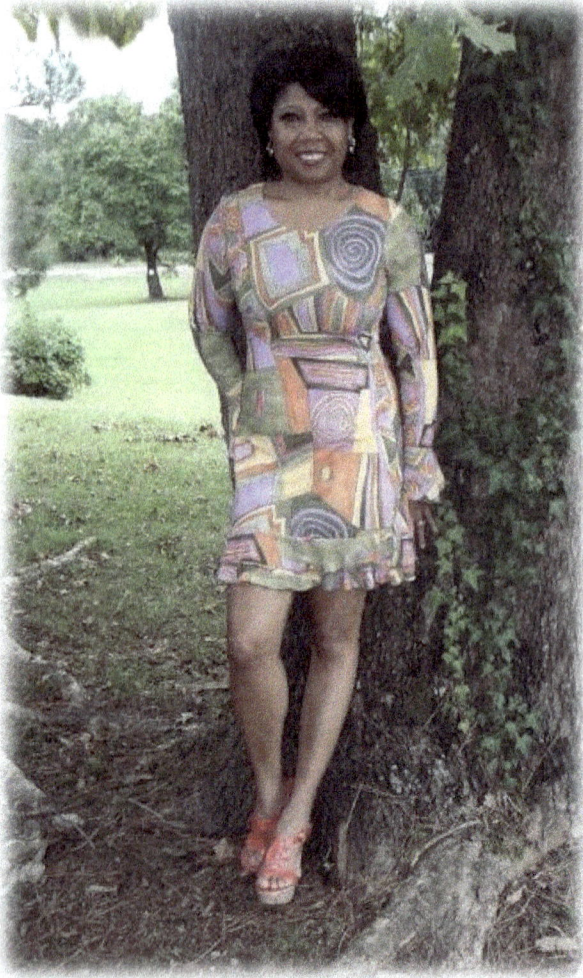

Geometric Retro Print Dress $1
Yard sale –Saltillo

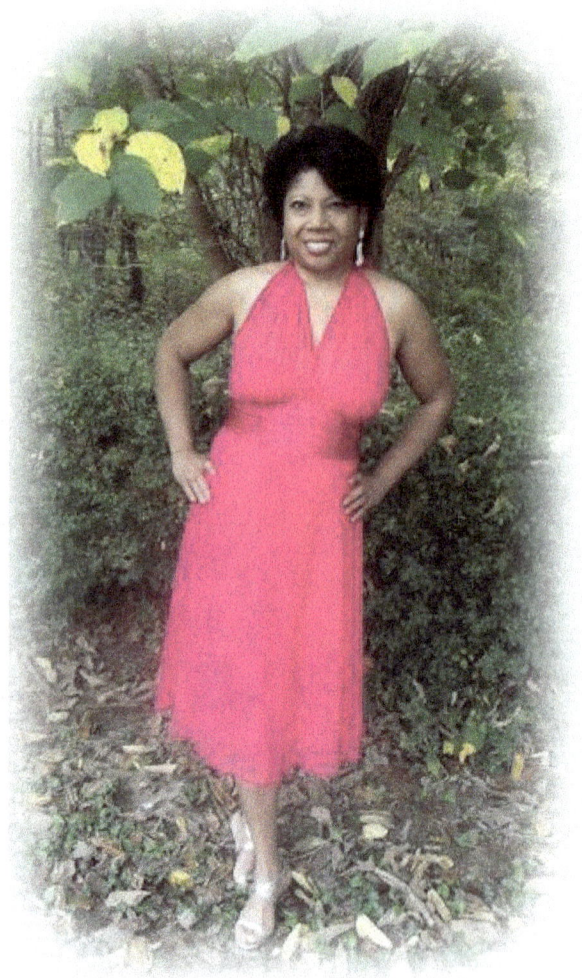

Rocking My Marilyn Dresses
$1 Yard sale

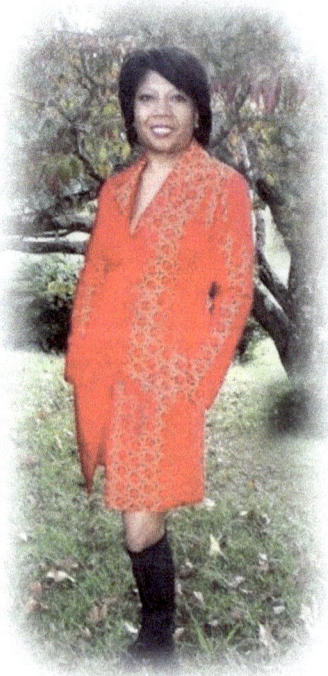

FAB Coat $3 Yardsale

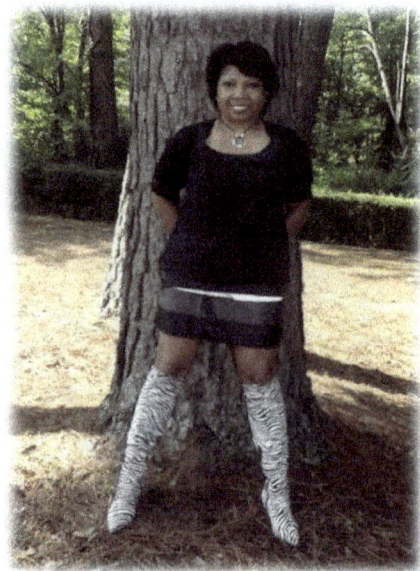

Boots $2 Top $1 Skirt $1
Found at three different yardsales
on the same day in Saltillo

July 24, 2019

Formal Dress -MONTAGE Boutique 50 Cents from Walls Discount Center - TUPELO

Courtesy of Hubby

That moment when you say:
Hmm.. Should I buy a pack of gum ...or a formal dress???
50 CENTS CAN GO A LONG WAY WHEN YOU ARE A THRIFTY SHOPPER !

Why do you KEEP saying you can't afford it? You can! This dress was FIFTY CENTS! Hubby brought home a bag of clothes for me from Walls. All new clothes with tags on them. Most cost over $100 from the back clearance room at Wall's South Gloster, Tupelo. All of the items were 50 cents each!

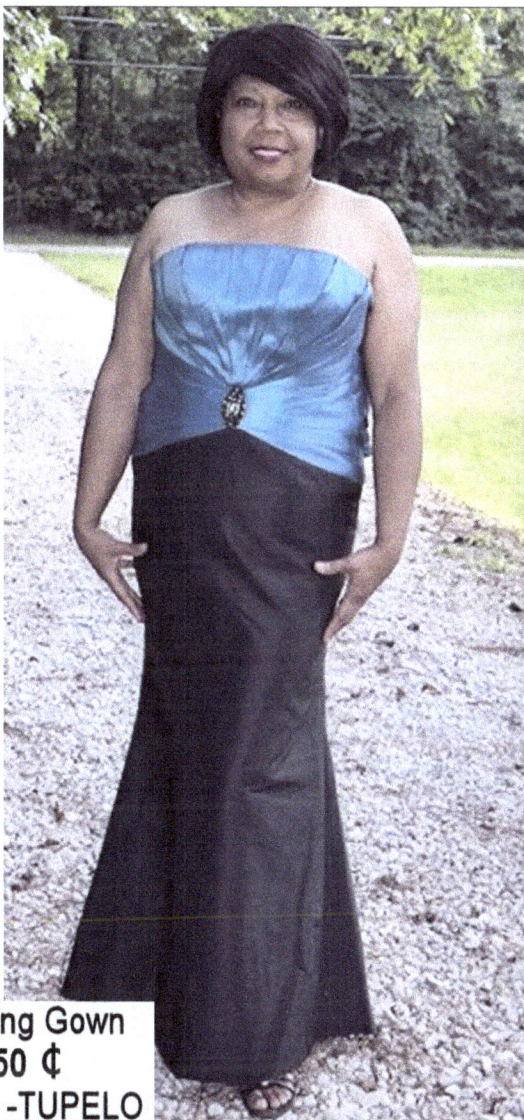

Evening Gown
50 ¢
Wall's -TUPELO

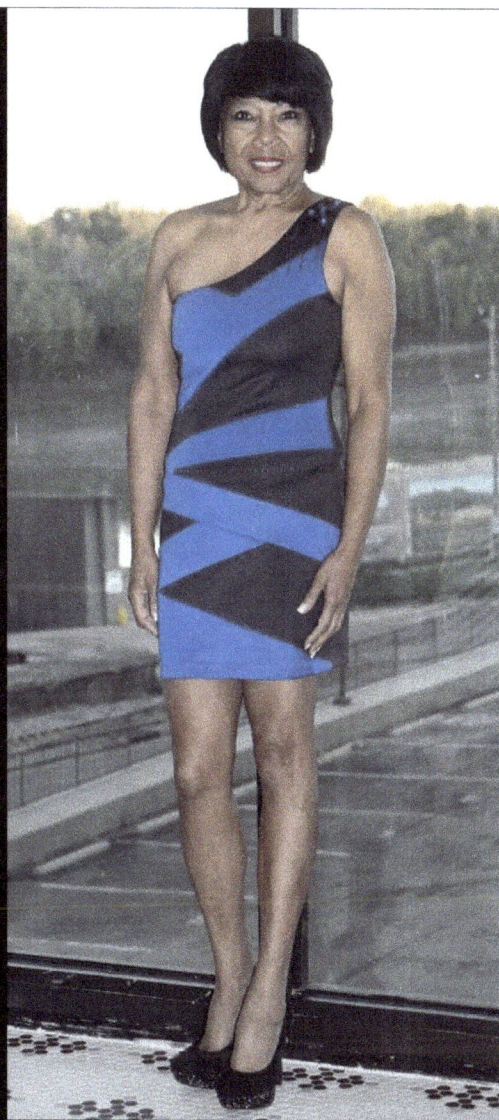

2019

2022

"Pageant Spray Tan Going On!"

FABULOSITY

I am ending this chapter with this picture, which is very much a perfect transition from the Fit and Fabulous fitness chapter to the Go Forth and Be Fabulous on a Shoestring Budget (thrift shopping , yardsaling building a fabulous wardrobe).

You see the very fluffy , biscuit middle and not so healthy or fit overall look, Even still, I thought that I was looking fabulous! Yes, I know the person should definitely wear the dress and not let the dress wear them. But, I was not doing this beauty justice at all. I wish that I had kept it so that I could have done a Before and After! This picture was taken at a time when my Dad was having major health issues and crisis medical situations during the later part of his life.

During 2019,he suffered a series of strokes. We were going back and forth constantly with doctor visits, several extended hospital stays (including intensive care), rehabilitation services, assisted living stays etc.

I was the Dad's primary care giver and the driver. As I was taking care of Dad's circumstances, I also wanted to make sure that Mom was stabilized and doing well. I was totally honored to be able to do so, for both of them. One wonderful thing that came from that time is that we became even closer and talked about everything imaginable!

My thoughts were nowhere near focused on my own health , diet or exercise. My Dad passed away in June of the next year. (2020) We miss him, dearly. For all of the care givers out there, I do want to say , that I do understand and sympathize with your circumstances. But, to be at your very best to take care of others, you have to make sure to take care of yourself .

To be able to be around to enjoy and take care of loved ones, you must take care of yourself. I had a little health scare of my own , about eight or nine months after my Dad had passed. I believe that it had a lot to do with my mind and body processing all that had gone on the previous year.

PND RANDOM RAMBLINGS
WARNING VERY, VERY LONG POST

Facebook Post: March 5, 2021

I have always considered myself to be special, unique, different and one of a kind. That is a wonderful thing in most circumstances, except when it comes to medical issues! Any medical encounter that I have is NEVER the norm! That is NOT a good thing! There might be someone out there who understands this problem. It is why I try to stay as healthy as possible and try to avoid any kind of medical interventions except for yearly check ups. So far at 57, I have done pretty good with the fact that I take no medications, have had no surgeries, no in patient hospitalizations except for the birth of my child , have only been put to sleep once for colonoscopy (a couple of years ago). So, my most recent medical ordeal was this week. On Tuesday night , I was having problems breathing! It was not just a little problem breathing but SEVERE! I thought that I was going to have to go to the emergency room, but because of COVID I really didn't want to be in a crowded emergency room or in a hospital period. I was not feeling sick in any way, I had no fever or vomiting or anything like that, I just couldn't breathe well AT ALL! .

I told Hubby I thought I could make it until morning! I must say, the hot lemon water that Hubby suggested I drink did help! I kept looking at my fingernails and my lips to see if they might be bluish for indications that I was not getting enough air . But, they were healthy , rosy and pink looking . (thought "Good!) I made it through the night and the next morning (Wednesday) I went to the urgent care clinic .

I saw the doctor He asked all of the questions to try to diagnose the problem. Blood pressure was fine and oxygen level was fine. Chest sounded good , Throat looked good. (Ok great. But I still can't breathe !!!) So the doctor says he want to get blood work and a chest x -ray to rule out any heart problems , see what the lungs are looking like and check blood-work /levels to see indications of possible blood clots. Of course just before the person was getting ready to draw blood, I warned her that I have VERY small veins. She did have to thump around , but she did very good! I was impressed. I thought I was home free with the needles! So, back with the doctor, he says the X-ray is clear ...no indication of any heart problems or pneumonia etc.. But, he says one level on the blood panel was elevated that could indicate blood clots, which can cause trouble breathing. So, he says that he wants to order a CT scan to see if there are blood clots. So I go to the imaging center to get that done. Here we go again with the veins and the needles. Believe it or not , there was a time in my life that I was very afraid of needles (actually petrified) That all ended when I had a baby . (late in life age 34) (More about that later)

Anyway, back to this week... So, for the CT Scan I was supposed to have an IV which requires a larger stick/needle) Of course I knew this was going to be a major problem. I was totally prepared for lots of sticks .tries and failures. The first technician tried twice . The first time she tried she was talking (too much) about how small the veins are and disap-pearing and all that and Ohh that one just blew (I did not need to hear you say that , real-ly) So she calls another person in to try and they talk again about how tiny the veins are, (and generally talking too much) Asking do I always have problems. I say of course. (Let's remember this whole time ..I can hardly breath !) They go to the other arm and the second person fails. So, the first person, says, we are going to call in the big guns. She must be the one who is great at sticks. So, she came and tried and failed. I was prepared for a lot of sticks but I was not prepared at all for no one being able to get the iv in.

The whole time, even though I can hardly breathe and want help, I am thinking this is too many people hovering around me , too close (even with masks.) I ask the technician: If there was an emergency situation and I had to have an Iv immediately and urgently what would they do. I am always curious about these things. She said something about a post or something. So, the thing that I dread the most has come to pass. They decide that they are not going to keep sticking me and will send me to the hospital for the CT where they have can find the veins with some kind of ultrasound or something. I am referred to the hospital outpatient with not sense of urgency or emergency with the fact
that...I can't breathe So...off to the hospital and of course we are stopped at Crosstown by the train. I burst out crying. Yes, we should have gone the other way on the expressway I guess but I am sure with my luck we would have been stopped by the train that goes across once you get off.

Anyway, I am checked in with all this paperwork and stuff and ... Still problems breathing! So finally the technician is doing the one where they find the vein with an ultra sound. He even has some problems. He seems a little baffled and flustered by it and I say there has to be another way. He asked like everyone always does. Do you always have these problems. He finally gets it in. I proceed with the CT scan.

The whole time through all of the procedures I was repeating my favorite scripture. Do not be anxious about anything, but in every situation, by prayer and petition, with thanksgiving, present your requests to God. Philippians 4:6(NIV) and Psalm 23 :Yea, though I walk through the valley of the shadow of death, I will fear no evil: for thou art with me; thy rod and thy staff they comfort me. (You can certainly feel like you are dying when you can't seem to get enough air) I asked God to take care of it all asking for good results , no blood clots etc.

I was sent home to wait for results. I am still having problems breathing, which does not seem a concern to anyone but me. I don't hear anything for a few hours and I call to check. I speak with the nurse and she says the Dr. says everything is fine on the CT scan ... no signs of blood clots.
(Thank You God for answered prayers and keeping me.)
I say, but I am still having problems breathing. (The reason for ALL OF THIS) She goes back to talk with doctor and he prescribes me ... AN INHALER
(almost 8 hrs. later and $5,000 worth or tests...AN INHALER)

Thank God for GREAT insurance!

#TryToStayHealthy
She said if I have more problems I can get a referral to a pulmonary specialist.
I said I would just try the inhaler. So, Thursday my breathing was progressively better And today (Friday), my breathing is much better. It is not normal but much better than the previous days. For what I can put together on the internet it could have been caused by some kind of allergic reaction or acid reflex condition. (I plan to have allergy testing done)

(Later thoughts: From reading some materials on grief, I have learned that it can cause breathing problems at times. Dealing with my dad's death might have played some part in the episode, along with anxiety from taking care of so many things following his death.)

(Update as of 2023: It has not happened again.)

I do believe that this incident had a great deal to do with my decision , in February 2022 to begin the journey to get into my Best Shape Ever by 60. (2024)

ELAINE– GRIEF

After the death of my husband , James Henry Neely, MD, I started to fully understand the term "grieving widow".

That is what I became.

I am the last survivor of my parents and seven siblings.

After their deaths, I was able to return to my normal routines of daily life.

After the death of my husband, I became a different person and was unable return to my normal routines.

I became concerned and decided that I had to learn as much as possible about grief.

I decided that I would read as much material as I could on the subject.

One of the first things that I noticed, during those early days, was that I did not cry at all.

This puzzled me.

After reading one of numerous books, I learned that watering eyes, draining sinuses, and colds often come as substitutes

for crying during grief.

I have had all of those symptoms. I have not shed a tear to this day.

I noticed that normal sleep patterns began to elude me.

I wanted to get in bed and sleep as much as possible.

I would fall asleep very early in the middle of the day, sometimes as early as two or three o'clock, and be awake all night and early in the mornings.

I learned that various sleep issues and insomnia can be serious problems, for many people, during grief .

I learned that proper nutrition is important during grief ,as many people have eating problems during this time.

I have had no problem in this area. My eating habits did not change and I have maintained a healthy diet.

I have learned that in most cases and especially for me, a grieving person needs someone to be there for them and by their side.

Thankfully, I have had that someone. Patricia and I live in the same residence.

She has been in charge of any and every issue that I have needed to address.

I am extremely grateful for this.

Overall, I have learned that there are many stages, symptoms and layers of grief and that people grieve in many different ways.

I strongly suggest that any grieving person learn as much as possible about this process.

PATRICIA—GRIEF

Being with my mother through the grieving process has been very much a learning experience on the extreme depths of grief. There was a poignant moment , during one of our conversations ,when we were talking about grief, which we do on many days.

My mother made the statement. "I am destroyed" It really shook me.

For her to say the words out loud stunned me , but did not surprise me at all, because I knew from every moment of being around her , that this is absolutely what she was feeling. It showed in every part of her being.

With all of her many attributes and accomplishments, for her to say those words, told of the extraordinarily deep level of grief that she was experiencing .

My father's death was devastating to her. The definition of the word explains it .

Devastating: highly destructive or damaging ; causing severe shock, distress, or grief.

I was very concerned about Mom's well-being during the first year after Dad's death.

I was always monitoring her closely, because I could see how crushed she was.

My father's parents had been married over 50 years when each of them died.

My grandmother had experienced a long illness. But, my grandfather died unexpectedly of a heart attack.

Within a year of his death, my grandmother was dead. I aways believed that she died of a broken heart/grief.

I believed that she gave up the will to live. I certainly did not want that to be the case with my mother.

So, I was always keeping a very watchful eye. I still do.

She had been married to my father 66 years, when he passed away.

That is more than so many people even have the privilege to live.

In many ways, her whole life was built around him. She even verbalized this , also.

When people would ask me how she was doing I would respond " She is just lost" .

I would often describe her as being a deer in head lights.

But, on further reflection, it is more like looking at a bewildered, helpless young fawn that has lost it's mother.

She had been with this man and depended on this man ALL of her adult life, and even before that .

She often talks about him starting to pay attention to her when she was in the eight grade, around age 14.

She was in jr high and he was in high school at Mary Holmes.

He went off to college at Kentucky State, when she was in high school. On one return visit from college , he gave her his Alpha fraternity pin. She said that he told her; "You know what this means" (you won't be dating anyone else) They were married April 19,1954. She was 18 years old . Mom said this was one of the happiest days of her life.

BUILDING A FRUGALLY FABULOUS WARDROBE

WARDROBE BUILDING TIP: Treat planning your wardrobe like planning a party, wedding, or big event. Have a budget, have a theme and have a color scheme.

Wardrobe Building : THEME
You should decide upon the picture that you want to paint and person that you want to portray...then put it together piece by piece. It could be sassy, jazzy, classy, sophisticated etc. Make a personal statement with your wardrobe. Make it add up to being TOTALLY YOU! When you have a good idea of your overall style the pieces will jump out at you and start calling your name!

Become a SPOTTER! Look for those favorite colors, style elements, name brands, etc. that you are continually/consistently drawn to and that flatter you. When you become good at SPOTTING at a glance, shopping is a breeze. You won't have to take the time to try to, somehow, sort through every single piece of clothing in the store. That becomes too overwhelming and exhausting.

Choose a COLOR SCHEME for your wardrobe. You cannot possibly buy and wear every color and every color will not wear well on you! Narrowing down your choices makes shopping so much easier! I suggest that you have about 3 or 4 core/basic colors that are the foundation of your wardrobe and four or five accent colors to jazz it up. If you look in my closet, you will immediately see that my core colors are BLACK, WHITE, and GRAY with accent colors of RED, HOT PINK , SOFT PINK and PURPLE. I also like mod color mixes!

Your brain is an amazing, extraordinary machine...a magnificent computer! It will automatically/effortlessly help you to edit your shopping selections for you if you give it the right input. If you have decided before hand what you are looking for (styles/colors/brands) those things will literally start to jump out at you! A perfect example is when you decide to buy a certain car. All of a sudden that car is almost all you see when you are driving! Whereas you never really noticed before, all of a sudden that particular car seems to be everywhere! Think of it like doing a search on your home computer. There is almost limitless information available at your fingertips but to find what you want, you must enter something specific into the search engine. *Narrow down your current and future wardrobe selections / style choices to only those type items that you have found to be consistently appealing to you and flattering on you .

EDIT, EDIT EDIT!!!

Experts say that most people wear only about 20% of the items in their closets. Reasons for this include: They are too big, or too small, they no longer fit into their lifestyle or in with the rest of their clothing, they need repairs that will never be done etc. The list goes on and on. Get rid of ALL such items! Keep only what you really love and wear on a regular basis.

Find a few accessories that will go with almost everything in your wardrobe. Scarves and belts can add a another dimension or a splash of color to your core selections. Blingy belts are an easy way to spice up any outfit in your wardrobe for special occasions!

WARDROBE TIP:

If it ain't broke..don't fix it!! Find your style. And stick with it! Stay with what works. Don't try to conform to every new trend that comes along. Everything just AIN'T for you!! Buy and keep ONLY that which makes you look/feel FABULOUS!!! If you always buy only what you love...You'll always love what you have. I have lots of favorite finds that I got many years.

I am always talking about how my fashion style and preferences have pretty much not changed at all over the years. When I buy something, I love it...and I love it for a long time! I have rarely ever looked at any piece of clothing that I have or have had and thought, that's not me! Mostly everything that I own was calling my name! If your clothes don't "talk" to you and connect with you, they are not for you.

With Thrift Shopping

You can be Frugally Fly and Fabulous In All Seasons.
You can be Frugally Fly and Fabulous For All Occasions.
Find core pieces that can take you to any occasion.
Once you know what you are looking for you will feel like it has been waiting there just for you! Guess what? It has!

A lot of people are still stuck wallowing in the fact that they might not look the best in a latest trend or what someone else says should look good on them when there is a world of fashion that will suit them perfectly. Narrow down your current and future wardrobe selections / style choices to only those type items that you have found to be consistently appealing to you and flattering on you . You will always open your closet with delight and those "I have nothing to wear" days will be far behind you.

COLUMN DRESSING

Column dressing is a way of putting outfits together where you layer a topper piece, like jacket or cardigan, over a monochromatic base. The column comes from the head-to-toe appearance of the use of one color as the foundation. Start by creating a column of color with your favorite neutral (like black, navy, grey or brown). You can use any combination: tank/skirt, top/pant or dress (a solid sheath) This "column" creates one continuous line and acts as a base. It's simple. It's stylish. It can be very slimming. With my column foundation of these two pieces (black pants and pullover top) with maybe 5 or 6 more pieces and some accessories (belts and scarves are key) I could easily have outfits for a month without wearing the same look twice. Actually, I could wear this very outfit every day for the rest of I have many foundation pieces and most cost me UNDER $5 very often only $1 or $2 dollars. And yes, often 25 or 50 cents my life and be completely happy! Truly!

1 Black Pants
2 Black Pencil Skirt
3 Black Dress
4 Black Camisole
5 Black Top ·short or 3/4 Length sleeves
6 Black and white print blouse that can be worn like a jacket
7 Red Trapeze /Swing sweater or jacket
8 Red Top
9 Red Pencil Skirt
10 Cobalt Blue top

From now on , you will never be operating in the space of lack, need or want where your wardrobe is concerned ! Even if you want to buy something new or don't feel you have the EXACT thing you want for a special occasion you now know exactly where you can find it , at the drop of a hat, at a moment's notice and at minimal cost ...the thrift shops will have it . An easy breezy formula dressing is to get a solid column in your best color and then just add ANY jacket or sweater. This will also work with a solid dress, a pair of pants and matching sweater or top Keep them all together at the end of your closet so they are easily accessible. When you do not want to match up anything with your various wardrobe items you can just throw on one for the columns and almost every sweater and jacket in your closet will match when you have found your best /core colors /your "season" !

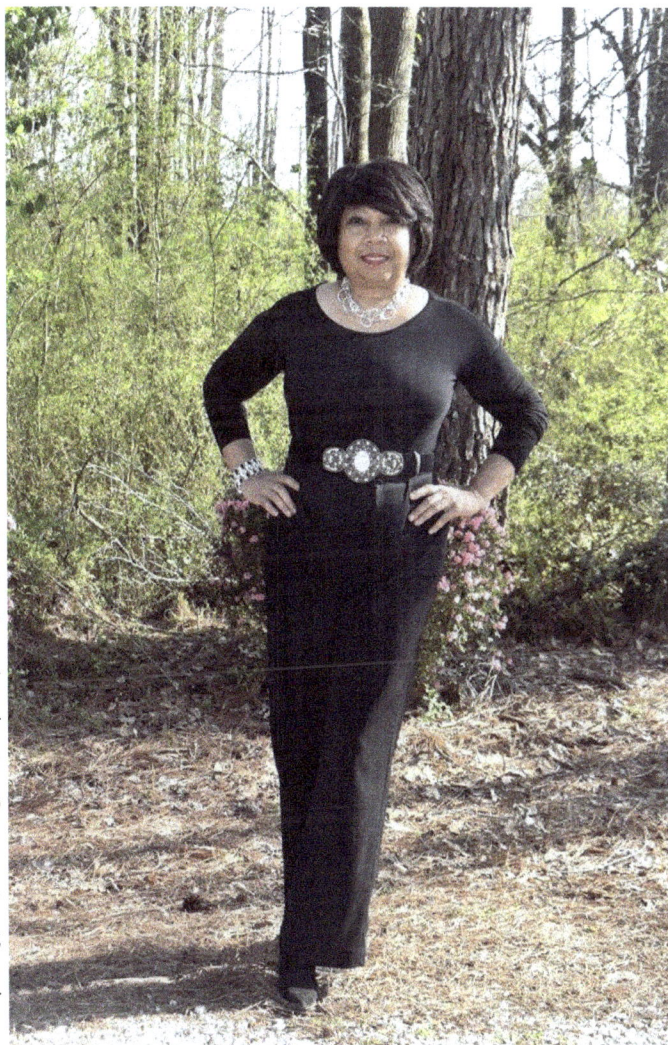

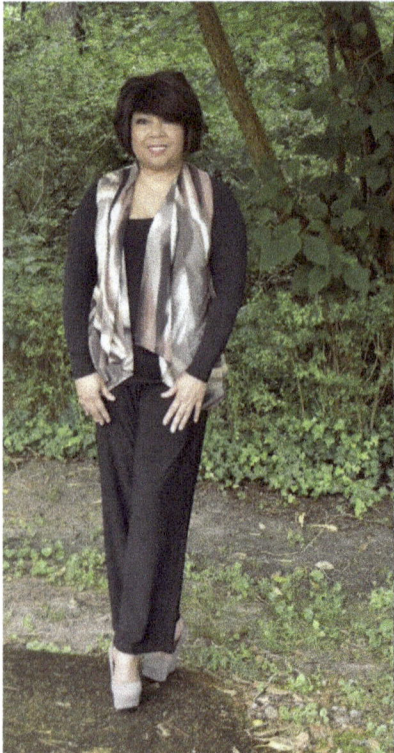
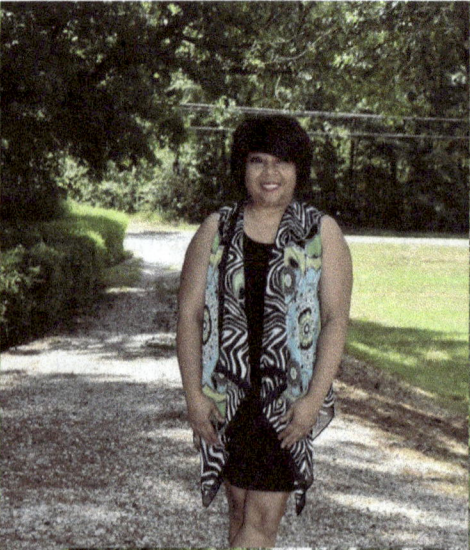
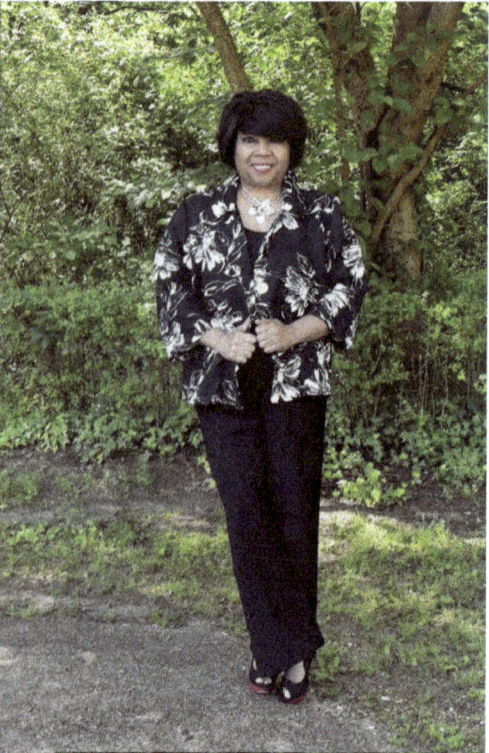
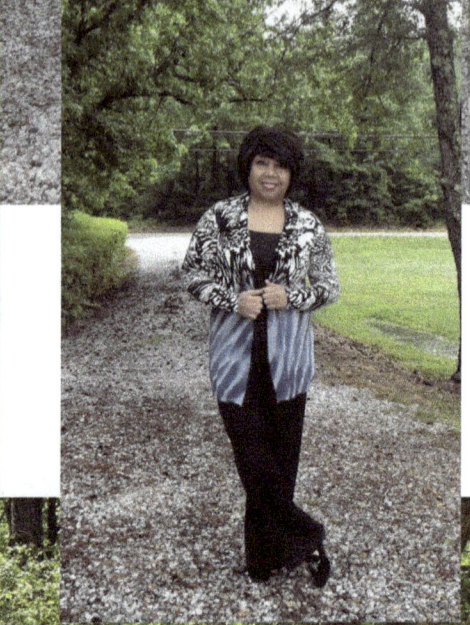
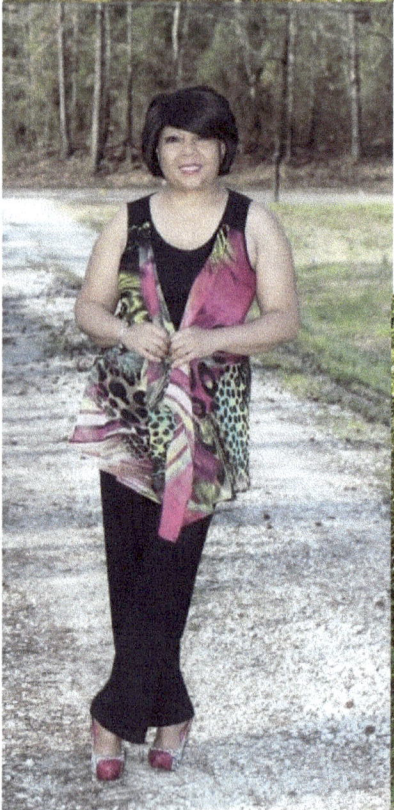
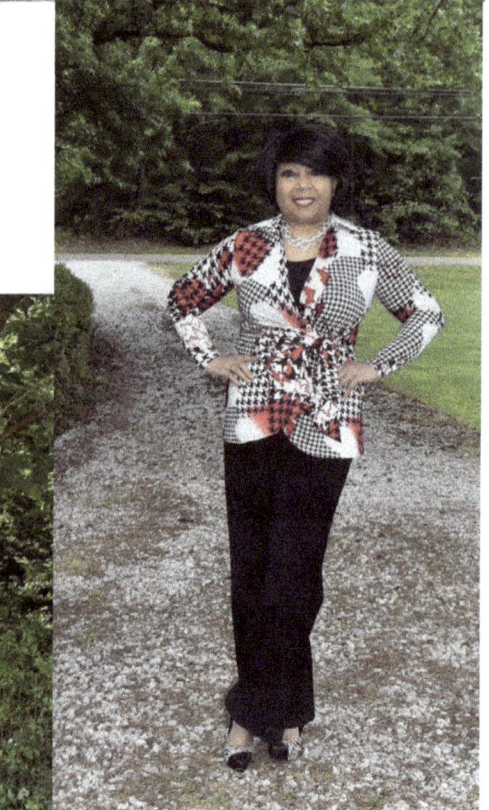
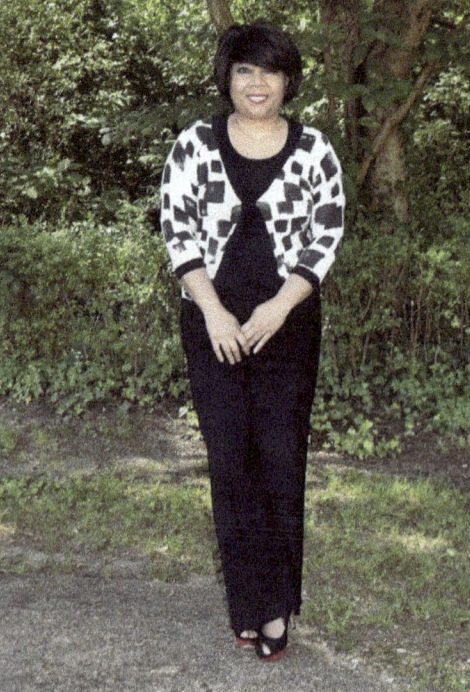

In perfecting your style, fit takes precedence over look. People are often disappointed because they see a look in a magazine or on someone else and decide they love the look and decide that they would love the look on them. It doesn't always work that way . You must consider your shape and how clothes fall on you in order to get the most perfect look. Something might be in your colors, and it might have the most amazing fabric or pattern, But. if it does not flatter your shape , it is meaningless .

You have to be able to pass up an amazing "looking" something for the perfect fitting something. That is what makes it amazing on YOU.

Go Forth and be Fabulous:
It's a Formula Not A Fantasy
1) Know Your Shape
2) Know Your Colors
3) Know Your Style
4) Know Your Size(s)
5)Know Your Designers/Brands/ Labels
6) Know Your Stores
7) Know Yourself

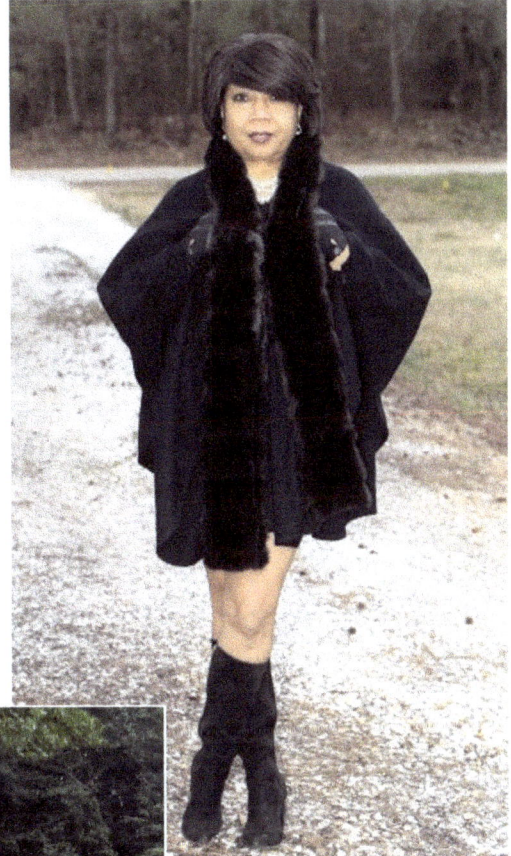

Faux fur trimmed cape
Under $10 Thrift Shop

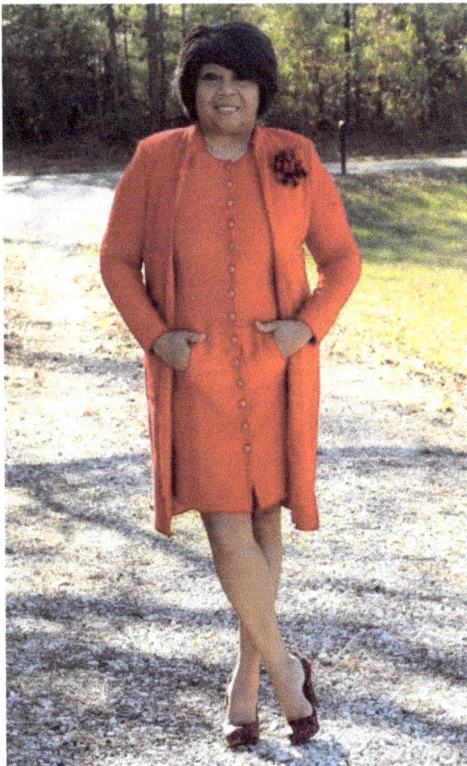

Red St. John Knit Suit
Under $10 City Thrift - Tupelo
JACKPOT!

St. John suits can retail for well over $1000

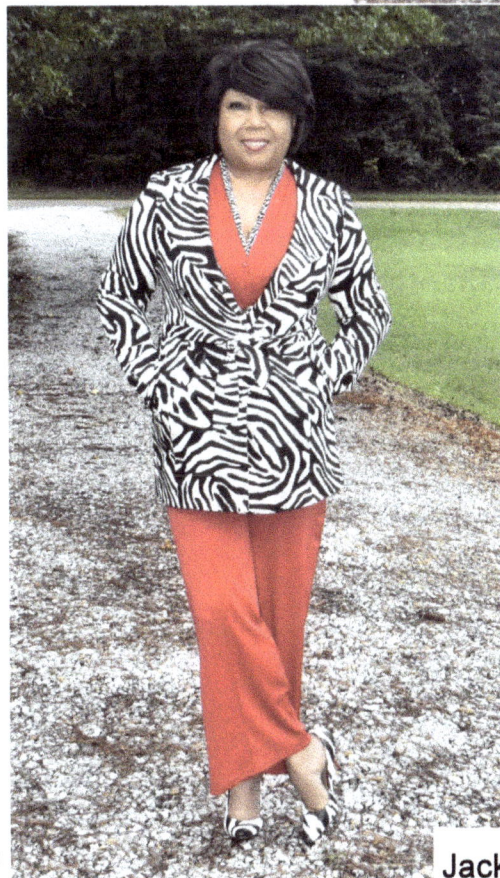

Jacket Under $5 Thrift Shop

The 1-10 rating system for your outfits can really help sharpen your skills and gives motivation to be more thoughtful in outfit selection. It automatically makes you think, what could I do to make it 10 or what makes it NOT a 10 . I am always happy to wear 7-10 , but love to know exactly what makes a 10. The 7 and above concept is a really important part of your style system. It takes the pressure off. Outfits don't have to be perfect. It creates margin and gives you a reason to celebrate when you find a 10. When you graduate from "Nice" "So Cute" Pretty" to Wow and "Stunning" you are on another level!

Find a Celebrity Style Role Model
Look for someone who has the same coloring as you
(hair, eye, hair color Type 3 , Autumn)
Look for someone who has the same stature as you
(height , build, not necessarily weight)
Follow their style choices/looks
Check out boards of them on Pinterest. Save favorite pictures/looks and use them as a guide
Celebrities pay hundreds of thousands of dollars for their clothes, their stylists, their perfectly polished looks ! It will be like having your very own celebrity stylist for FREE!

WARDROBE BUILDING TIPS:
 In your closet look at the top 10 pieces that you reach for again and again.
Find the common theme in those pieces.
Notice the colors, the textures, the fit, the shape , the style, of these pieces.
Find 10 pieces in your closet that you have not worn in the past 12 months.
Ask yourself why you haven't worn them and make a note of that.
Find three-five words that you would like associated with your look/style.
Note the clothes that represent those words.
In the future look for those types of clothes.
Take note of the brands that show up repeatedly in your closet.
Those will be the ones you will want to look for when you shop .

Know Your Style ~ I Love Pencil Skirts !!

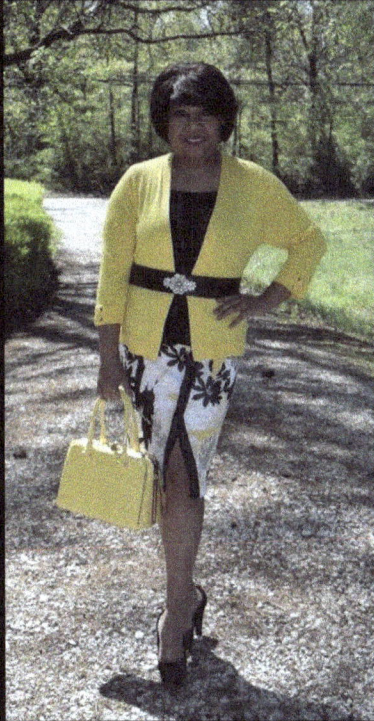

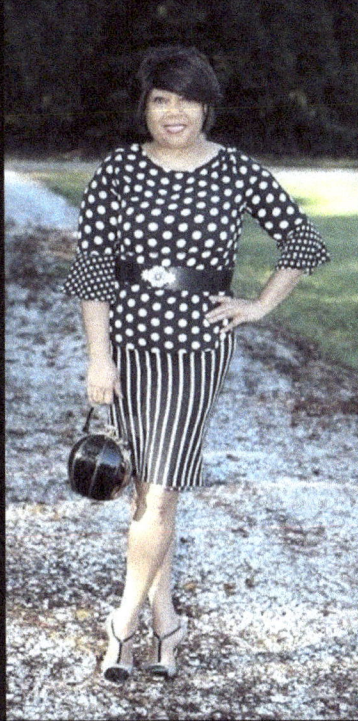

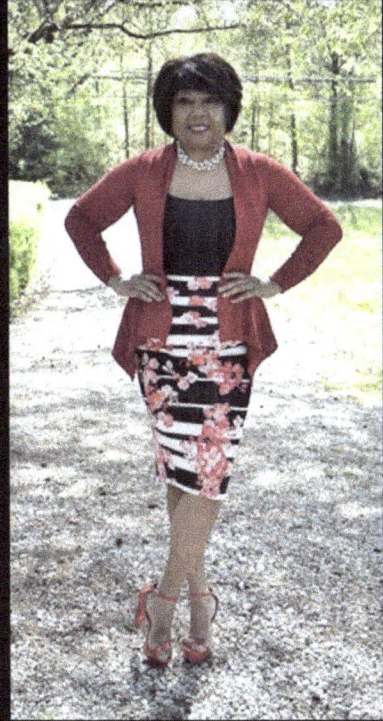

Diva on a Dime

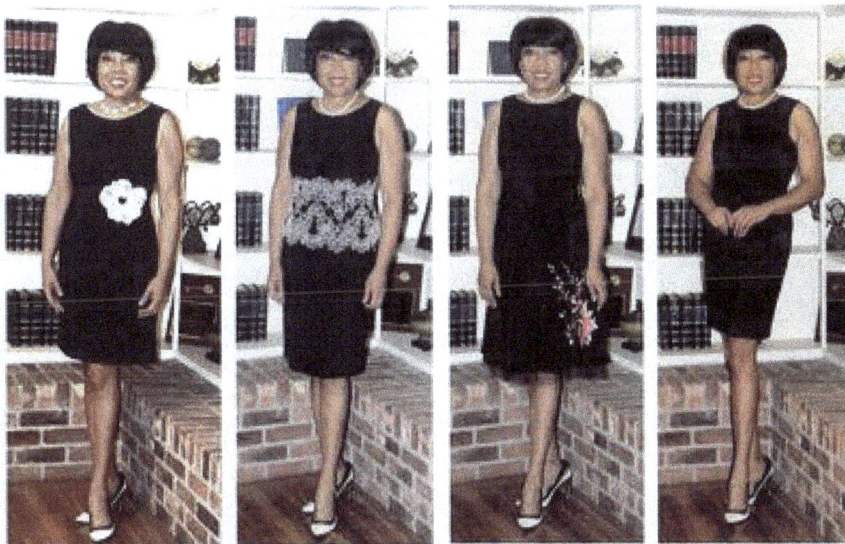

*Do you have a pair of shoes that
you wear over and over again ?*

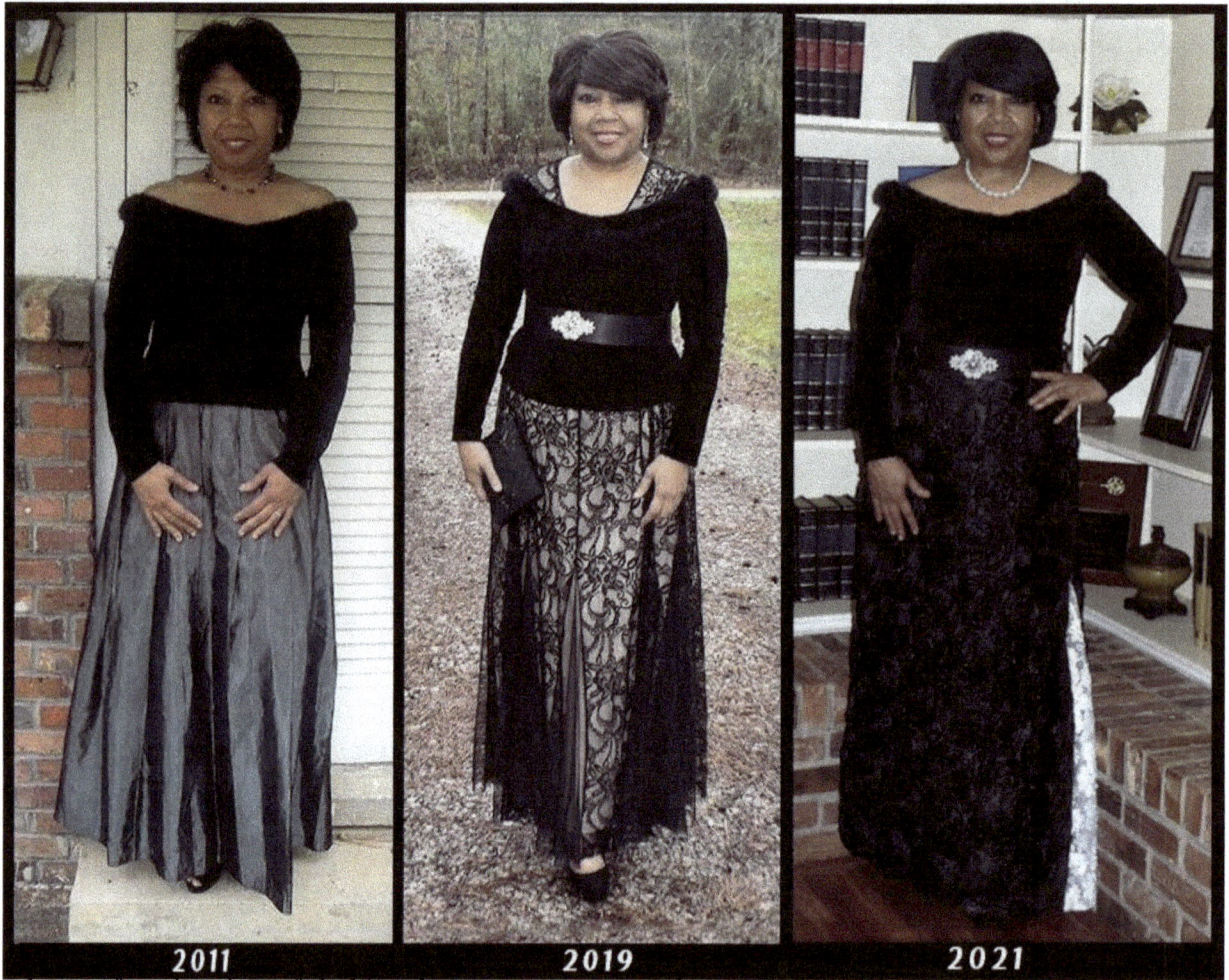

2011   2019   2021

Do you have a favorite piece of clothing that you wear over and over again...for years and years ?? One of mine is a velvet faux fur trimmed top I have worn it over and over through the years

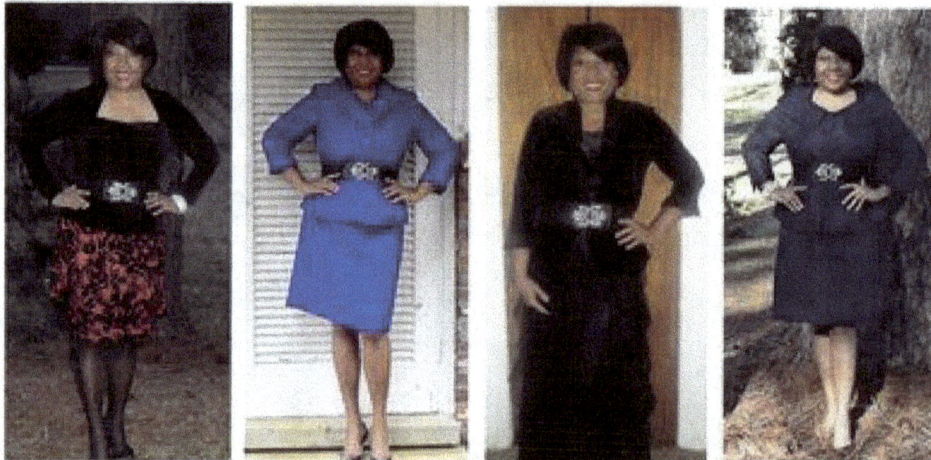

Diva on a Dime

Do you have a favorite accessory that you can wear with almost anything ?

MIXING PRINTS

As you can see in the pictures, the majority of my wardrobe centers around black and white and a few brights (mostly red and yellow) And, I LOVE MIXING PRINTS ! People are always complimenting me on and asking about my pattern mixing. Most people say that they could never do it....or are too afraid to try it . If it's black and white , I'll mix and match with no questions asked ! When you are thrift shopper you can experiment on all kinds of styles. Just give it a try. If something doesn't work for you, donate it back, pass on to friends or have your own sales. Whatever the case , you will never be out of any significant amount of money . Have fun ! Experiment ! Explore! I love the saying" Life is too short to wear boring clothes! You can start with as MUCH mixing (like here) or as little as you are comfortable with. It's as simple as that ! #MissionAccomplished

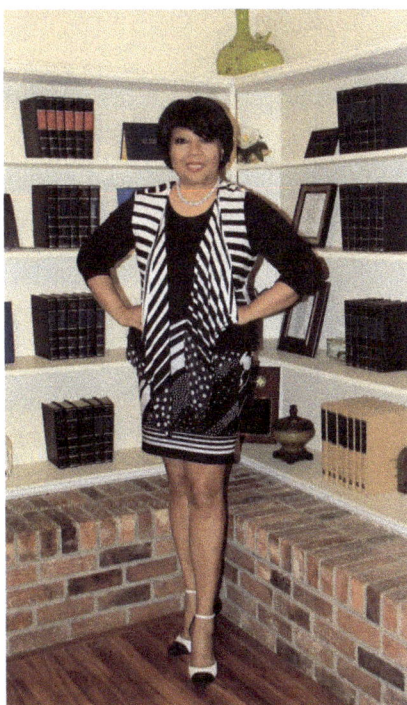

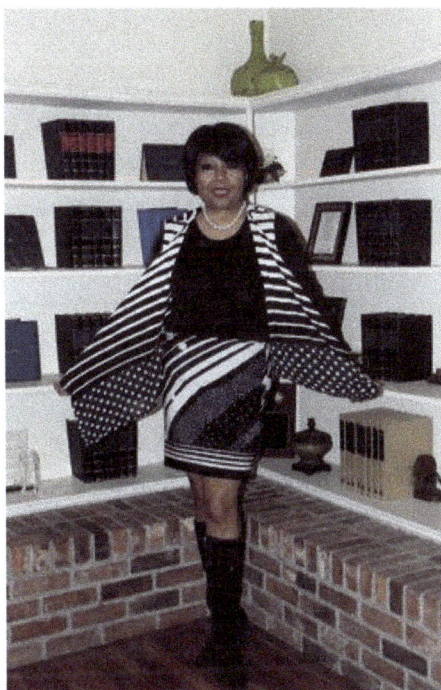

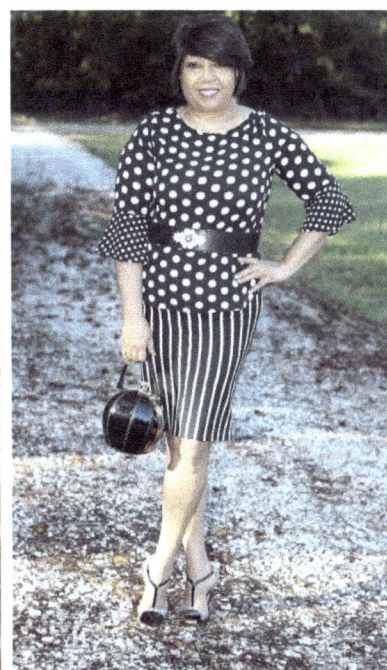

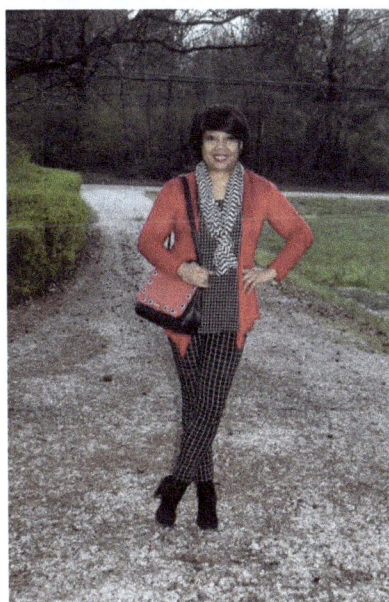

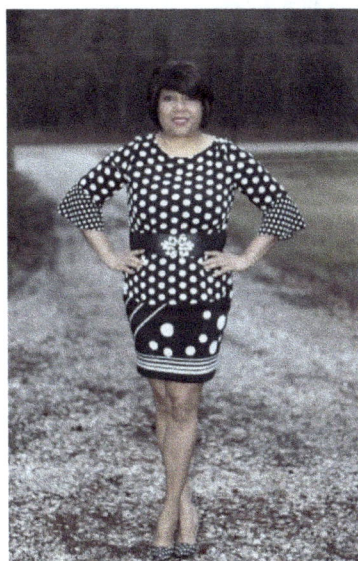

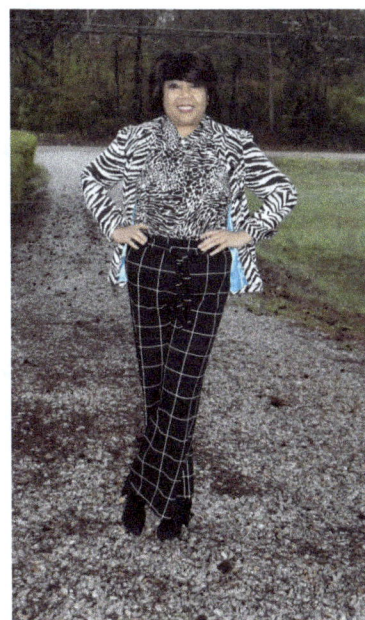

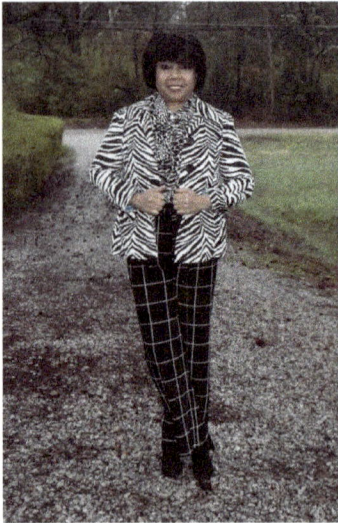 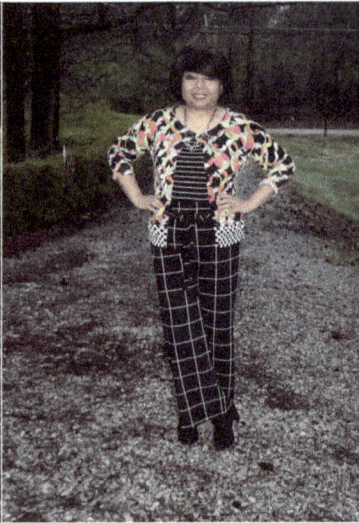 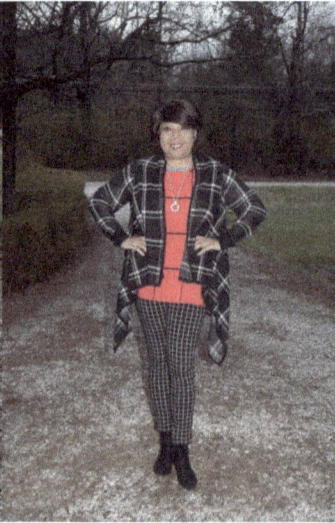 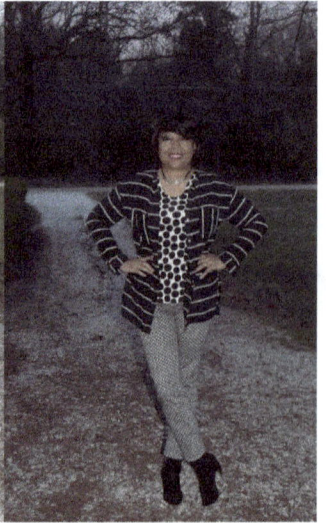

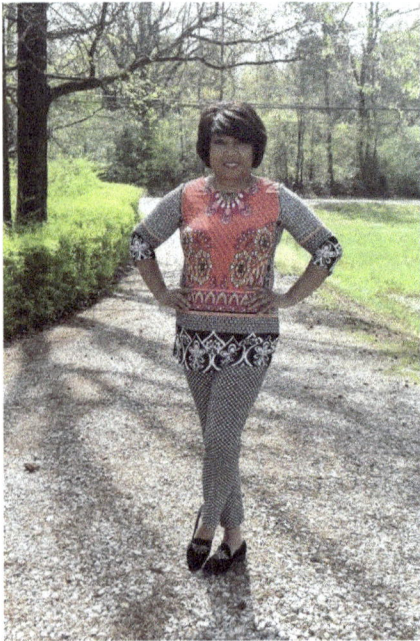 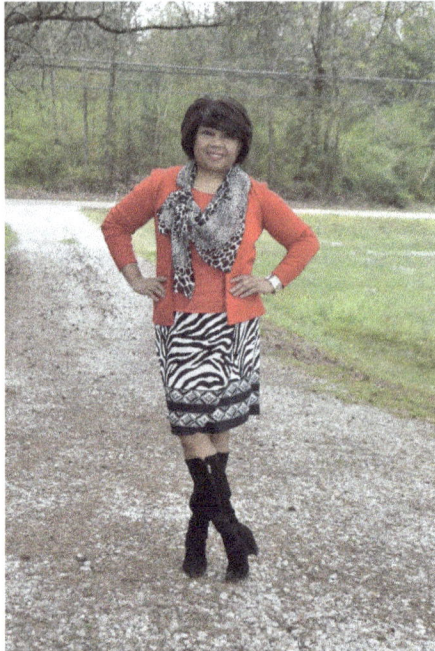 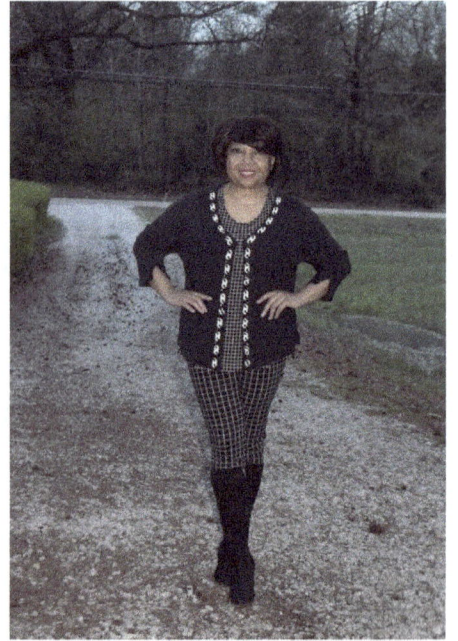

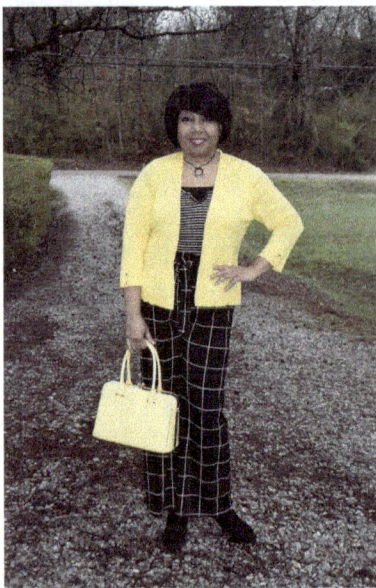 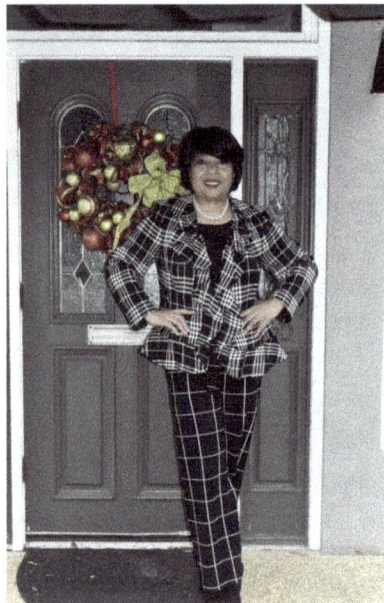 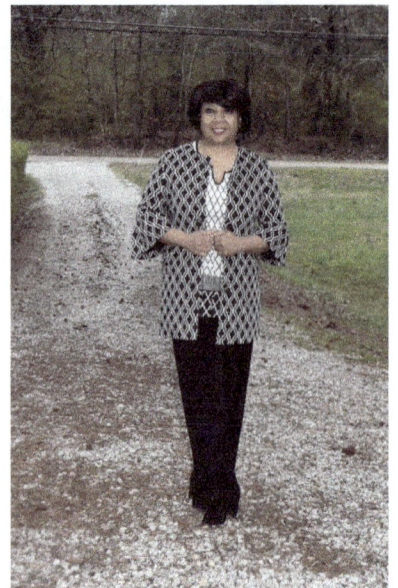

What is my favorite color to wear???

Black, Black , Black with Black and Black on Black! Did I say BLACK??? Since my early 20's black has been my favorite color to wear. I probably got my love of black from my mother . She loves to wear black, especially in her later years. She has told me many times that her mother had a certain black dress, black shoes and black purse ready for special occasions. My mother does the same. She keeps a certain black dress and black suit that are her go to outfits for special events. Her "uniform" is a simple black dress or a dressy black pant suit with a broach or flower pin.

Flashback picture from 2011. There's NOTHING like a LBD "little black dress" !!!

THIS DRESS IS OVER 40 years old.

I bought this dress when I was in the 8th grade...Actually I BEGGED my mother to buy it for me! (LOL) My Mom said that it was too old/grown up for me and that I didn't have any-where to wear it...which I guess was pretty true. But, I just HAD to have it!! It was SOO me!!! (Well it is isn't it??!!) The saleslady at Pryors (Tupelo) helped me talk her into it.

(Thanks Lady!!) (Thanks' Mom!!!) I think it was $80. It turned out that I didn't wear it in public until several years later in the 11th or 12th grade...for a modeling segment in a Black History Program at school (My nickname and "stage name " was G. G. Glamour Girl!) Since that time, I have worn it MANY, MANY times and STILL wear it today !

WHAT DO I ALWAYS SAY ??!!!!

1. You can NEVER go wrong with black .

2. When ALL else fails...wear black !

3. Black is the new Black !!!

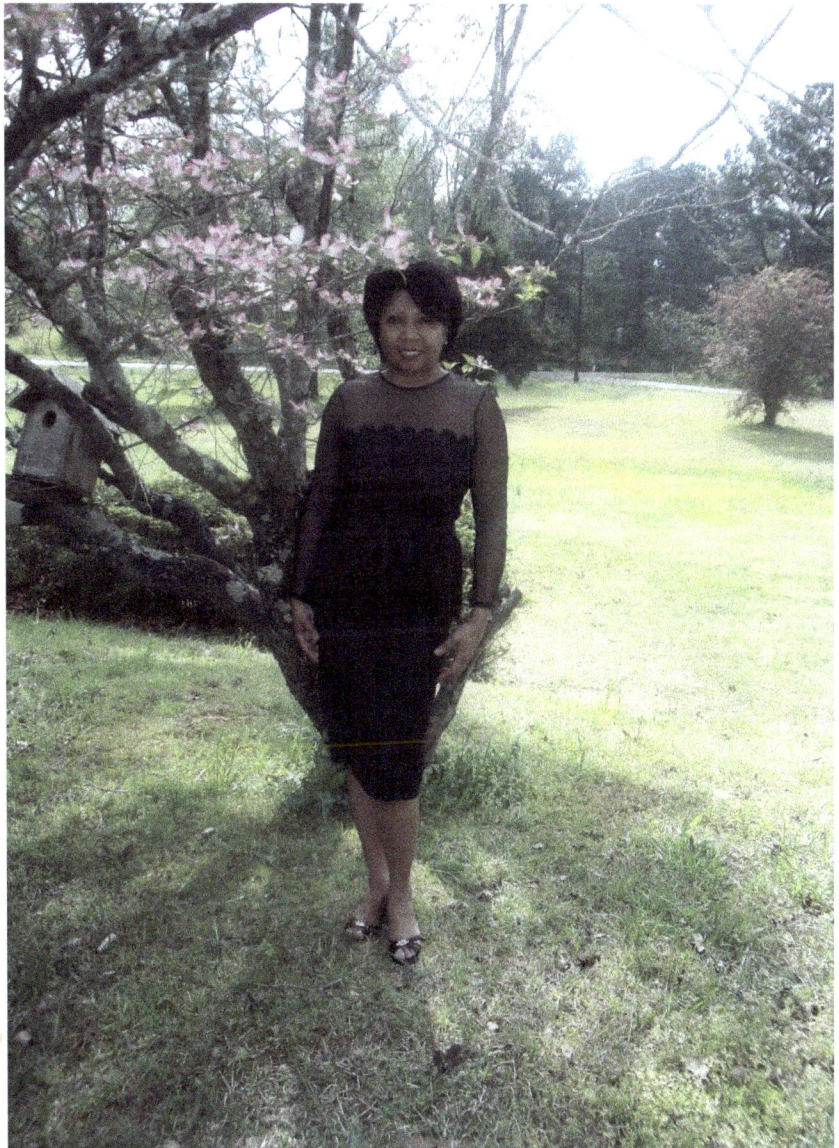

When I love something I really love it!

Here is my over 40 year old Little Black Dress.. Escorting Toni Seawright-Miss Mississippi and 4th Runner Up to Miss America on her visit to Tupelo,MS-1987

Yep, that's a picture of me and fabulous friend Toni Seawright who was the first African American to be crowned Miss Mississippi. Friend Yvonne Fields and I were her escorts for her visit to Tupelo that year. I was 23 or 24 and Yes, I'm wearing that black lace that my Mama bought for me when I was in the 8th grade! I begged and begged for it .! She thought it was too mature for me, but, as you can see I got it.

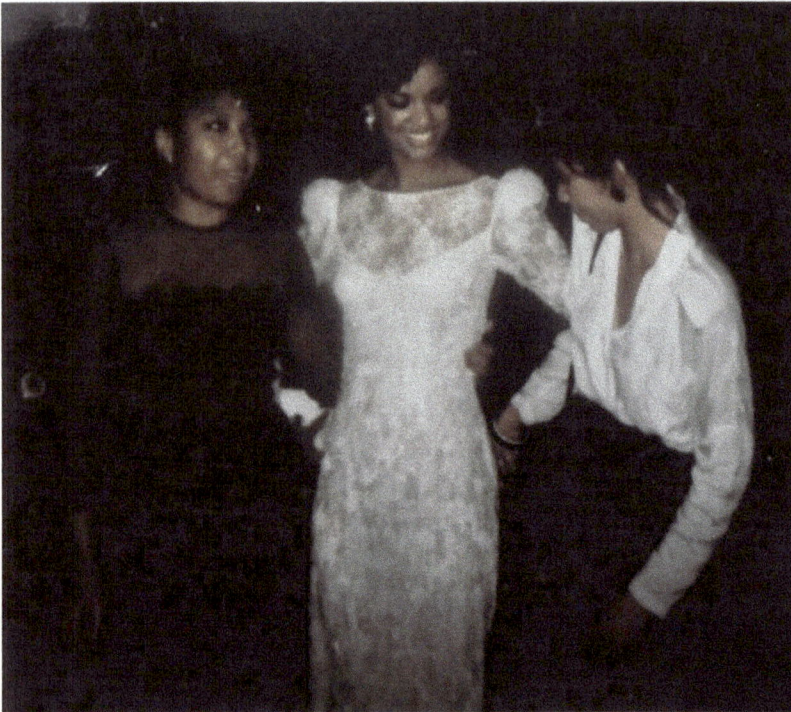

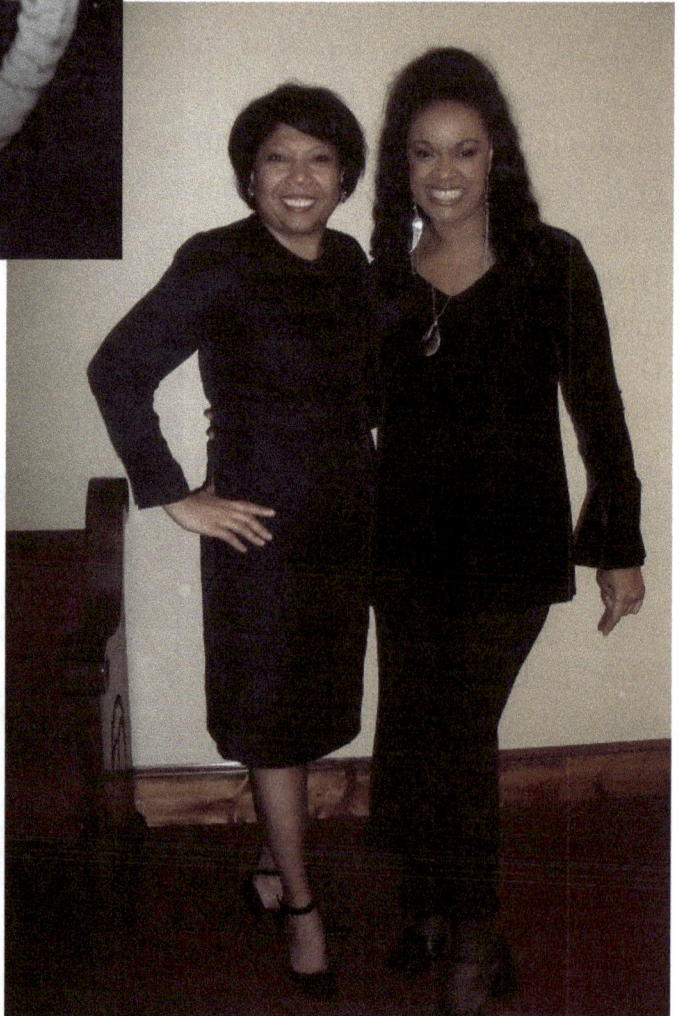

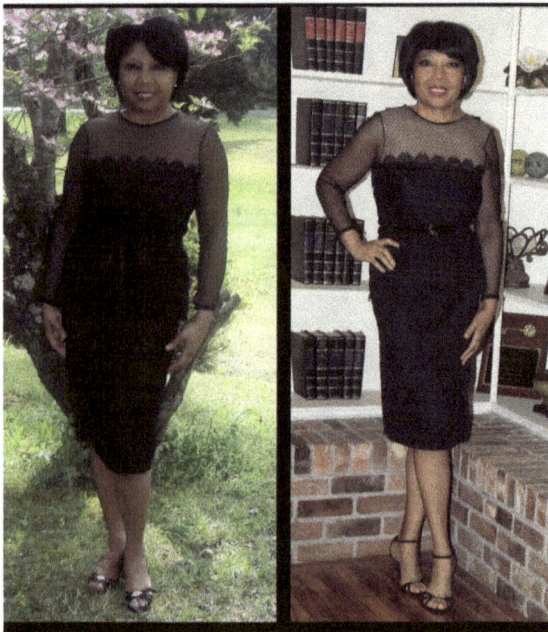

2011 (47)   2023 (59)

That Little Black Dress

WE LOVE WEARING BLACK

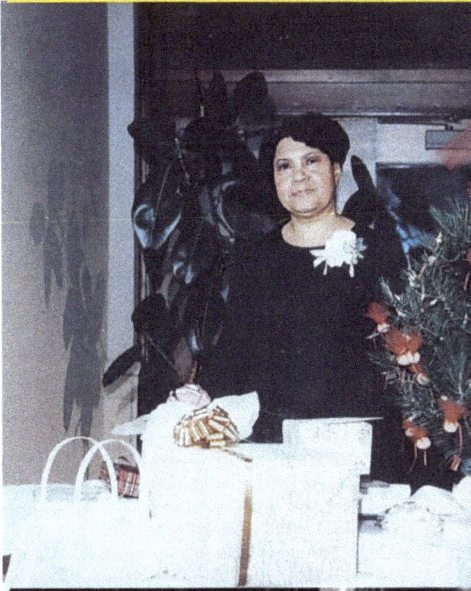
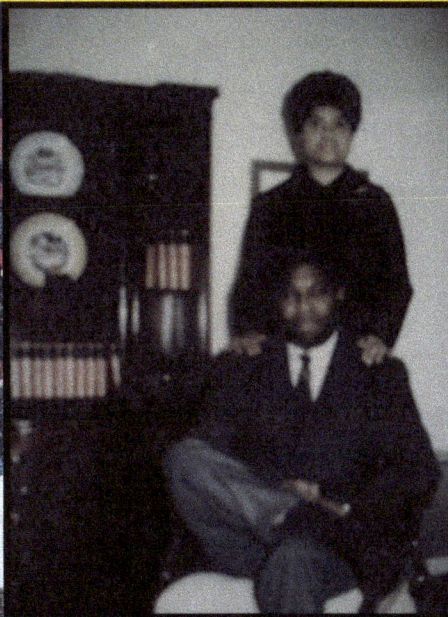
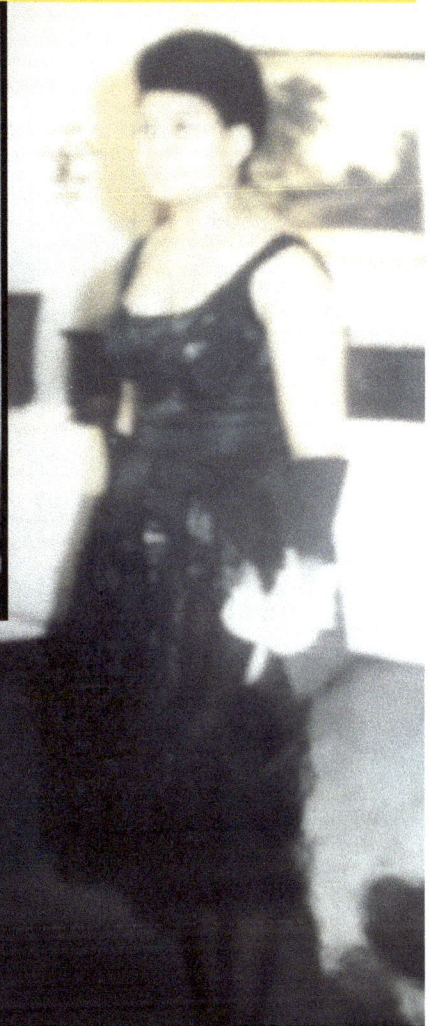
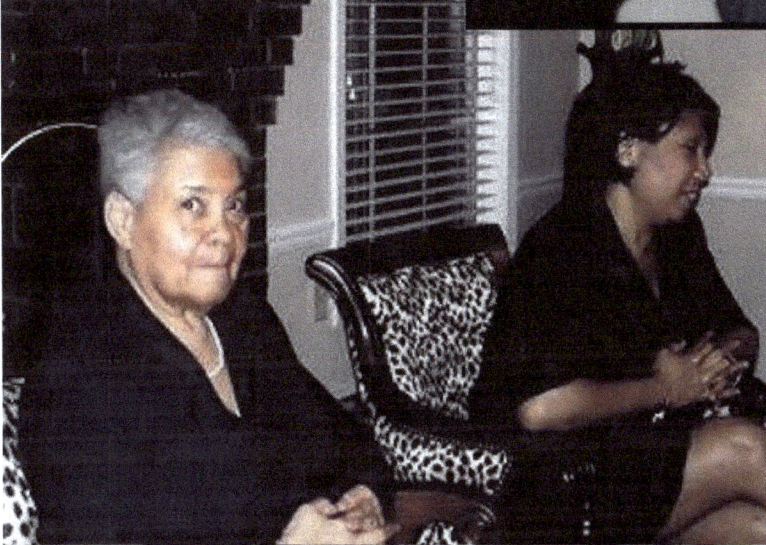
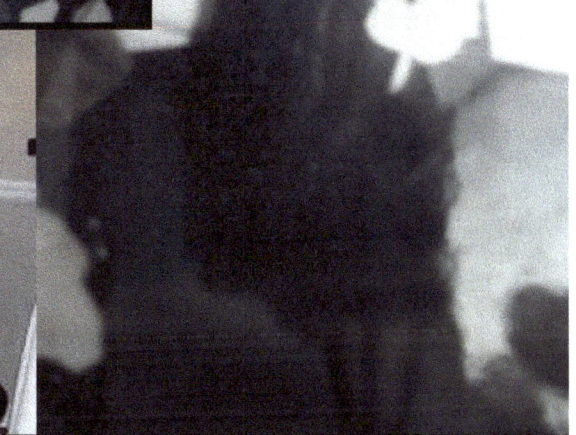
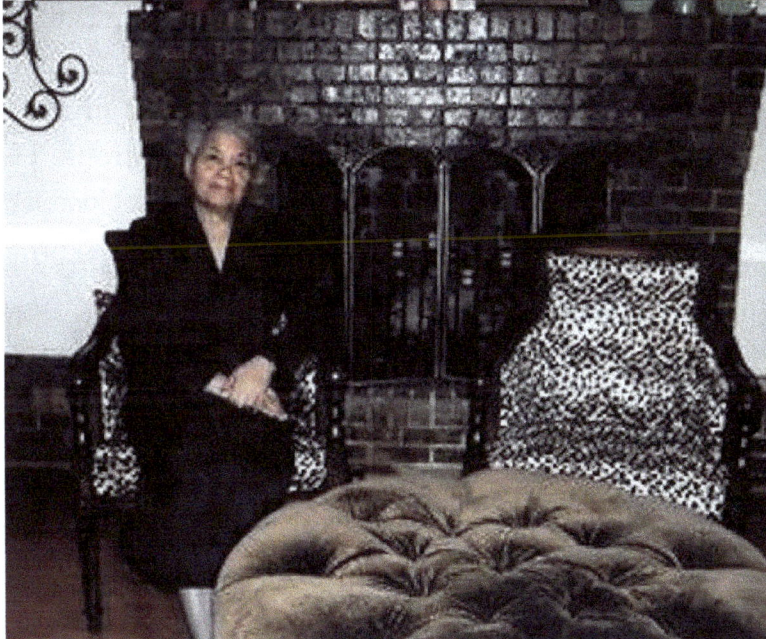
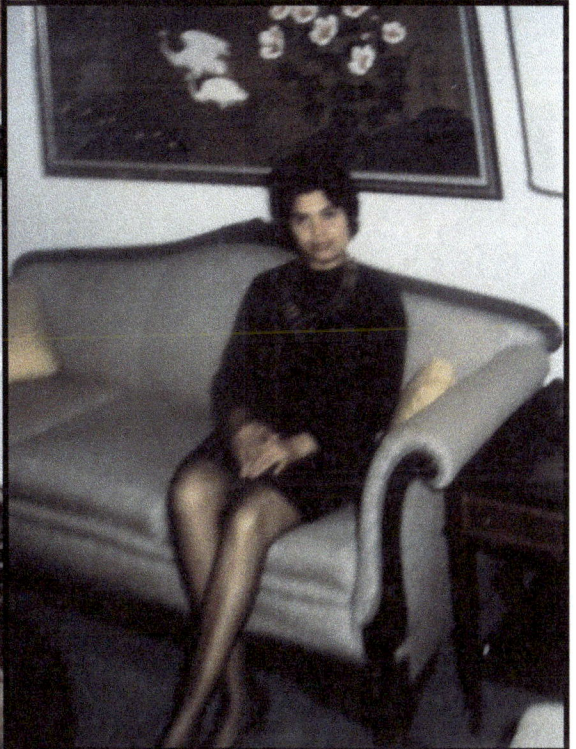

When I was growing up, EVERYWHERE we went my Mom held my hand, She did it all through the years until I was probably 18 or 19. One day , in the mall , she was holding my hand. I told her , "Mama , I think I am too old for you to be holding my hand all the time. " ...And, we stopped. #Teenagers Many years later ...I am in my 50's and she is in her 80's. Now, everywhere we go, where there is any kind of crowd or with a lot of people, I always hold her hand. So happy. So proud ...to be able to hold my Mama's hand! #Tears #Blessed

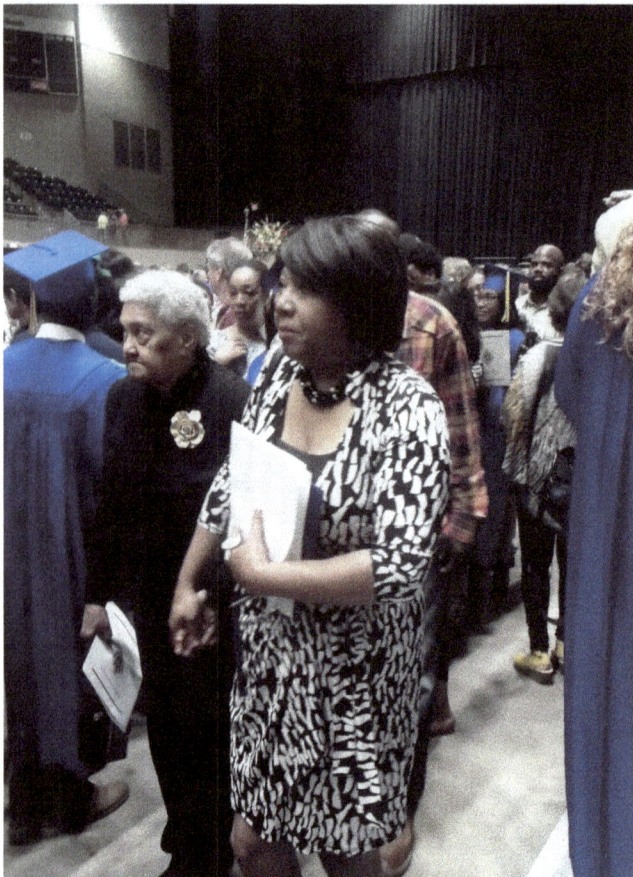

THIS PICTURE IS FROM MY SON'S HIGH SCHOOL GRADUATION MAY 2017

Mom is wearing her "uniform"

Facebook Post May 19, 2017

Headed out of the graduation last night, I had a flashback moment. When I was growing up, EVERYWHERE we went my Mom held my hand, All throughout high school my mother loved to hold my hand when we were in the mall of walking anywhere. I think she just wanted to keep a certain kind of connection...and her way of keeping me close. One day , in the mall , she was holding my hand, I was probably in the 11th or 12th grade I told her , "Mama , I think I am too old for you to be holding my hand all the time. " ...And, we stopped. #Teenagers Many years later ...I am in my 50's and she is in her 80's. Last night, in the mad crush of trying to exit the arena, I grabbed my mother's hand, to keep her close.

FAST FORWARD TWO YEARS 2019 Henry's ICC Graduate "Associate's Degree" #olemissbound, 2022 Ole Miss Grad

We wore almost the same thing and I held her hand as we navigated through the crowd to exit the building.

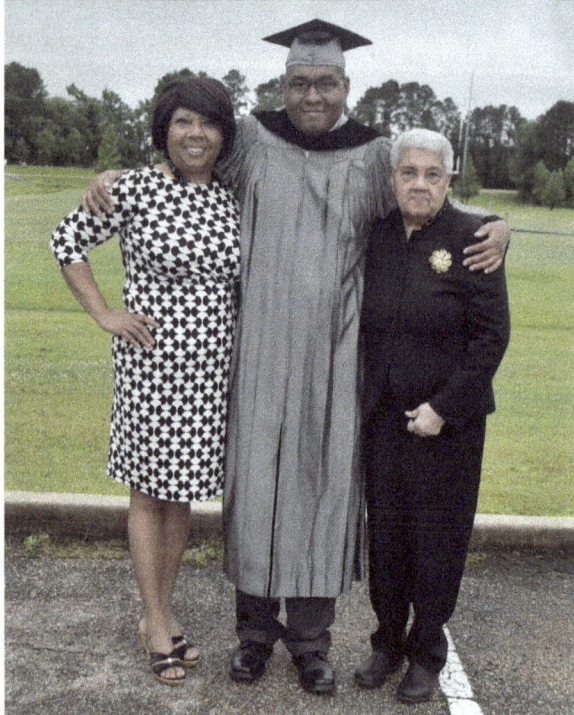

Facebook post May11, 2019

Everyone told me that I was going to have a complete emotional melt down at my son's high school graduation. I was like really??? No way! I was so glad for him to get out of High School, I didn't know what to do! Everyone kept warning me! I kept poo pooing at the ridiculousness of it all! I was like PLEASE ! Stop The Madness! You just don't know!!! The day came! I sat by a bestie church buddy. Because of their last names , Henry and her daughter have been sitting next to each other in school ceremonies since grade school. We laughed and talked the whole time! We had the best time ! Not one tear! I acted, felt exactly how I thought I would ...Completely Giddy! Fast forward ,,,ICC graduation. No expectations of any unusual feelings except for pride. We took a few pictures outside...and as he was walking away to go into the building, in his cap and gown ...I was blindsided I had a complete melt down.

I was suddenly overwhelmed with emotions! The flood gates opened! I just stared at him walking. In my mind, I was saying ..On my goodness. That's my BABY!!! My BABY is graduating from COLLEGE! I was in complete Mommy melt down mode for about a minute just blubbering , then I was fine. The rest of the day was blissful! All Mom's beware ,those meltdown moments are lurking around any corner . Trust Me! PS. Don't think that I'm NOT crying (again) as I type this, when I certainly AM December 5, 2019

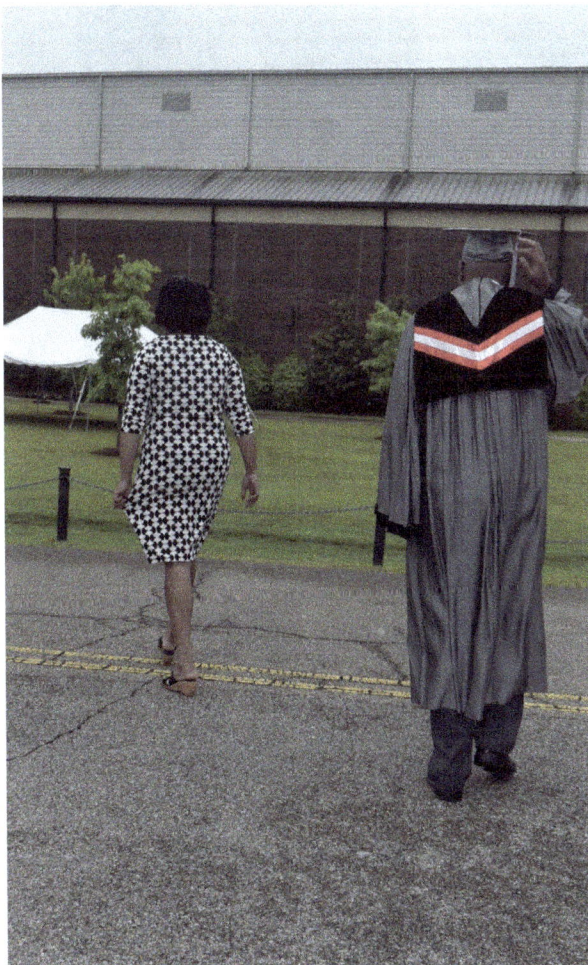

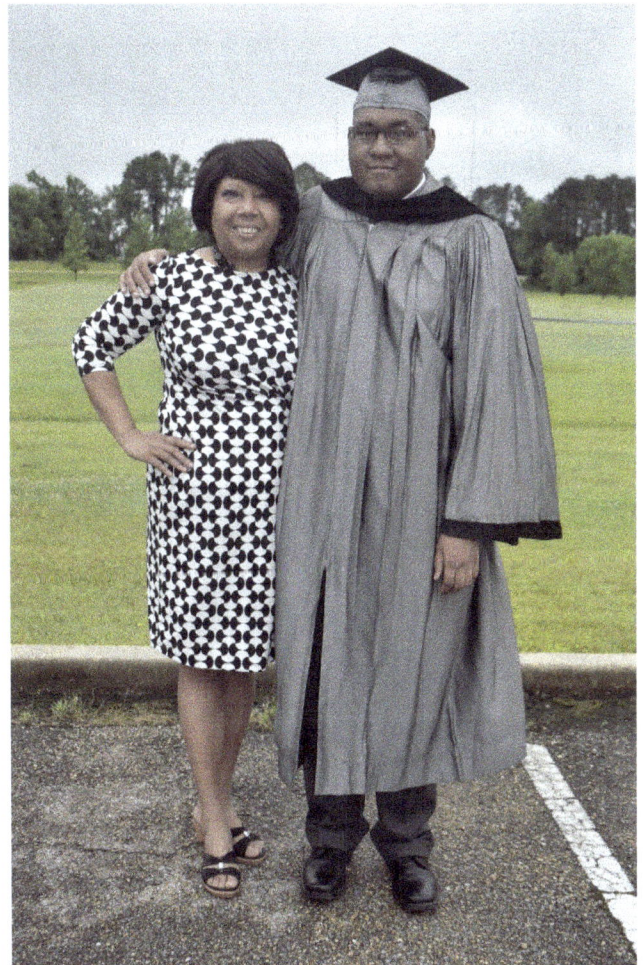

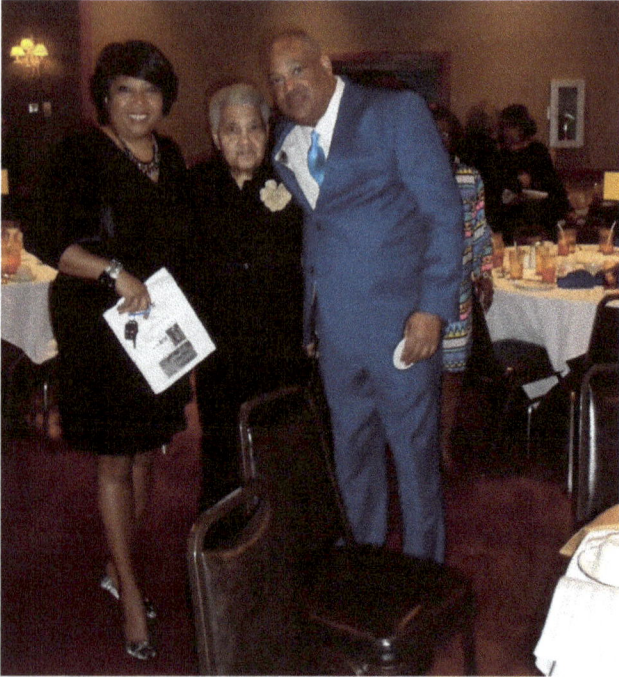

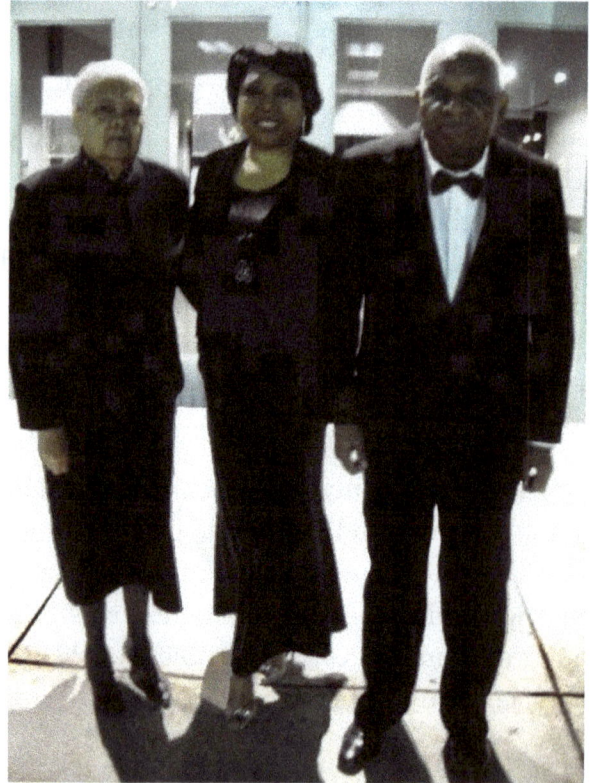

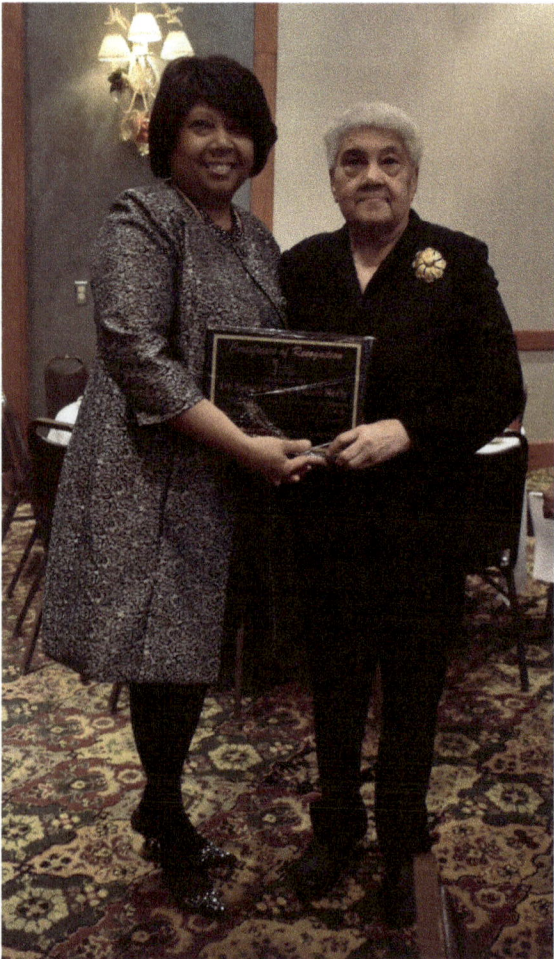

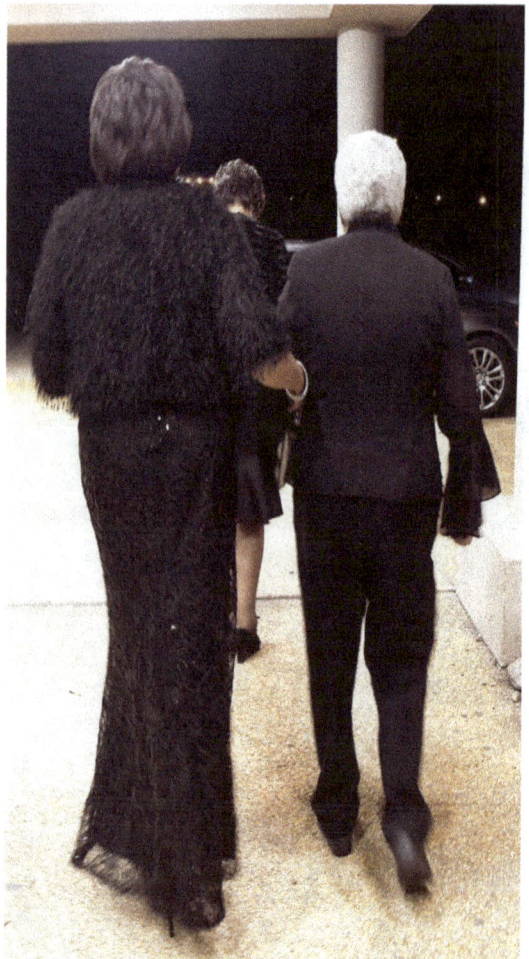

You will be greatly missed Mrs Delores Lagrone! My Diva Friend!

Whatever event there was, we would always find each other and take a picture ! She added a certain light and LIFE wherever she went! As my mother's beautician for over 40 years. we laughed and talked about EVERYTHING!

—June 2020 PND with Mrs. Delores Lagrone

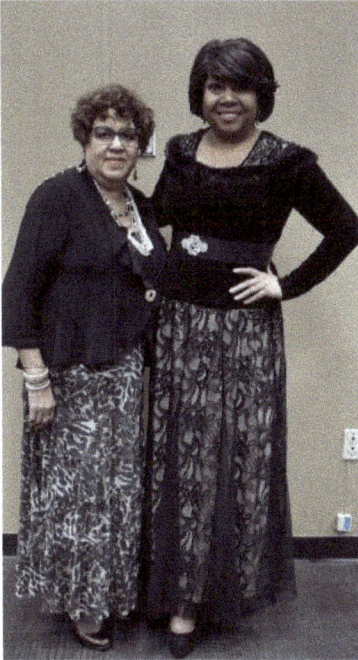

An original Diva and the definition of FABULOSITY from way back When I was growing up we couldn't wait to see what Mrs. D would step in the door wearing! She never disappointed! I think many times, the highlight of the event was her outfit! I've had some great role models in the "game"... and still learning!

January 18, 2020 I wrote

This picture of Mrs Delores Lagrone, BELOW, kind of sums up the deeper part of what an influence and mentor she was to so many! Yes , we always joked about fabulosity and being divalicious . We always talked about fun and fashion, But beyond that she was always giving insights and pointers and thoughts on every subject imaginable. She was truly a woman who loved life and living it to the FULLEST. She was no shrinking violet, or sidelines Sally. She jumped right in the middle of everything with great passion and gusto. I would often tell her that she made ME tired just looking at all of the things she did and places that she went. She just laughed.

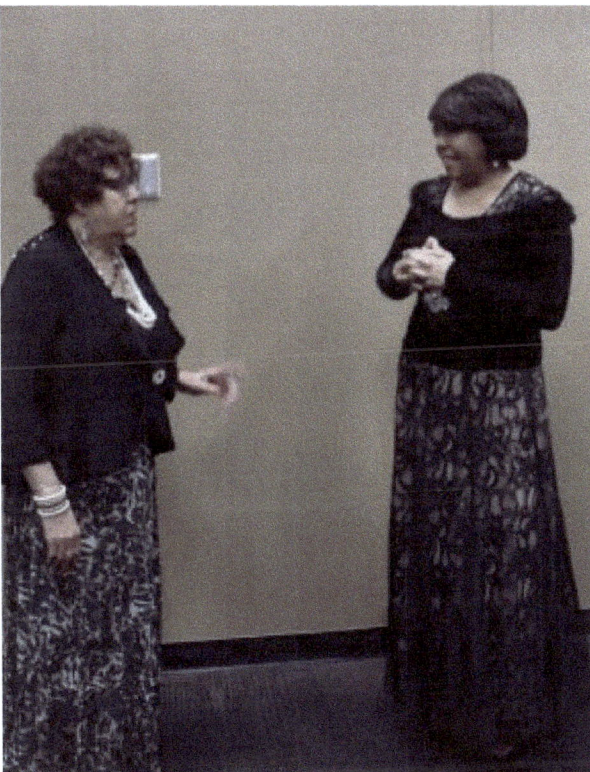

THAT laugh ! She was my Mom's beautician from the 1970's. We would chat without ceasing as she did my Mom's hair and always laughed at what kindred spirits we were, Mom was/is very low key, quiet and subdued ... and we were NOT!:)

If there was an event , she was there! She knew that I was always looking for the blow by blow, whenever I wasn't there (which was often!) She never missed a detail. Thanks Mrs. D for adding such color and excitement to the world! You lived out loud in living color and we loved it! She was the epitome of my motto: Be You ! Do You ! SHINE!

Taking pointers from the master

#Divalicious

33rd Annual Dr.Martin Luther King,Jr Banquet 2020 A Black-Tire Affair" Moving Towards
The Dream of Love,Compassion,Respect and Harmony for All People

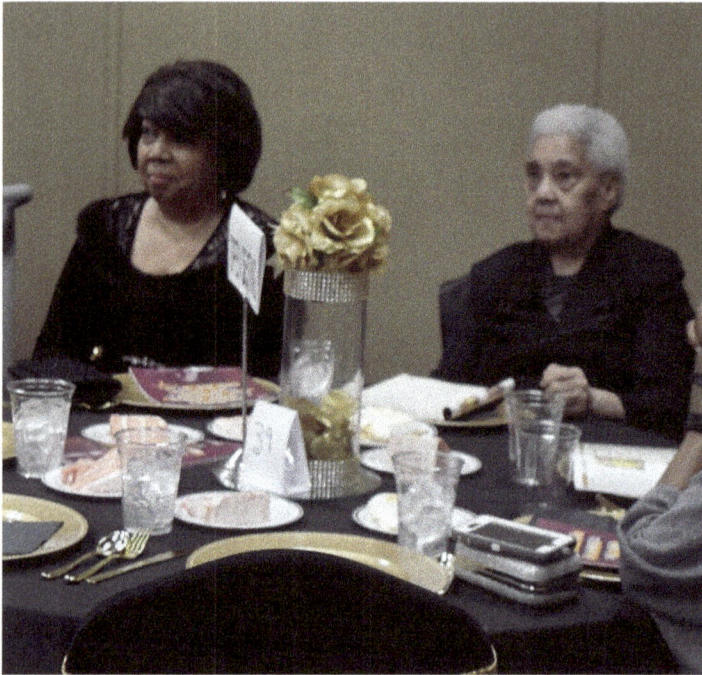

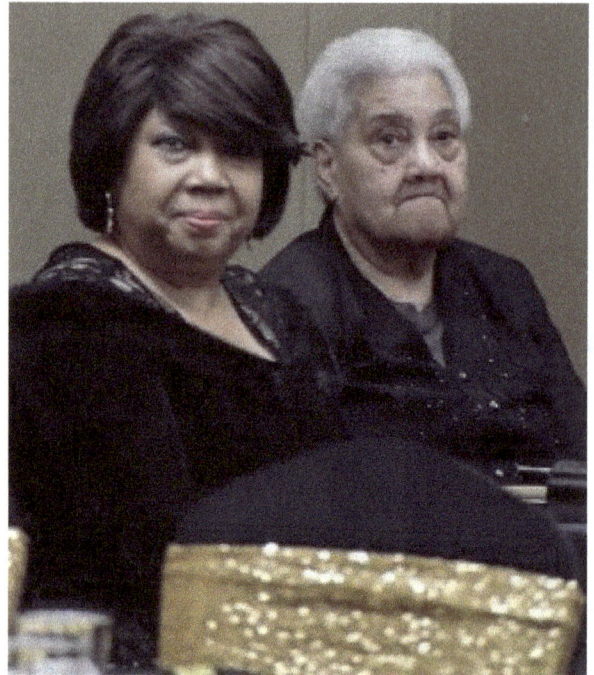

January 2017
Celebrating 109th Founder's Day Alpha Kappa Alpha Sorority,
Incorporated with International President, Dr. Dorothy Buckhanan

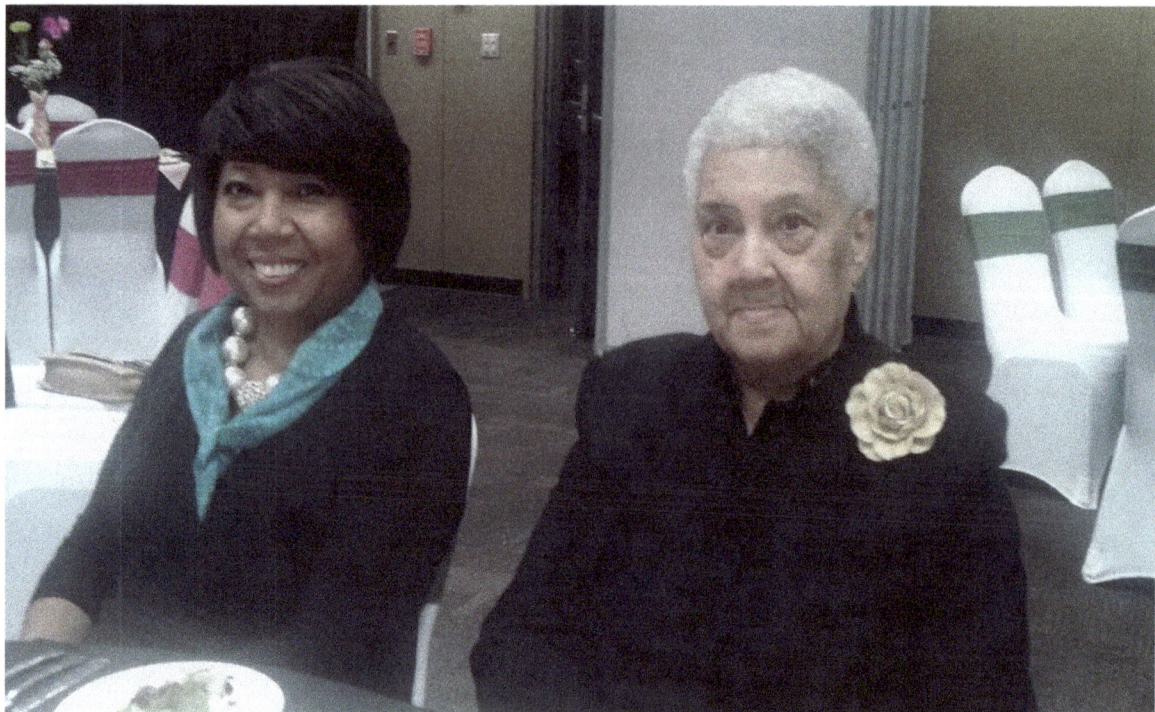

Me, Mom, and my brother Brian
MLK Banquet
January 2017

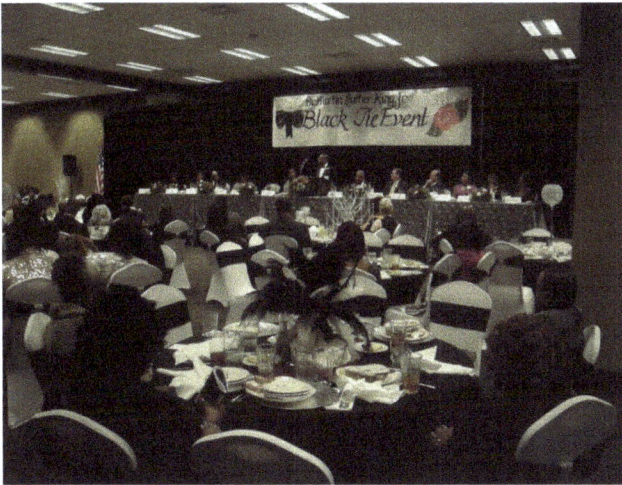

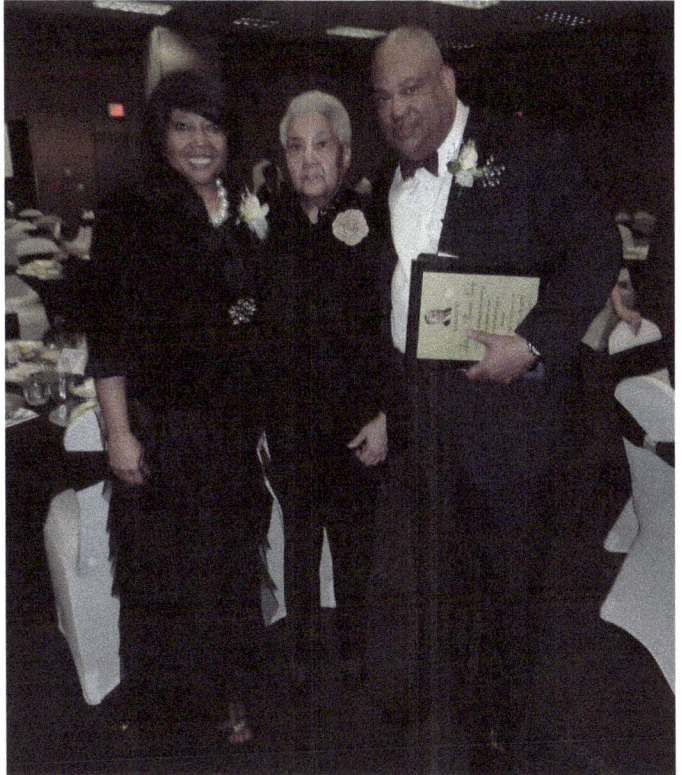

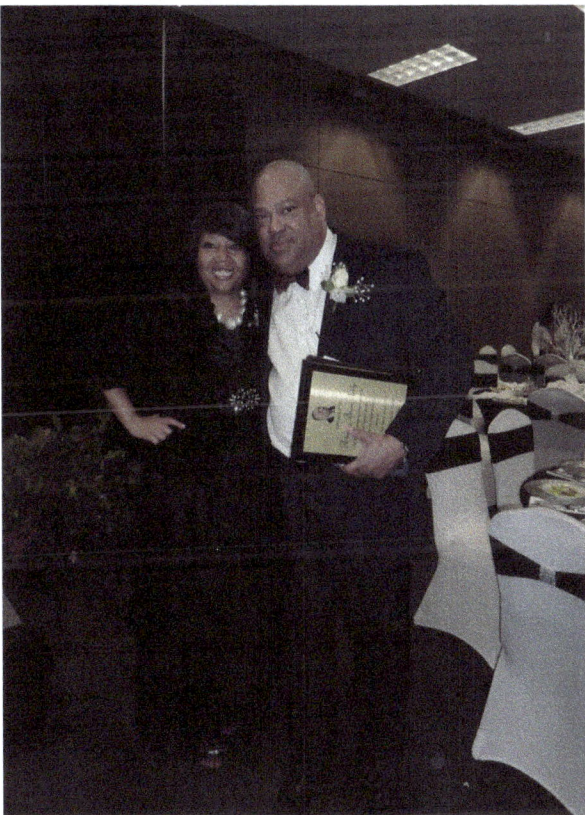

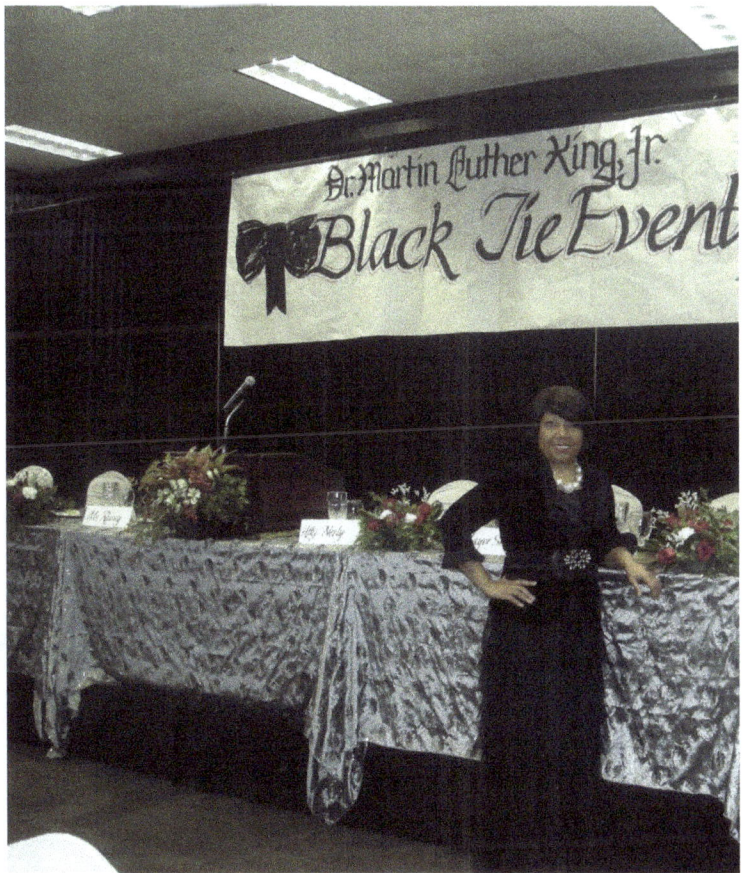

December 5, 2019 UNCF Banquet

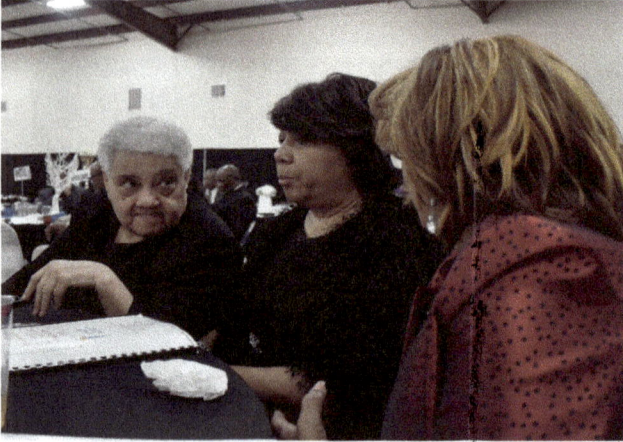

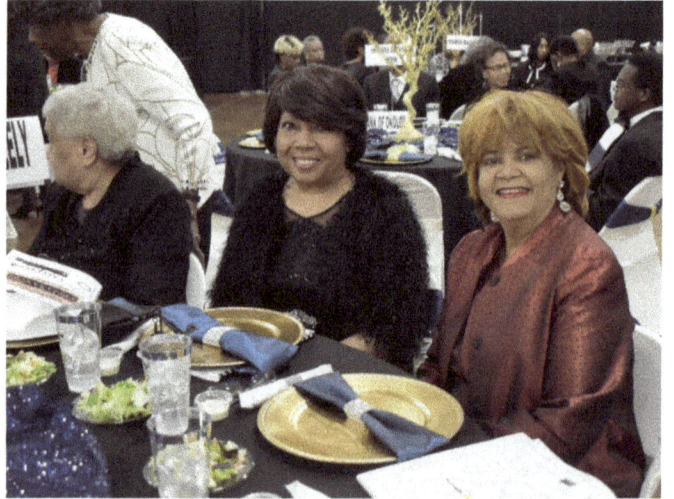

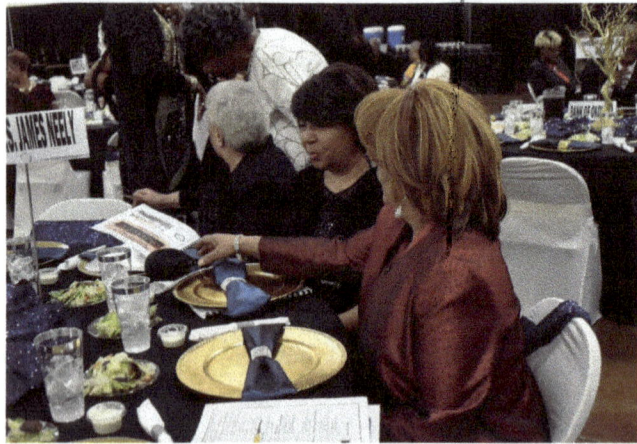

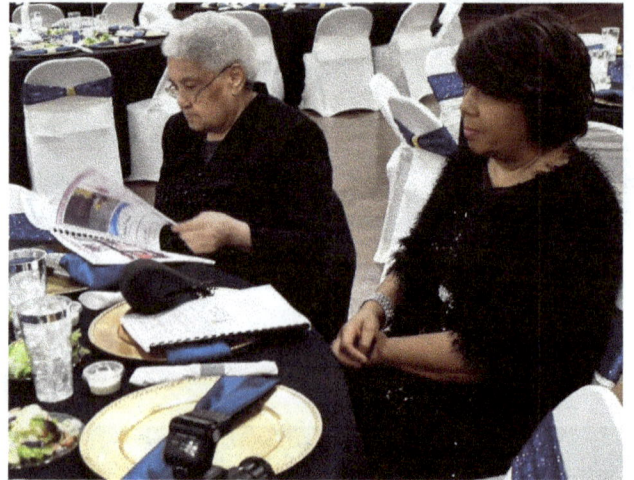

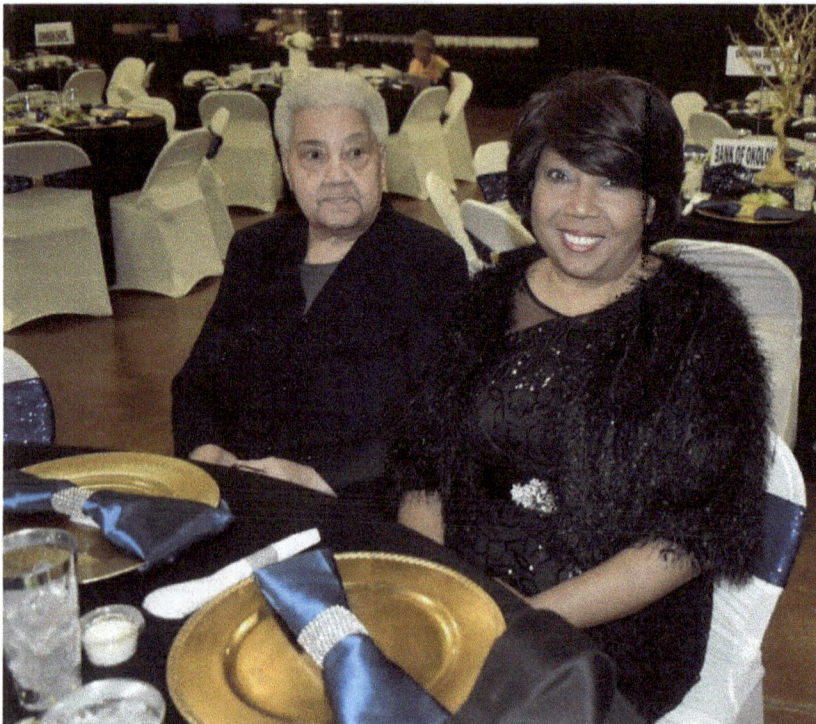

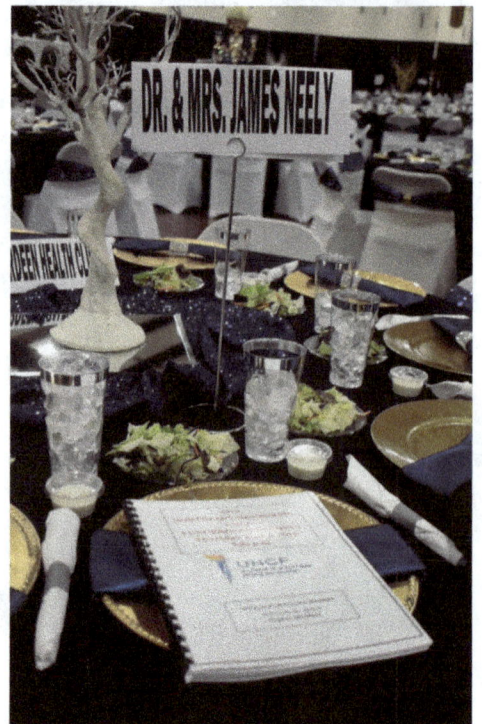

One is never over dressed or under dressed in a "Little Black Dress"

-Karl Lagerfeld

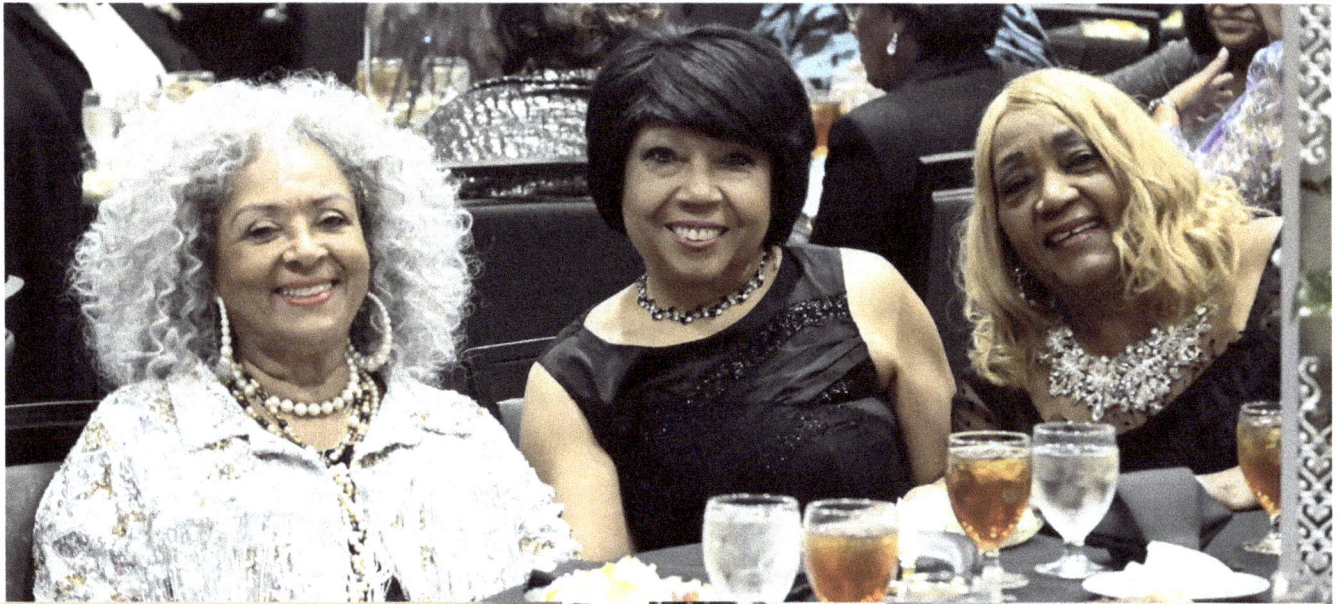

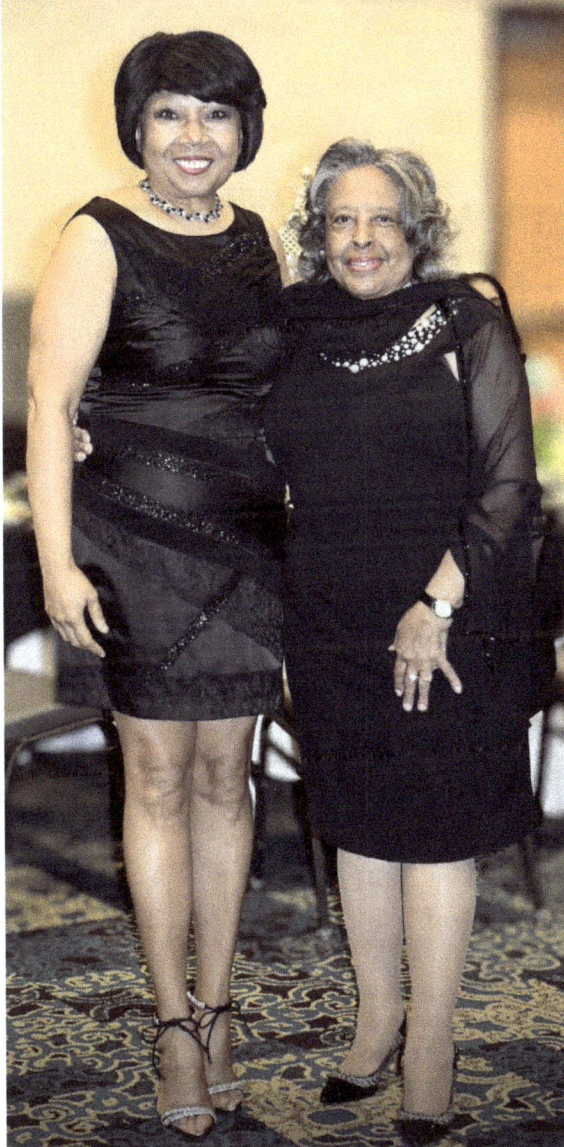

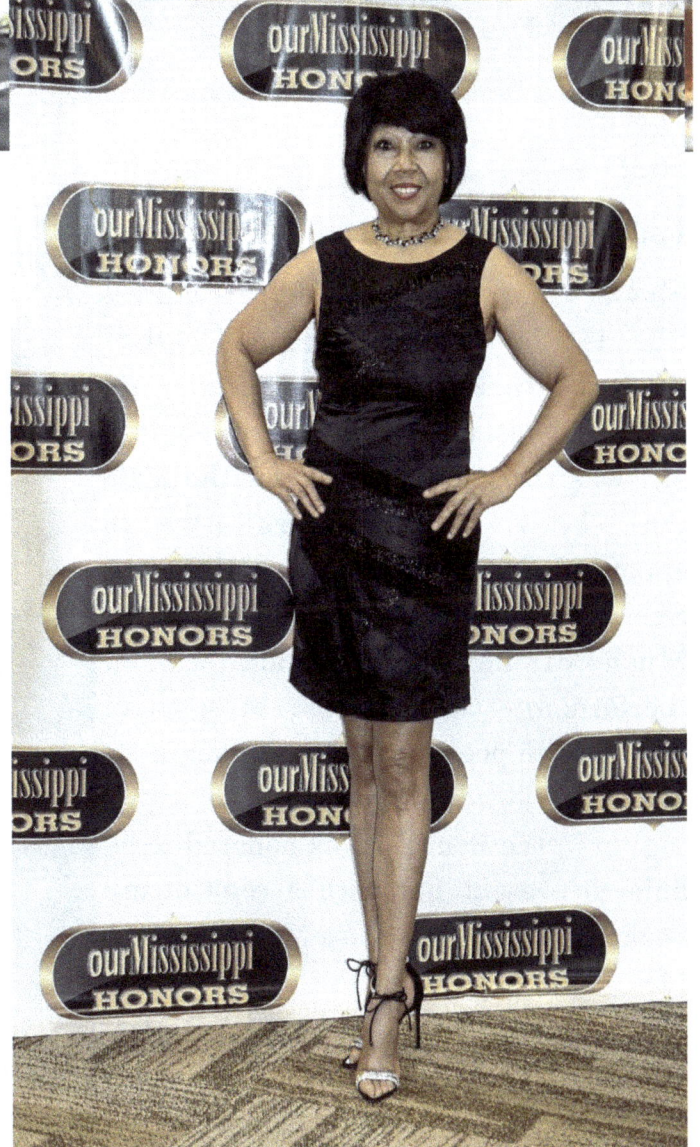

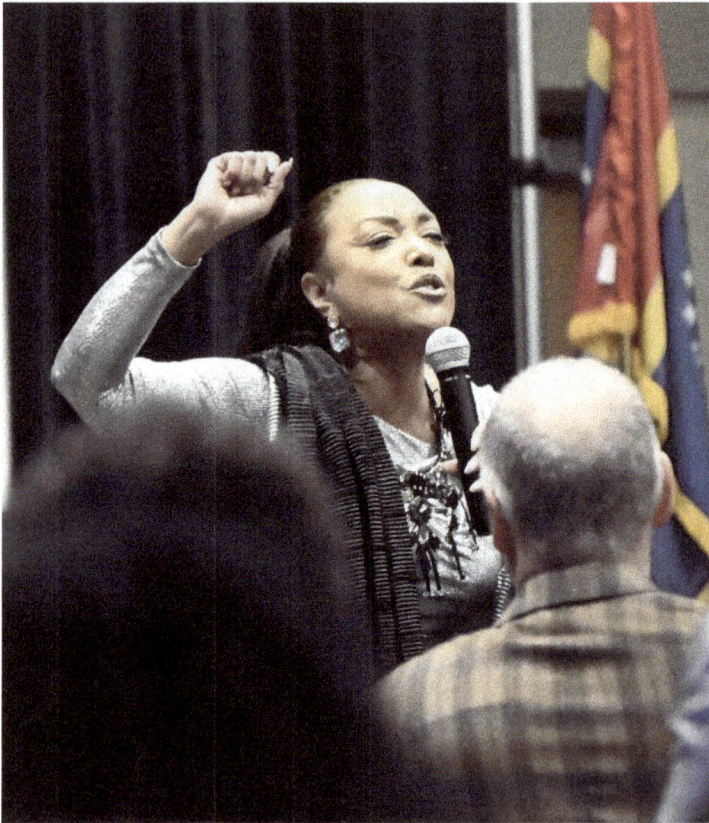

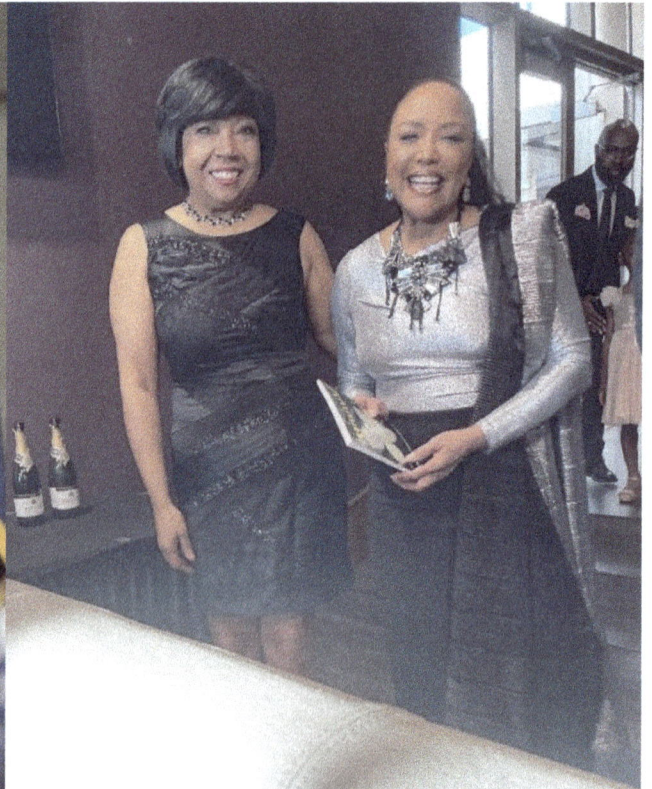

I adore Lynn Whitfield !

She is class and elegance personified! She is the epitome of FABULOUS! #FebruaryGirlsRock(Born February 15, 1953) I was more than overjoyed that she was the guest speaker for the 2023 Our Mississippi Honors Awards Program! The program was outstanding! She was amazing! She loves poetry. Much of her presentation was a "performance"/spoken word of some of her favorite poems. She also talked a lot about the joys and advantages of growing up in the South. I was honored to be able to present her with a copy of my book of southern poems, Mississippi In Me.

Photos by James Dorsey (Hubby)

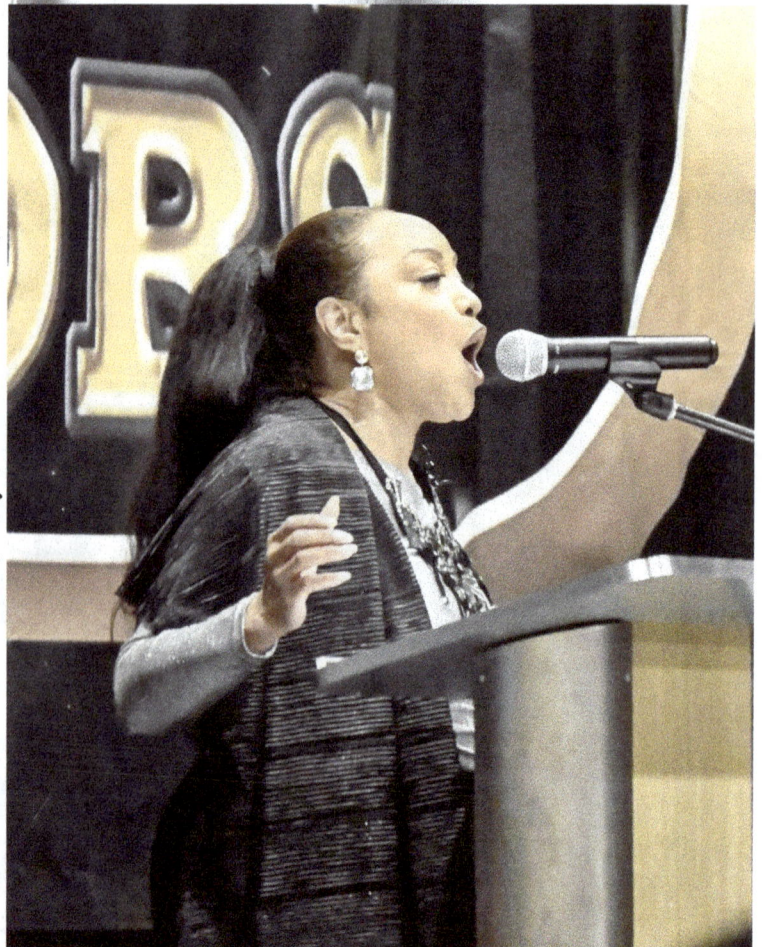

OFFICIAL RESOLUTION-STATE OF MISSISSIPPI

Adopted January 19, 2015

A resolution commending and Congratulating Talented Poet and Native Mississippian , Patricia Neely-Dorsey for her many achievements as a writer and extend best wishes for many more years of success

WHEREAS Patricia Neely-Dorsey is not only a talented poet, who is loved by many , she is also a native daughter of Mississippi and WHEREAS she is a 1982 graduate of Tupelo High School in Tupelo , Mississippi , and she received a bachelor of arts degree in psychology from Boston University in Boston, Massachusetts and

WHEREAS , after living for almost 20 years in Memphis, Tennessee working in the mental health field , she returned to her hometown of Tupelo, Mississippi in

August 2007, and

WHEREAS, Mrs. Neely-Dorsey published her first book of poetry Reflections of a Mississippi Magnolia-A Life In Poems in February 208 and her second book My Magnolia Memories and Musings -In Poems , was

published in February 2012 and

WHEREAS. , she continues to live in Tupelo with her husband James, and son Henry and miniature Schnauzer Happy , and she is a proud member of Alpha Kappa Alpha Sorority Inc, an avid reader and

passionate writer and

WHEREAS, Mrs, Neely-Dorsey has always considered herself a "Goodwill Ambassador" for Mississippi and the South , and she believes tht we can bridge many gaps of misunderstanding across regional , racial , cultural ,

generational and economic lines by simply sharing our stories and

WHEREAS, it is the policy of the House of Representatives to commend the success of talented , humble, hardworking , Mississippians, such as Mrs. Neely-Dorsey , who have earned positive recognition and who claim their Mississippi heritage proudly with a

badge of honor throughout this great nation :

NOW, THEREFORE, BE IT RESOLVED THE HOUSE OF REPRESENTATIVES OF THE STATE OF MISSISSIPPI , That we do hereby commend and congratulate Mrs. Neely-Dorsey for her many accomplishments and extend best wishes to our native daughter for many more years of tremendous success .

BE IT FURTHER RESOLVED That copies of this resolution be furnished to Mrs. Patricia Neely-Dorsey and the members of the Capitol Press Corps.

DAY AT THE CAPITOL
Jackson Mississippi
February 6, 2015

$1 Yard Sale Dress

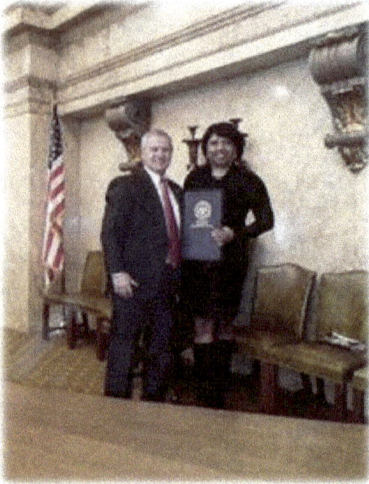

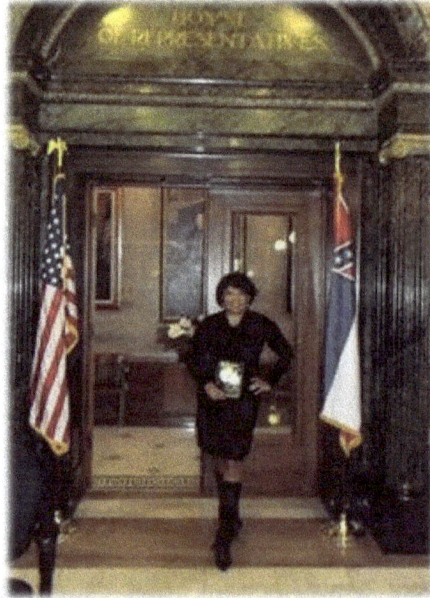

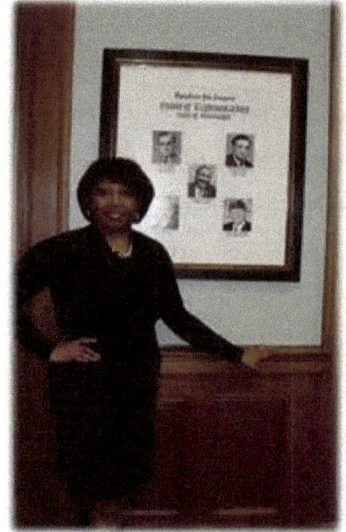

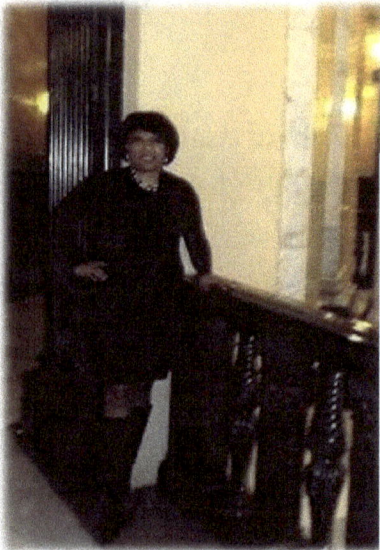

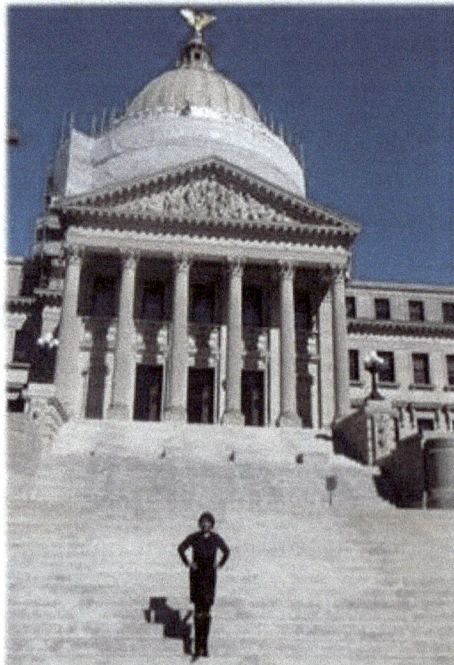

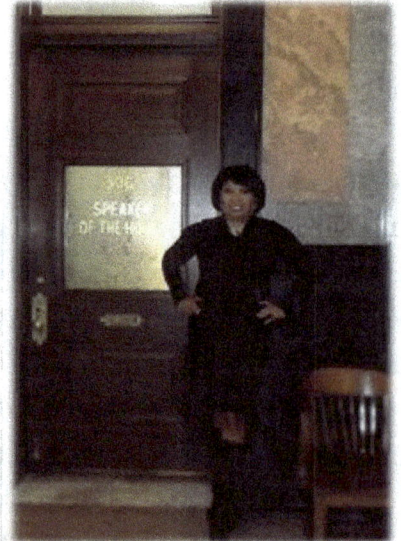

Patricia Neely-Dorsey
Always, Always Celebrating the South and
Promoting a Positive Mississippi

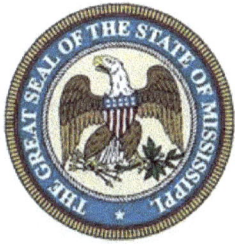

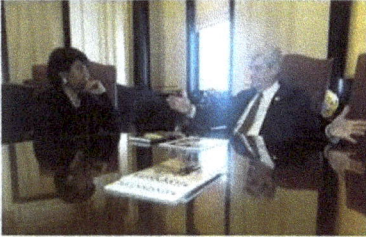

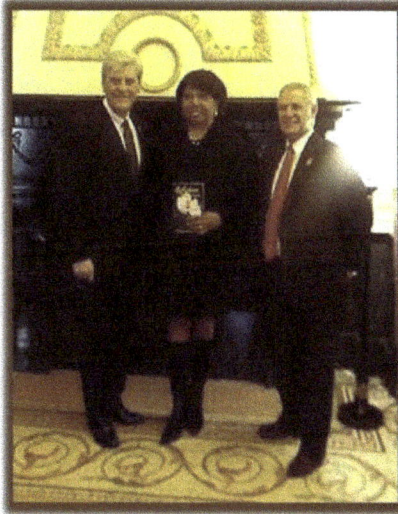

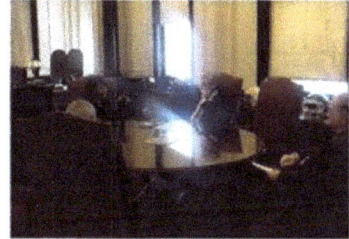

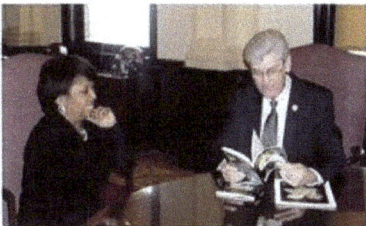

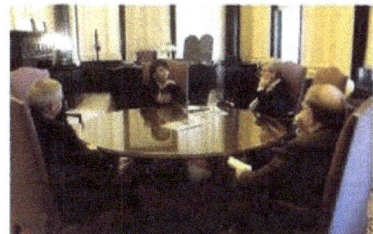

Patricia Neely-Dorsey Private Audience with Governor Phil Bryant
Always, Always, Celebrating the South and Promoting a Positive Mississippi!

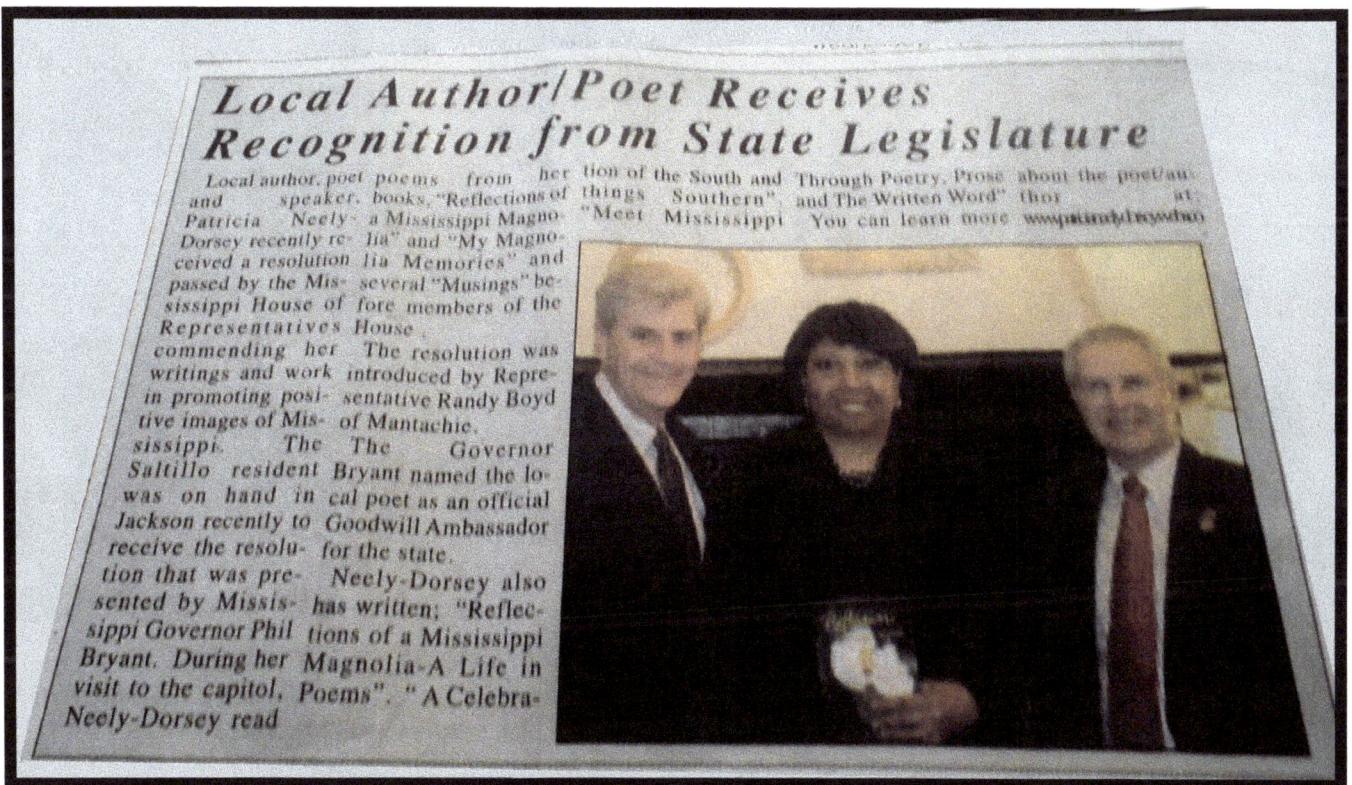

Local Author/Poet Receives Recognition from State Legislature

Local author, poet and speaker, Patricia Neely-Dorsey recently received a resolution passed by the Mississippi House of Representatives commending her writings and work in promoting positive images of Mississippi. The Saltillo resident was on hand in Jackson recently to receive the resolution that was presented by Mississippi Governor Phil Bryant. During her visit to the capitol, Neely-Dorsey read poems from her books, "Reflections of a Mississippi Magnolia" and "My Magnolia Memories" and several "Musings" before members of the House.

The resolution was introduced by Representative Randy Boyd of Mantachie.

The Governor Bryant named the local poet as an official Goodwill Ambassador for the state.

Neely-Dorsey also has written: "Reflections of a Mississippi Magnolia-A Life in Poems". "A Celebration of the South and things Southern" "Meet Mississippi Through Poetry, Prose and The Written Word" tha........ at "Meet Mississippi" You can learn more www................

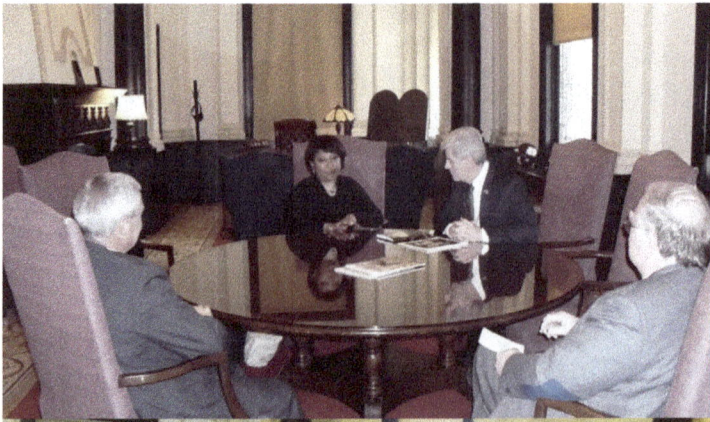
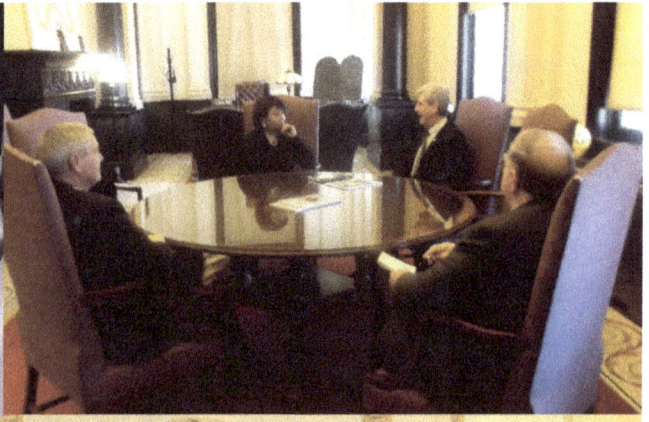
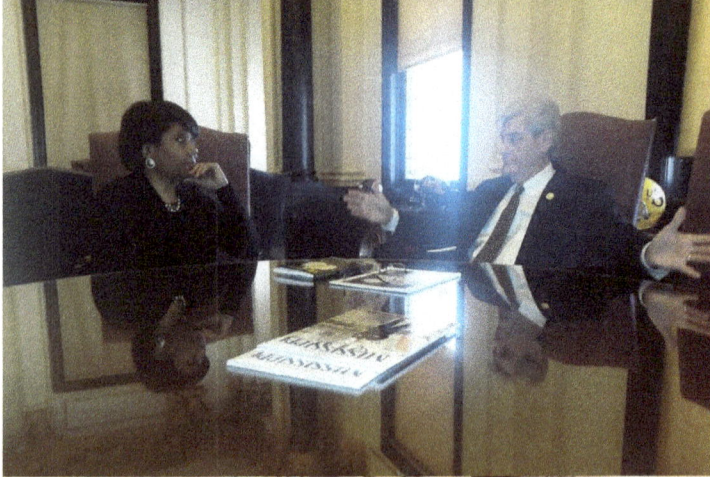
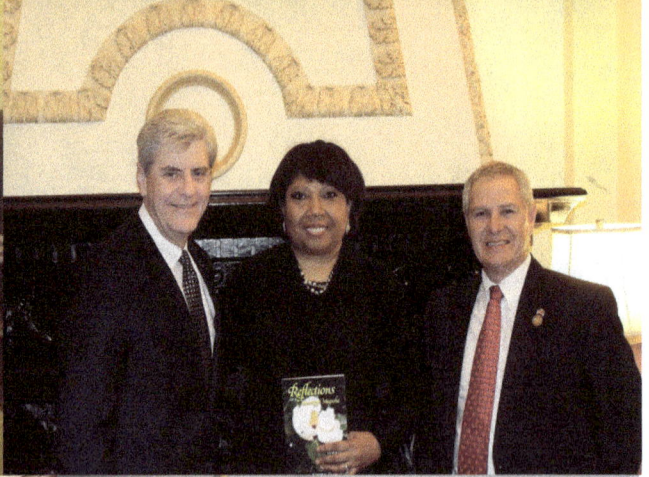
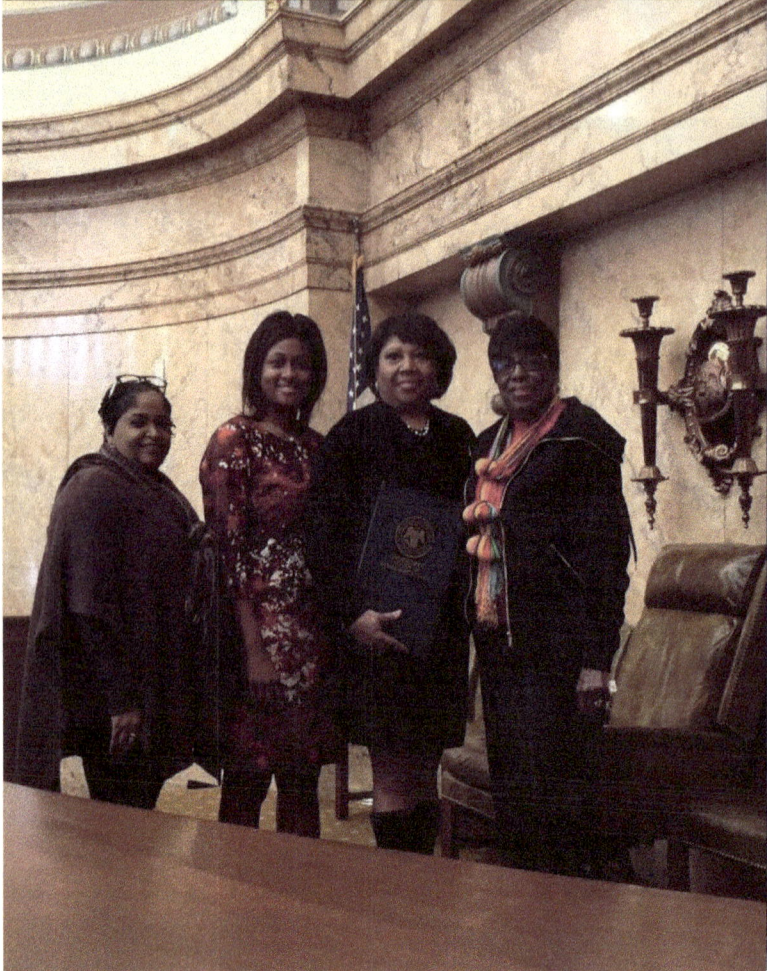
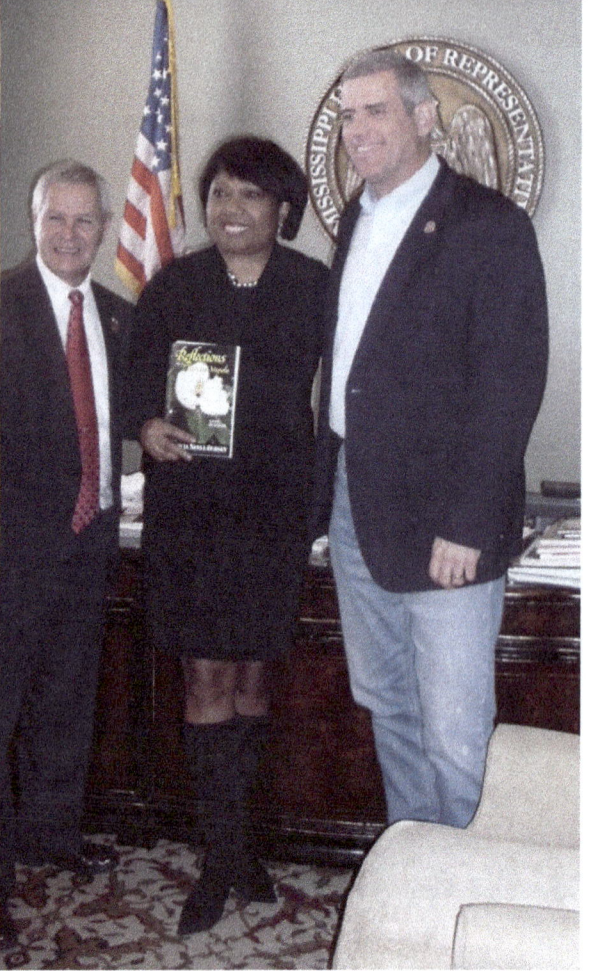

Very honored to receive Humanitarian Award ...in a $5 Thrift Shop Dress
35th Anniversary Banquet-February 2019
Tupelo Alumnae Chapter Delta Sigma Theta Sorority Inc.
Thrilled to have the support of my sorors from Alpha Kappa Alpha Sorority, Inc

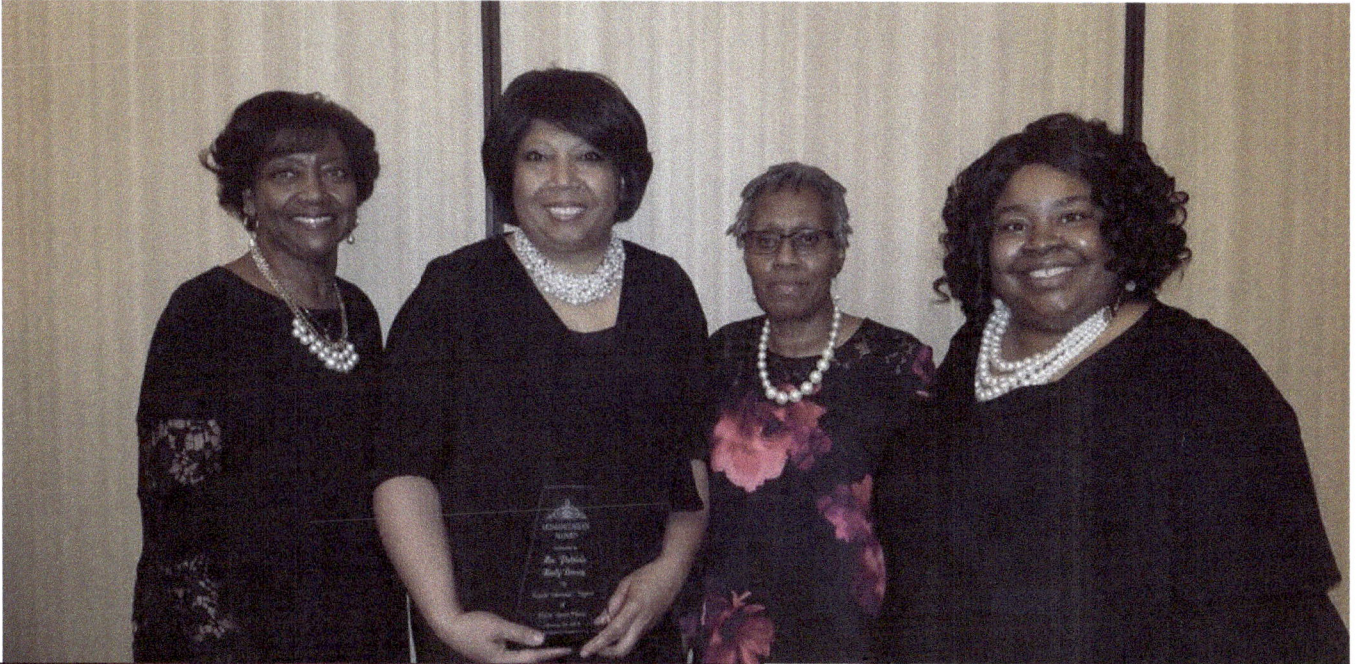

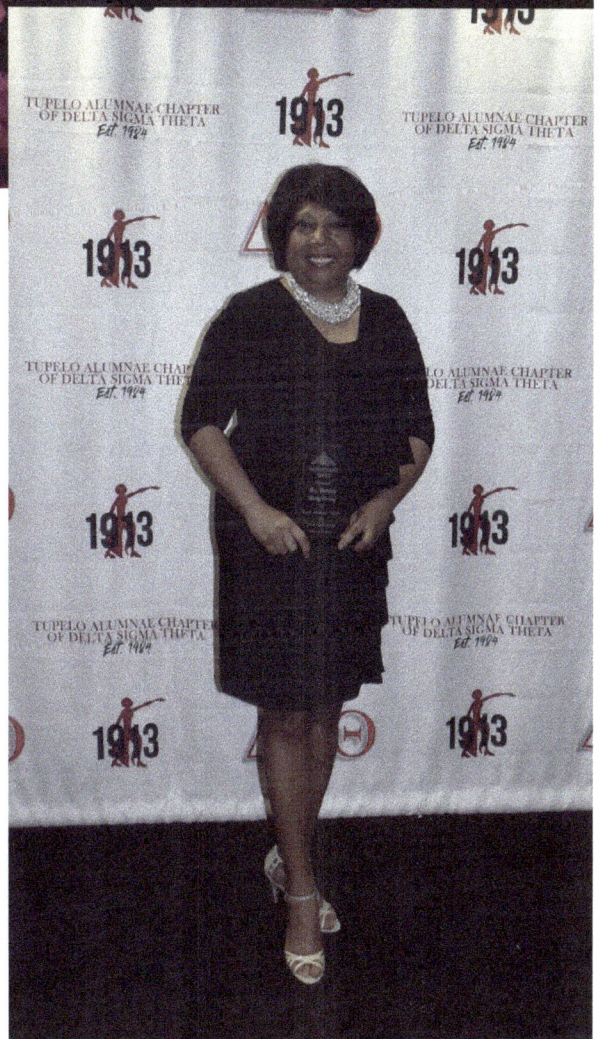

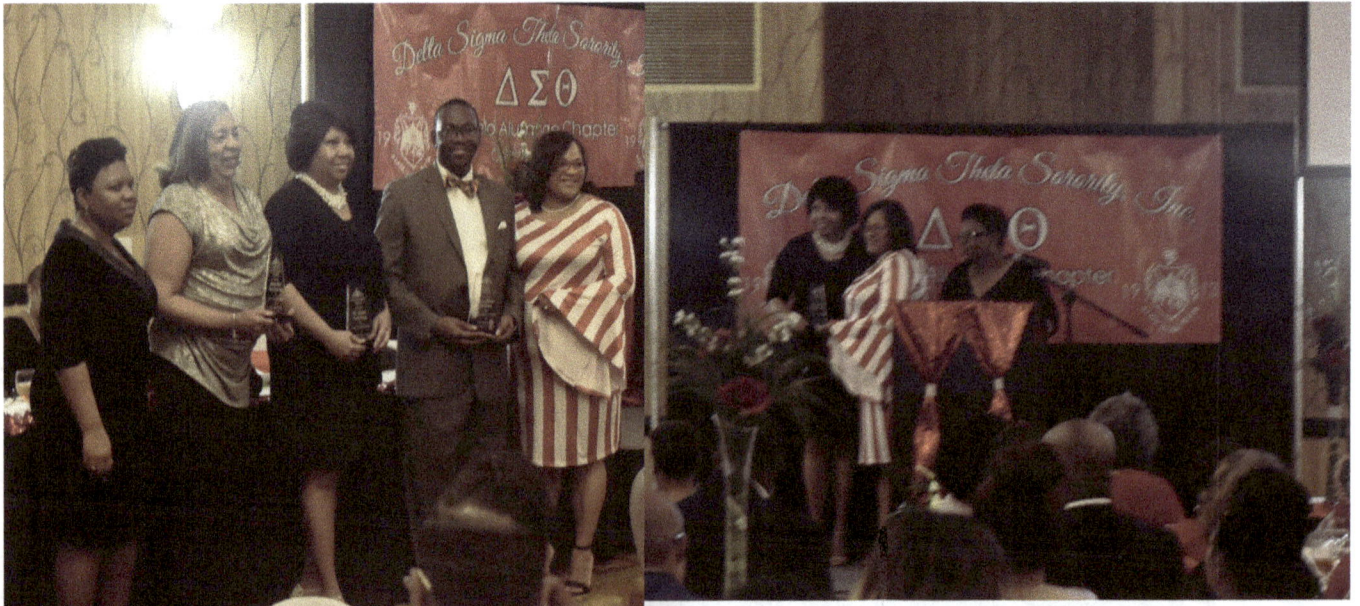

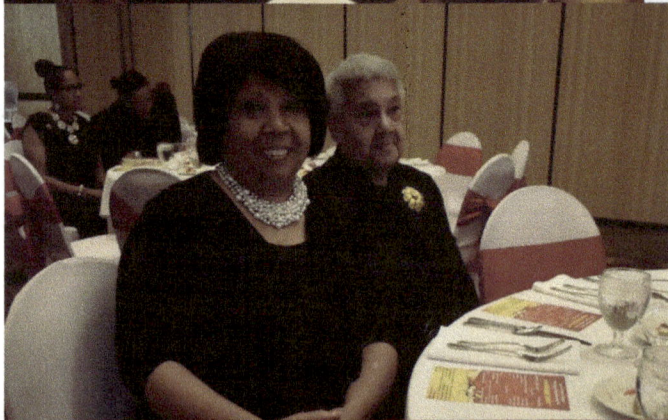

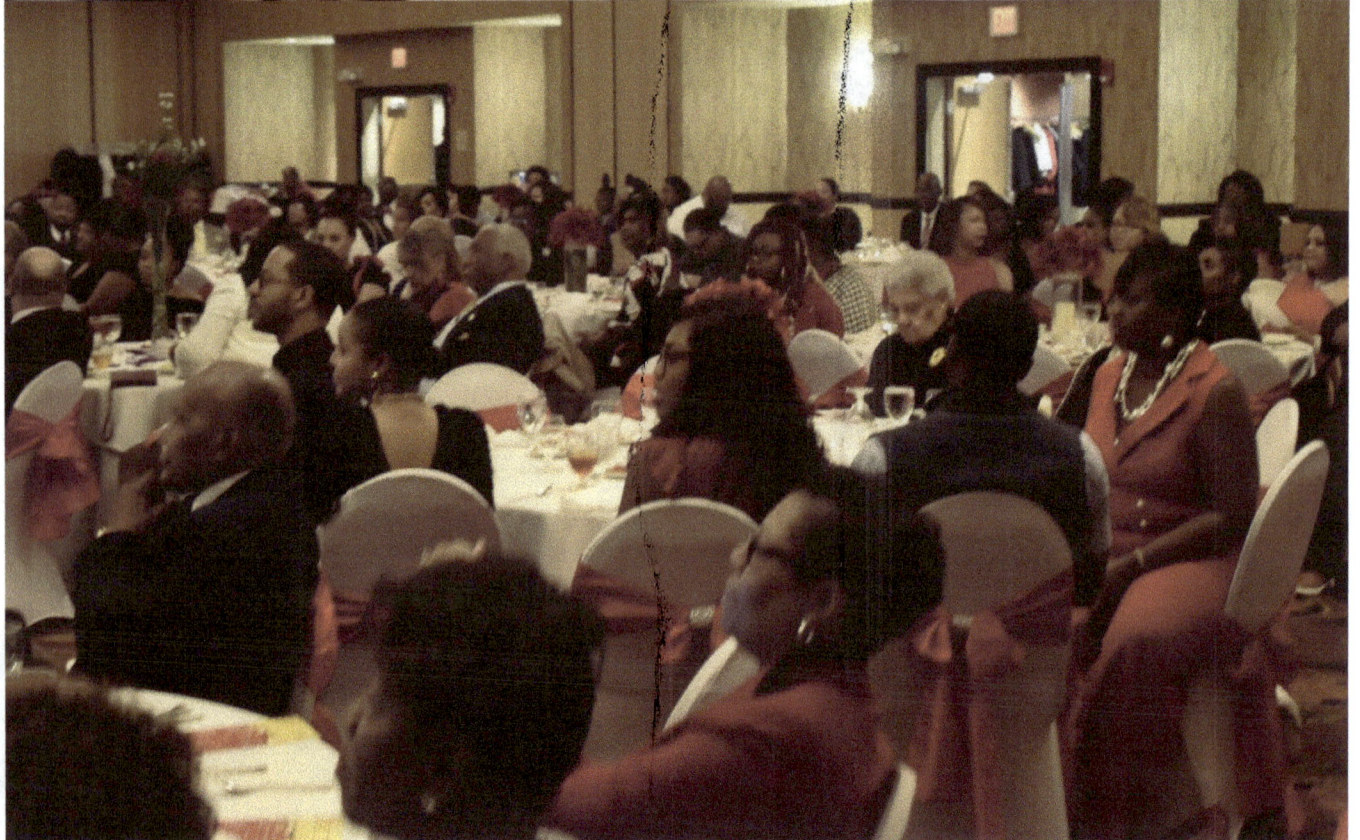

Facebook post April 14, 2020

Just the beginning of a style journey. We start with the clothing to hone in on the exact style, next hair makeup and accessories. All clothing thrifted items and straight from my closet.

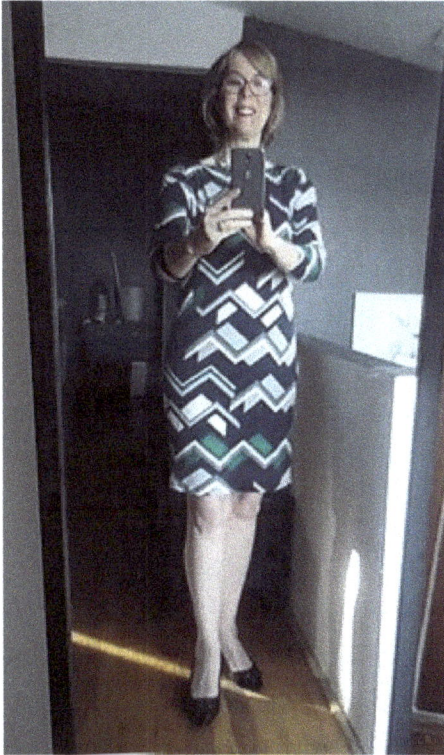

How it began... April 14

That moment when a total stranger in Pennsylvania who is in one of the fashion groups that you are in, makes some really sweet comments on your pictures about loving your style then sends you a message saying I honesty would like to hire you. What do you think? I'm a professional and would live a wardrobe similar.

Do you have time or the desire to take on clients?

PND: WHAT DO YOU DO ???

Hook her up, Work Your Magic, of course !

Give some feedback and thoughts on the looks in the comment. They will be valuable to her.

Facebook post: Styling Client coming along nicely !

May 5, 2020

Pennsylvania

Yep, that dress is a perfect 10 on her Ralph Lauren straight out of the PND Perfect 10 wardrobe closet !

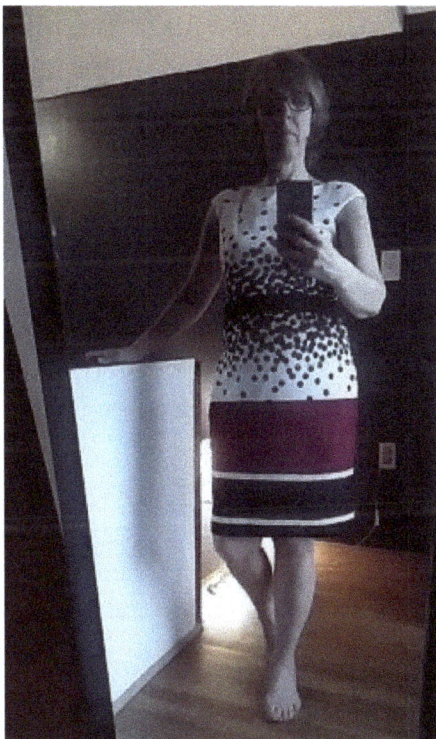

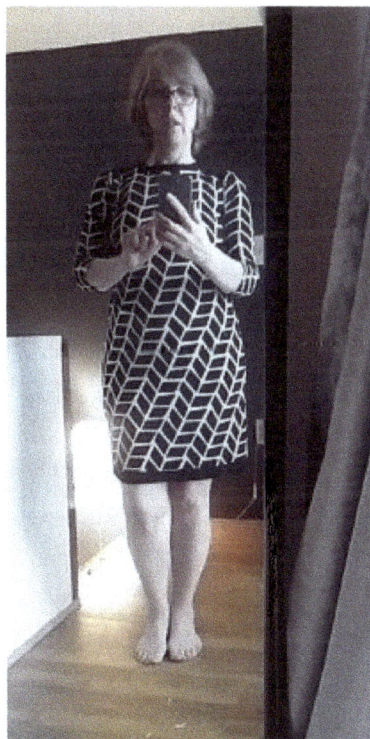

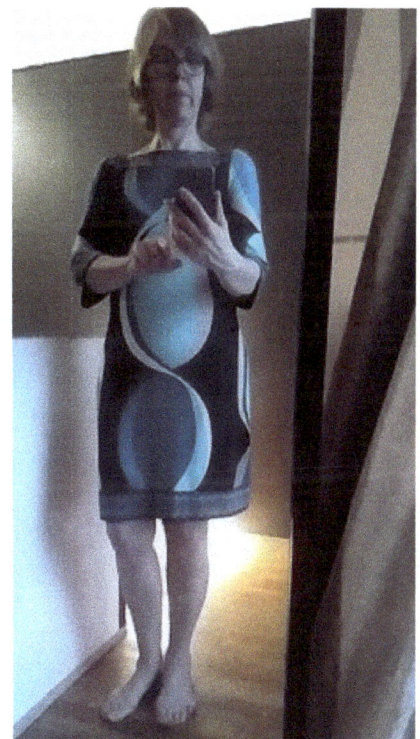

Facebook Post : October 19, 2020

I met a new friend (from Texas) in a group that I am in for Apple Shapes. (We tend to be more round around the middle, especially when we gain weight) She made a post that said: After lurking here for months being especially inspired by Patricia Neely- Dorsey's styles, I decided to get some waterfall jackets, wide belts, and try some bold patterns. I'm having fun with my clothes for the first time in a long time.

She posted a picture wearing a waterfall sweater , polka dot skirt and wide belt . She did a great job with the look! Some time later she posted this picture and said how much she loved the blouse. You can tell by the smile. She didn't quite pull the look together to make it the most flattering. But her fashion journey is a work in progress and it is supposed to be more or less a support group . Some of the comments were not very kind. Several told her that she should never wear large prints or animal prints up top with the body type. They told her that she should not wear wide belts. One person said whoever told her she could wear wide belts needs to stop it. Anyway, I sent her a private message.

I told her that she could ABSOLUTELY wear wide belts and she could ABSOLUTELY wear that top that she loved, I gave her some pointers on how to tweak the look (a little PND magic) She posted this before and after with a message: With some pointers from Patricia Neely-Dorsey, I found that I can absolutely wear wide belts and this top that I love, it's just how I wear it. She advised me to push up my sleeves and wear a center piece that would break up the pattern so that it will not be overwhelming. She also advised a wider leg on the bottom. It makes all of the difference! (Which is awesome because I love this shirt!!)

She received tons of compliments ! (Of course !)

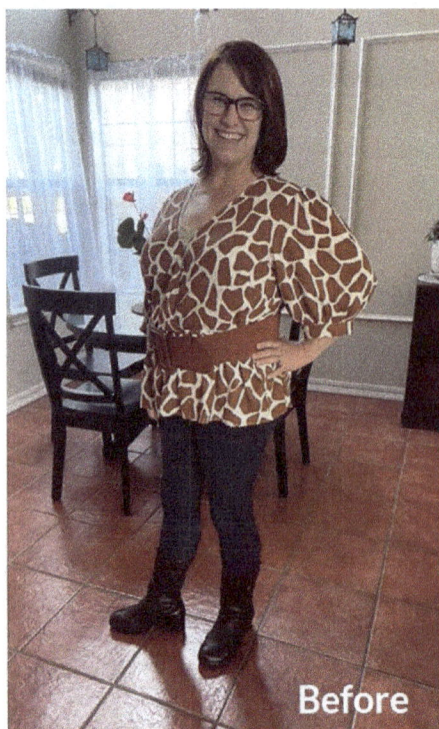

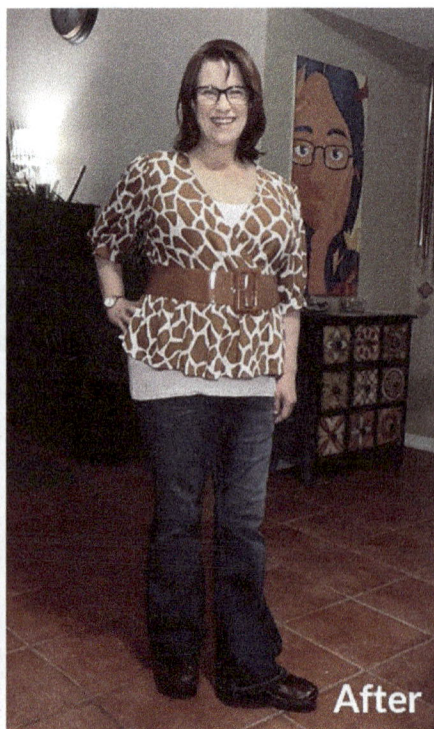

Before

After

Cathy has such an infectious ,bubbly personality . We bonded immediately. Cathy said that she had always felt lost when it came to fashion. Over the next several months, I gave Cathy style and shopping tips. Of course, to get her jumpstarted on her fashion journey, I sent her boxes of clothes in the colors and styles that I knew would fit her perfectly, to give her a concrete idea of what she would be looking for when she became confident in doing it on her own. When you are a thrift shopper , it's super easy and inexpensive to do things like that!

October 30, 2020

Cathy posted on Facebook: I'm learning that you can tweak an outfit into working. I got some help on this one from my favorite coach, Patricia Neely-Dorsey. I got dressed this morning and wasn't happy with the result, so I sent her a pic and she told me some things to try. Patricia told me this morning that most women over 50 (like me) are apple shaped (damn cortisol). This journey is making such a difference in how I feel about how I look.

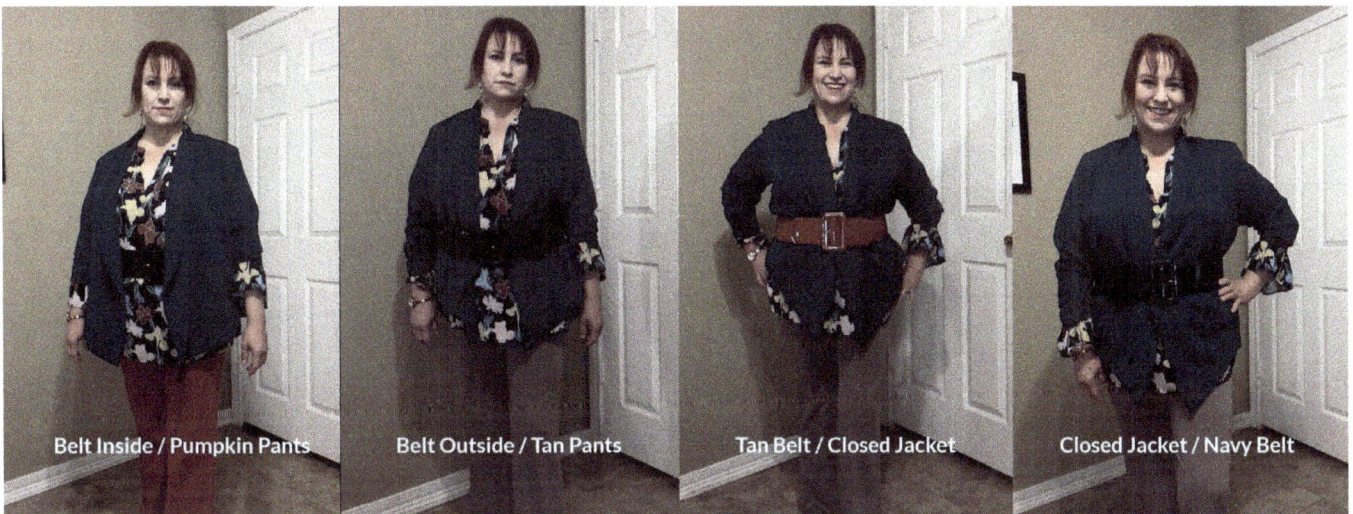

Belt Inside / Pumpkin Pants   Belt Outside / Tan Pants   Tan Belt / Closed Jacket   Closed Jacket / Navy Belt

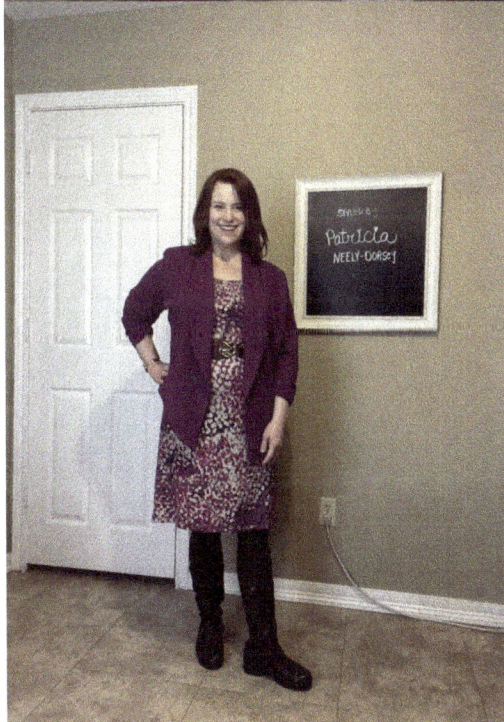

March 18, 2021 Cathy Posted on Facebook: Style Journey Cathy wrote: Until I met Patricia Neely-Dorsey, I NEVER wore printed dresses. Now they are my favorites!!

December 8, 2020

Cathy is enjoying her style journey! She is an Autumn in the seasonal coloring category. The deeper, more vibrant , more saturated colors absolutely make her SHINE!

She writes:

In this new clothes adventure, I've discovered that the brighter, richer colors make up better looks for me. They also feel better on. More like they fit. I have friends that look beautiful in pale shades, but I'm finding I feel more like me when the palette is richer.

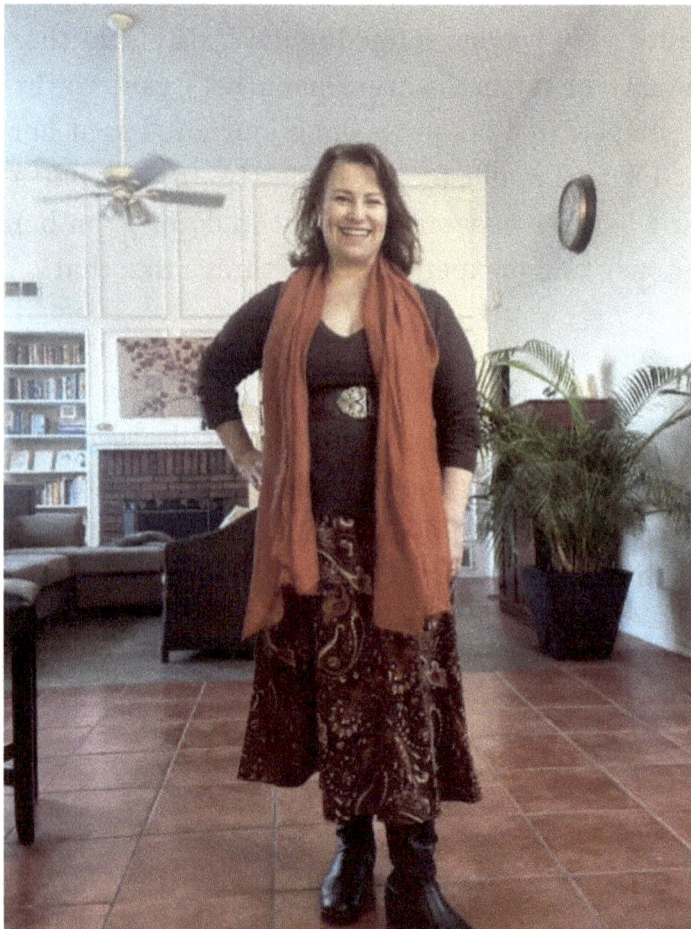

September 23, 2021 Style Journey
Cathy (Facebook friend in Texas)
Wrote: Patricia Neely-Dorsey has THE
BEST EYE!! She spotted this skirt at a
thrift store for me Today has the bar-
est hint of chill and I got to pull out my
boots and try it. The long scarf creates
a column for the eye.

September 30, 2021
STYLE JOURNEY
Cathy Hutchison posted:
One of the new things for me this year
thanks to Patricia's coaching is refining my
colors. This is essentially the same outfit,
but one has a cool pink and the other a
warm pink. In one photo, the outfit stands
out, and in the other photo the color balanc-
es with me, then I stand out. Learning my
colors has been a really big deal.

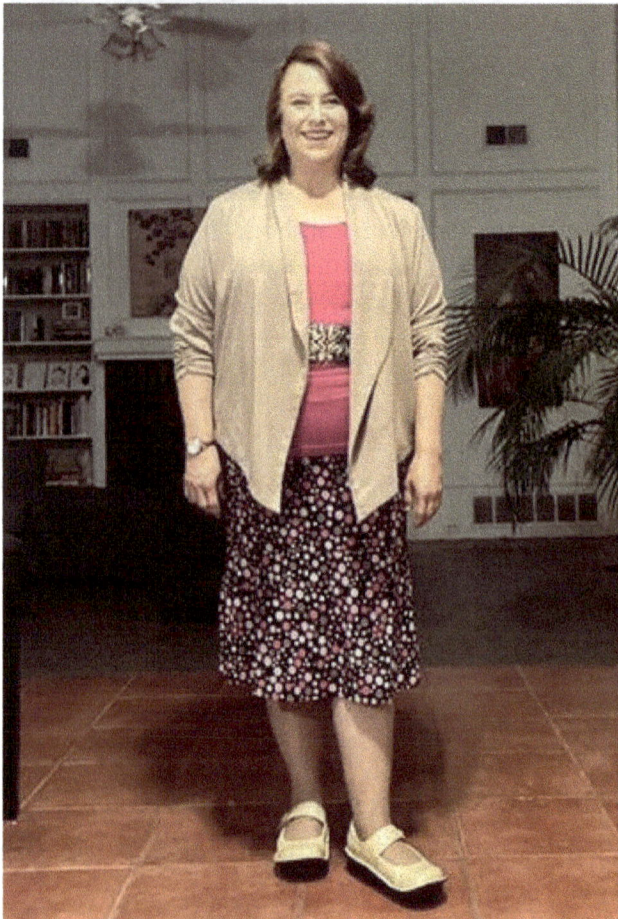

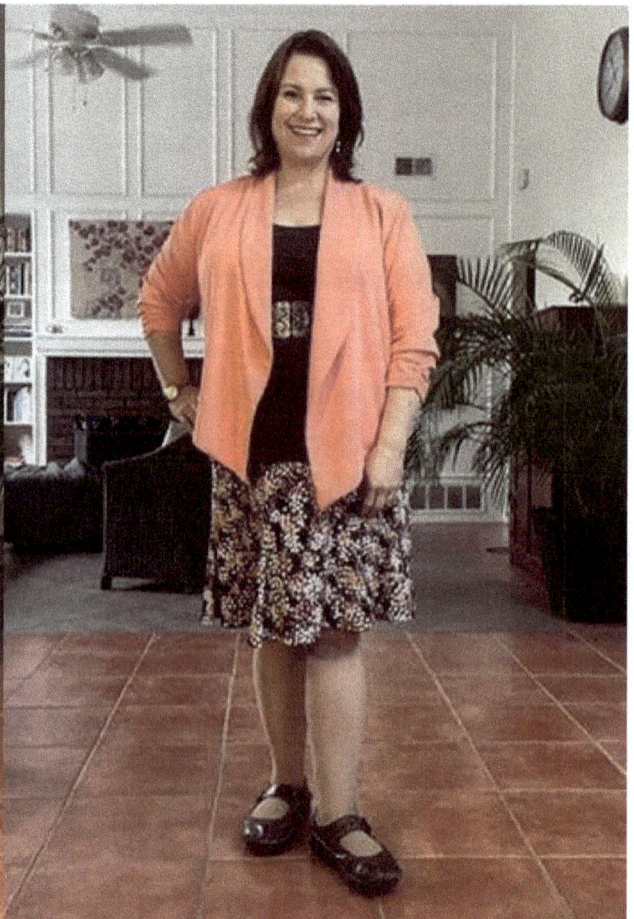

Message July 3, 2021 from Cathy

I would still love to come to Mississippi in the fall for a weekend. I definitely want to meet you in person. You have completely transformed my relationship with clothing. I want to get to talk in real life.

Message July 13, 2021 from Cathy

Here are some dates. I'm not sure yet if I'll drive or fly, but I can figure out details once I know what works for you: Oct 1-3 Oct 8-10 Oct 15 - 17 Nov 5-7. I could come for one night and we just grab dinner or I could stay the weekend and we can thrift shop, see Tupelo and maybe I could even go to church with you. Let me know what works best with your life! I got a flight to Memphis and am renting a car. That means I will get in Friday afternoon, and need to leave Sunday afternoon to drive back to Memphis catch a 4:30 flight. My friend, I cannot wait to meet your Mississippi. (And to meet YOU live and in person.)

PND We chose this coming weekend Oct 15-17/ I am looking forward to a weekend filled with FOOD, FASHION and FUN! She will fly to Memphis and drive to Tupelo on Friday. She will check into her cozy Airbnb in downtown Tupelo around 3:00 PM.

October 2021

I had the extreme pleasure of showing My Tupelo to my Facebook friend and now MUCH MORE than Facebook friend , who flew all the way from Texas just because she wanted to meet me in person! She had never been to Mississippi. She flew to Memphis and drove to Tupelo. We had a blast! We first became acquainted on Facebook in a Fashion/Style group that we are in. She tagged me in a post that said she had been stalking my pictures and trying to imitate aspects of my style. I was flattered! It was so neat seeing her attempts at PND styling.

She wrote

"After lurking here for months being especially inspired by Patricia Neely- Dorsey's styles, I decided to get some waterfall jackets, wide belts, and try some bold patterns. I'm having fun with my clothes for the first time in a long time." Of course fashion can be trial and error One day , she posted a new find that she was thrilled about. The execution wasn't complete-ly on point, but the 100 watt smile was! Some of the comments were not so nice! Several were telling her she shouldn't wear that style or wide belts as the case was in the outfit. I sent her a personal message and told her she could absolutely wear it and gave her some tweaks on how to do it. She reposted and the outfit was a hit. We started personal messaging and I told her I would help her with her personal style. Over the next year she learned the joys of thrift shopping , Poshmark deals , waterfall sweaters and column founda-tions! P.S. Before our styling friendship began , she says that she almost NEVER wore dresses and skirts! Now, she wears them almost EVERY DAY (Like Me) ! Proud " Style Mom "LOL!

October 2021 Cathy posted on her page :

THE PND EXPERIENCE. So, I wanted to come meet my amazing mentor, Patricia Neely-Dorsey, in person. You would not believe how much life this incredible woman packed into a single evening. Seriously, it was the best! Checked into the cutest guest house airbnb ever. We went to the Tupelo, MS visitors center. Saw Elvis's birthplace. Touched the names at the memorial at Veterans Park. Walked around downtown Tupelo. Went to the hardware store where Elvis bought his first guitar. (The man behind the counter was an amazing storyteller.) Had a fried brisket sandwich with amazing coleslaw and candied jalapeños. AND WENT THRIFT STORE SHOPPING. But the best part was getting to spend time in Patricia's presence. We've had a virtual friendship, so it was really cool to hear her voice and walk and talk.

Update: Now, Cathy is an expert thrift shopper and has perfected her personal style!

Cathy Wrote:

I'm an unlikely fashionista. Clothes have always felt hard. Those women who walk into a room looking put together? I wish! I've spent most of my life feeling like my body is the wrong shape. This was true even when I was a size eight. I hired a personal stylist once, and while buying trendy clothes made me finally feel like I was "doing it right," she was focused on trends — which meant she dressed me like a skinny girl. When I mentioned how uncomfortable the clothes were, she told me I should "buy Spanx." Have you ever tried on Spanx? Nothing implies your body is the wrong shape more clearly than pulling on the nylon and spandex version of a sausage casing that cuts off your respiration. I should have walked away from the experience feeling like the clothes simply didn't fit, but instead, I felt like I was the one who didn't fit. I tried again a few years later with a personal shopper from Nordstrom and wound up weeping in the parking garage as stabs of guilt tore through me over the ridiculous amount of money I'd just spent on a trivial pair of jeans. Nope. Fashion was not for me.

Still, I kept binge-watching makeover shows, wondering if there was some secret way to experience the transition I saw the people on television experience. Fashion seemed to be something I had to enjoy from the sidelines. That is until Patricia Neely Dorsey took me under her wing. Our friendship started in a Facebook group. Patricia was so elegant! She would post these photos of fabulous outfits then post the price.

Often she would look runway-ready sharing that the whole outfit–which she snagged at a thrift store–cost $12. I began following her posts, learning as I went. (I initially thought she was a professional stylist because of the great advice she gave, but it turns out she is a poet who lives in and writes about Mississippi.) When I was finally brave enough to try something, I posted myself in an outfit I'd assembled that mimicked one of hers. She told me how to tweak it to make it even better.

I tried another new look and posted it to the group. I knew it wasn't working, but I didn't know why. The discussion in the comments devolved into a deliberation over the pros and cons of belts with a few unkind words about how I looked. Patricia messaged me privately and offered constructive advice. She then made an offer I hadn't expected:

"Let's do this journey together! Ask me any questions — and when you pick an outfit, send me a picture, and let's discuss how to make it absolutely fabulous for you! We want every outfit to be at least a 7 or above on a scale of 1–10. Show me some pictures of your favorite wardrobe pieces. Let me help you complete your look! I love your enthusiasm and your 100 watt smile! You rock!"

Not only did she make me feel glorious, but she had also just invited me to 30 days of what turned out to be style boot camp.

Those next 30 days completely changed my relationship with clothes–and my body. I learned that when you wear clothes that are authentic to you they look good. Your confidence rises. You feel amazing. You no longer feel like you don't fit. The fashion industry creates a design template for a limited season, then produces it in volume. But we are different shapes and sizes. We have different lifestyles and live in varied climates. One size never fits all. Patricia showed me that I wasn't a mismatch for the clothes that didn't work for me. The clothes were a mismatch for me, and it was up to me to learn which shapes and colors worked, and which didn't. This knowledge gave me the power to break the media-based templates to find what made me feel confident. (She can do the same for you too.) Once I'd made peace with my body—and my closet—I learned Patricia had more to teach me. I was watching her drop sizes online. She had told me she was going to get into the best shape of her life by 60. And she was doing it! After a business trip where I felt fashionable but tired, I called her. "What are you doing? I want to do it too!" Patricia shared her journey with me. I joined her on the path. As I'm typing this, I'm 20 lbs lighter than when I made that phone call four months ago. I'm incredibly grateful for Patricia's influence in my life. She shines and helps others do the same. Ready to feel beautiful? Do what she says! Patricia is the best possible mentor!

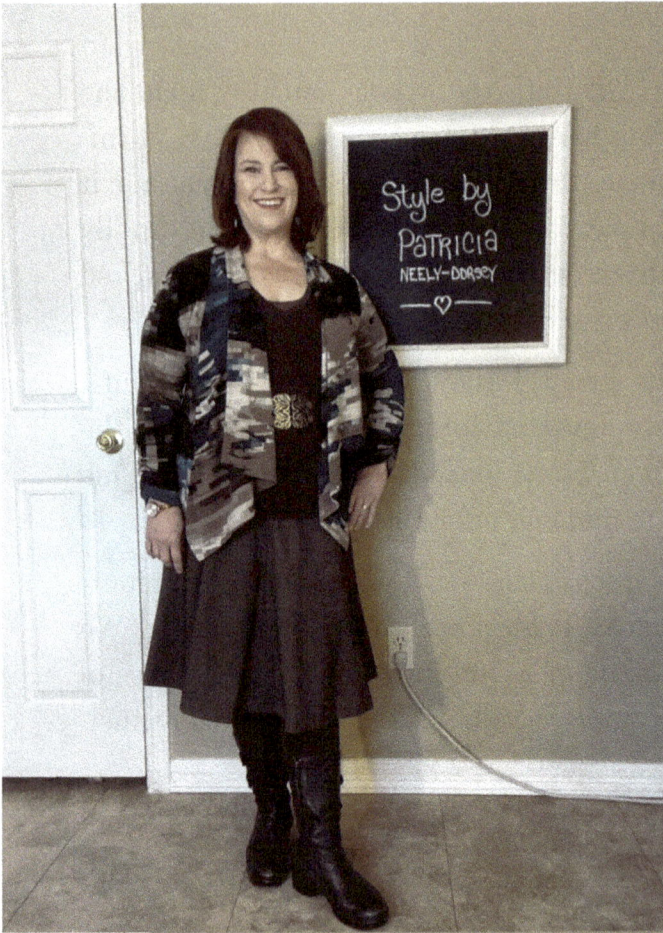
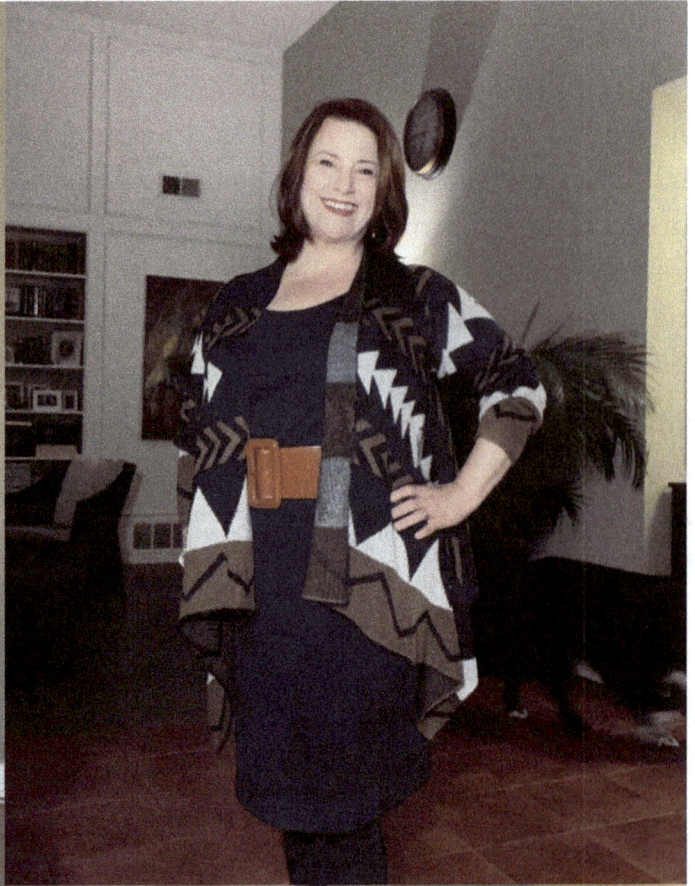
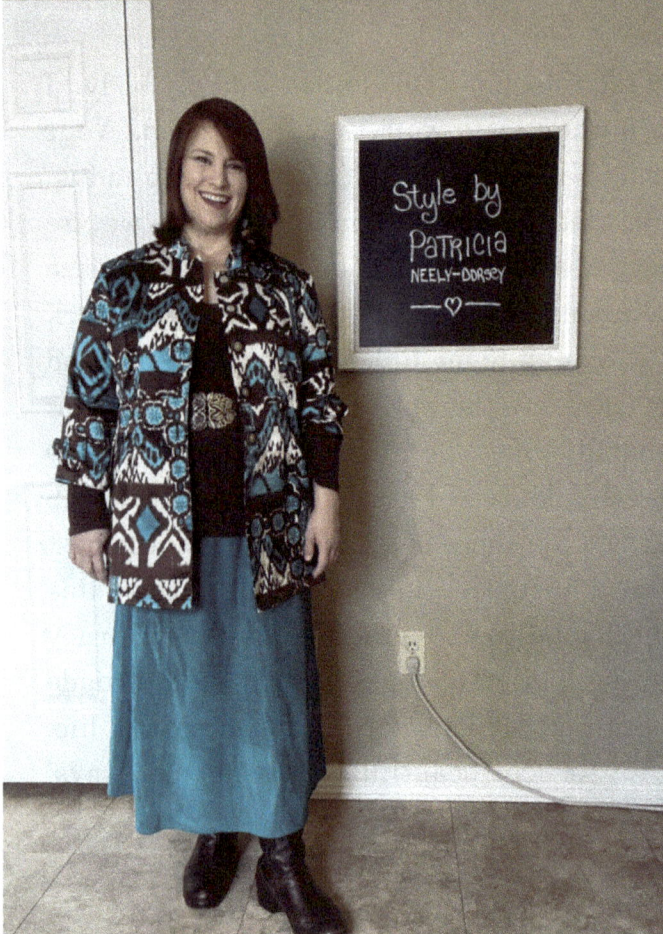
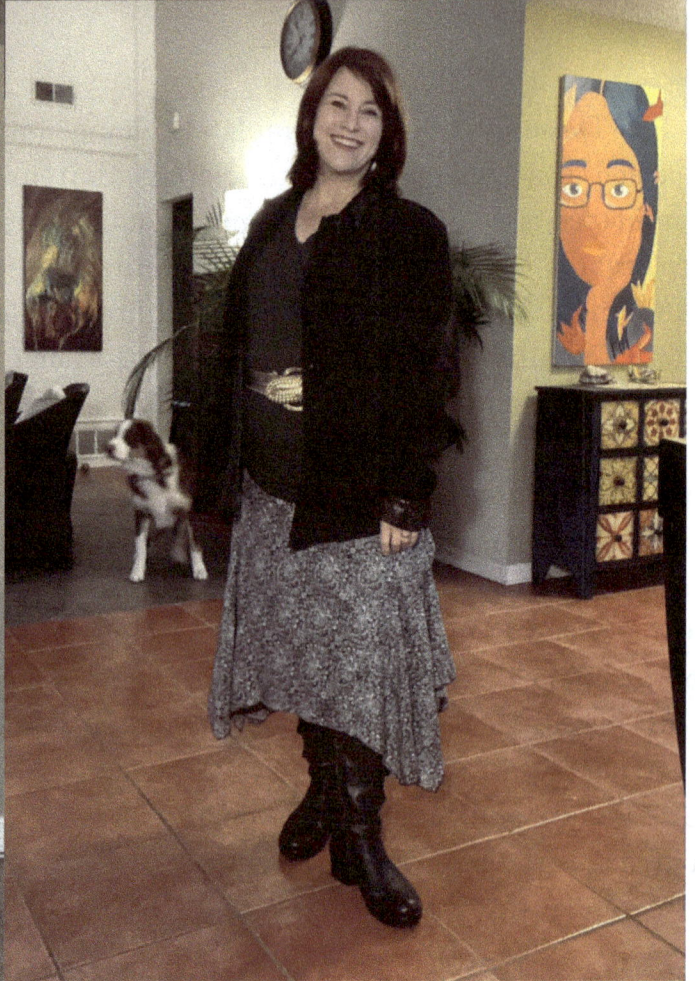

I had planned a whole fabulous weekend to show Cathy around My Tupelo. But ,near the end of our first day's visit , she was contacted by family that her husband had experienced a health crisis. After monitoring the situation throughout the night, she made plans to leave the next morning.

October 2021 Cathy posted on her page:

THE PND EXPERIENCE. So, I wanted to come meet my amazing mentor, Patricia Neely-Dorsey, in person. You would not believe how much life this incredible woman packed into a single evening. Seriously, it was the best! Checked into the cutest guest house airbnb ever. We went to the Tupelo, MS visitors center. Saw Elvis's birthplace. Touched the names at the memorial at Veterans Park. Walked around downtown Tupelo. Went to the hardware store where Elvis bought his first guitar. (The man behind the counter was an amazing storyteller.)Had a fried brisket sandwich with amazing coleslaw and candied jalapeños. AND WENT THRIFT STORE SHOPPING. But the best part was getting to spend time in Patricia's presence. We've had a virtual friendship, so it was really cool to hear her voice and walk and talk.

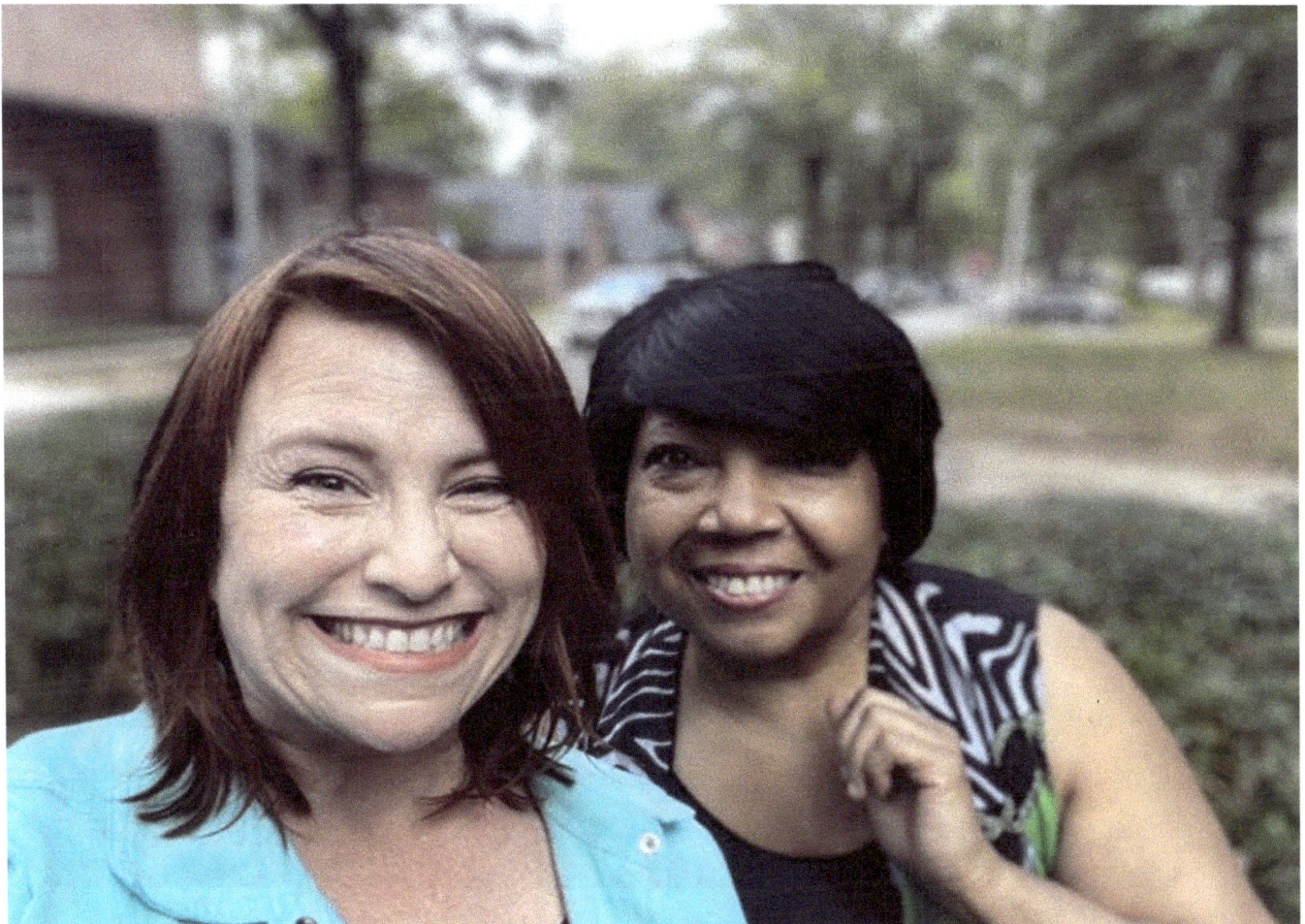

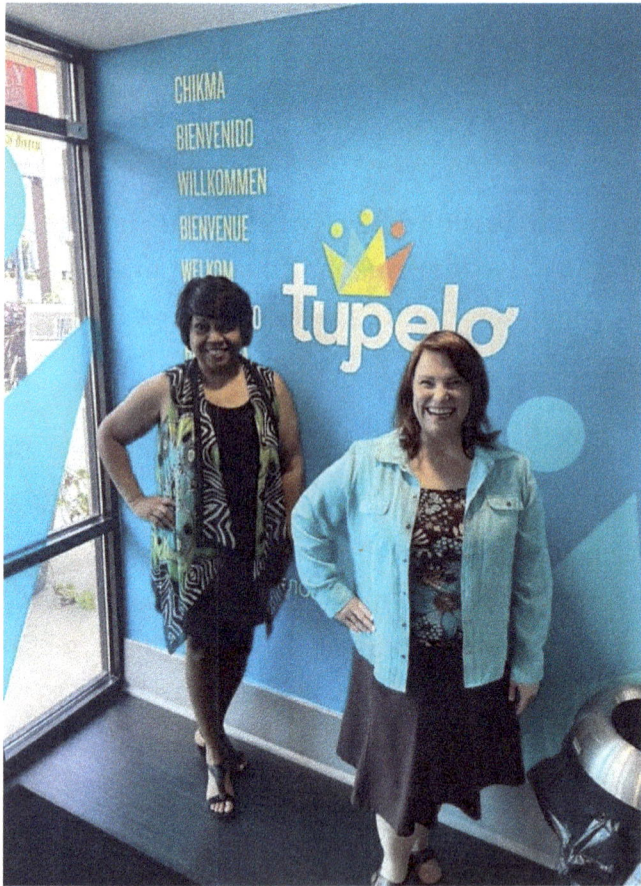

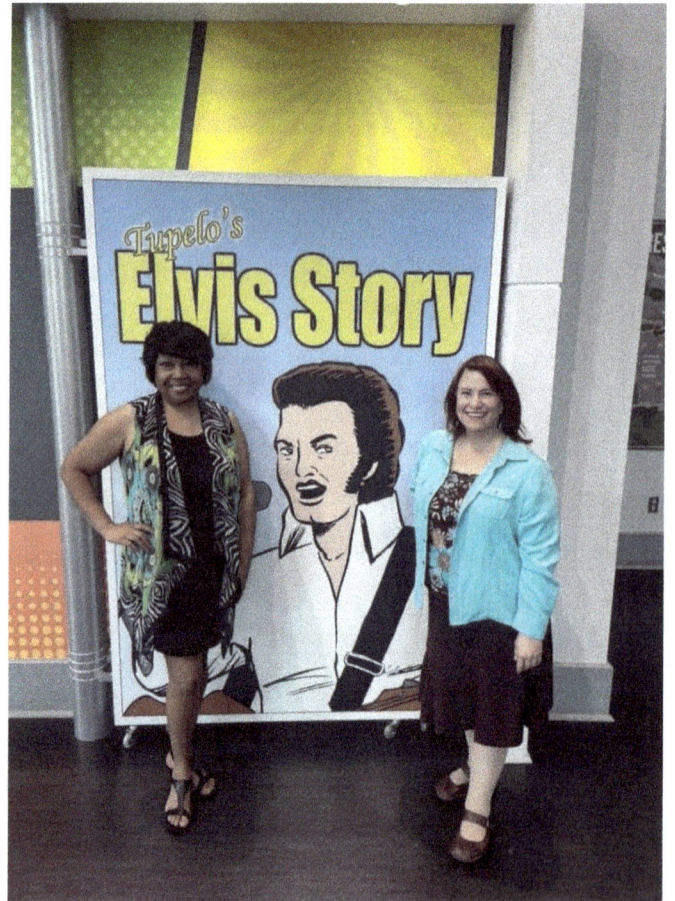

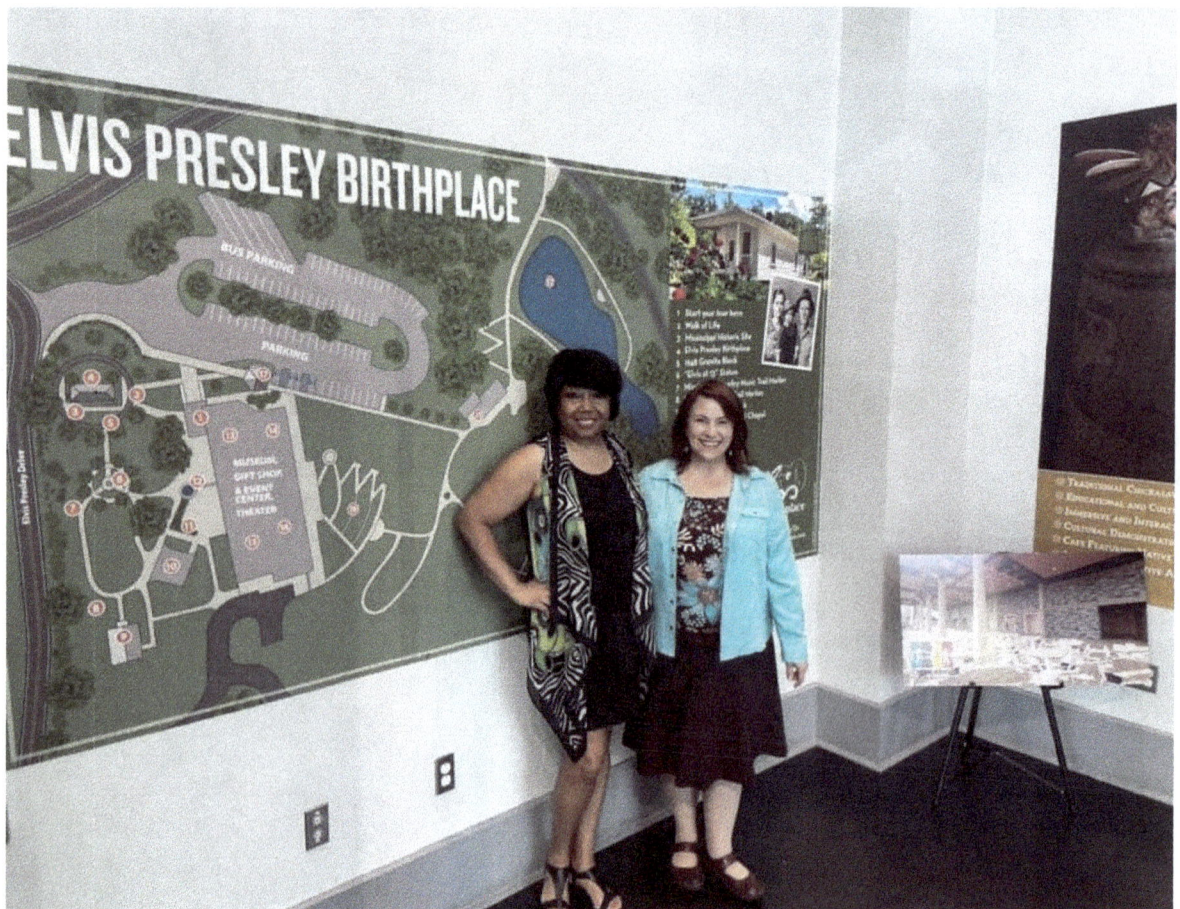

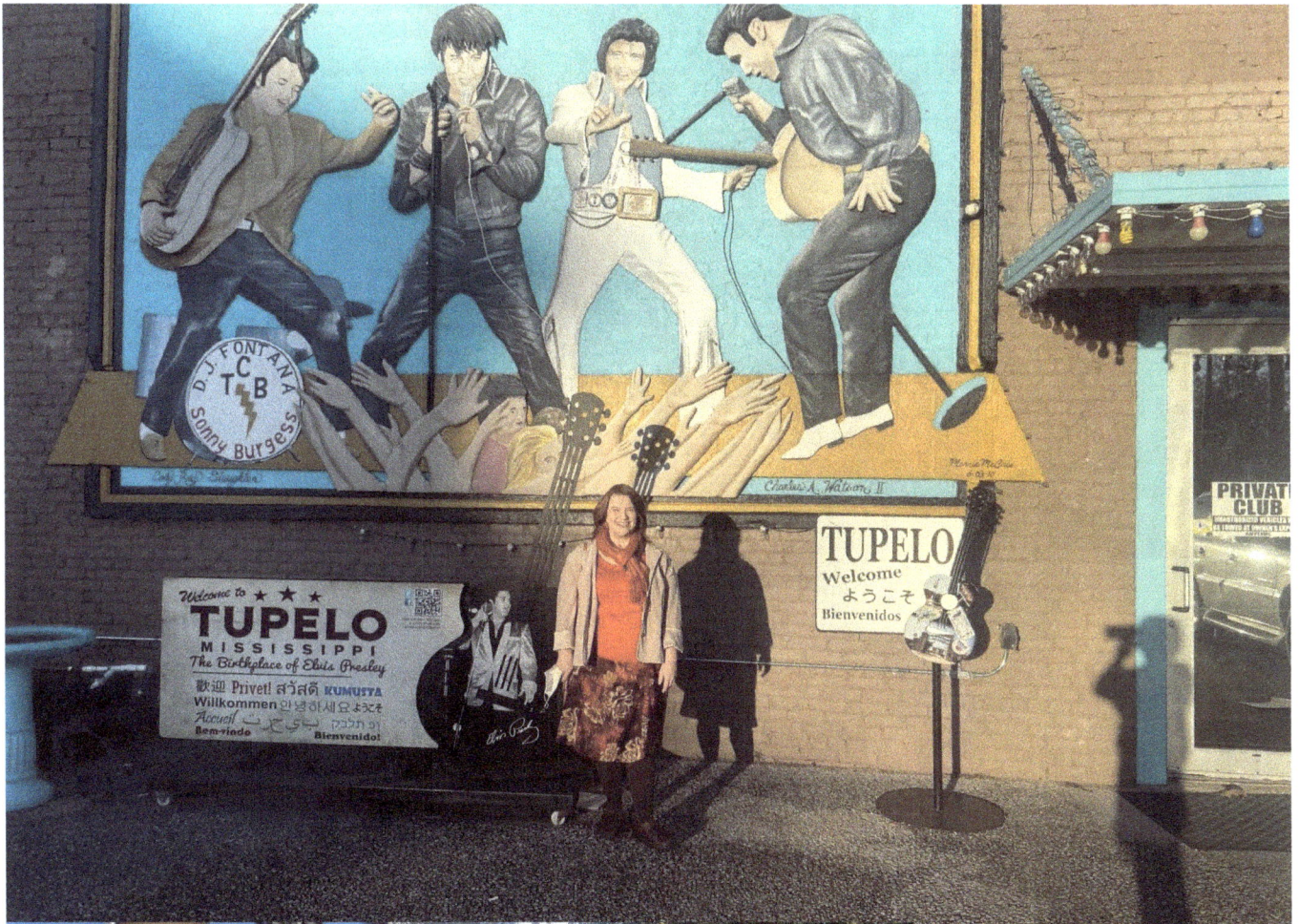

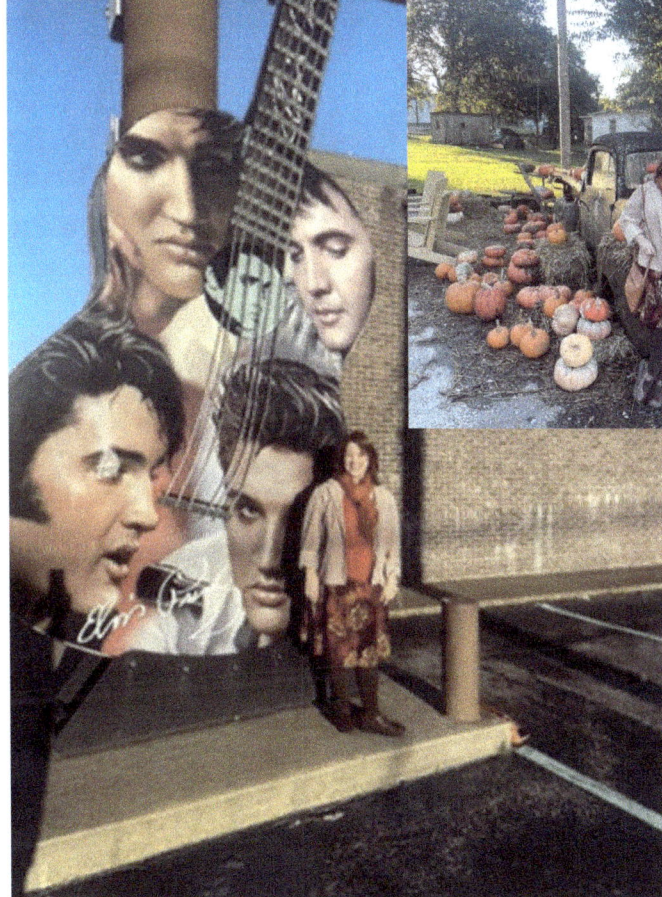

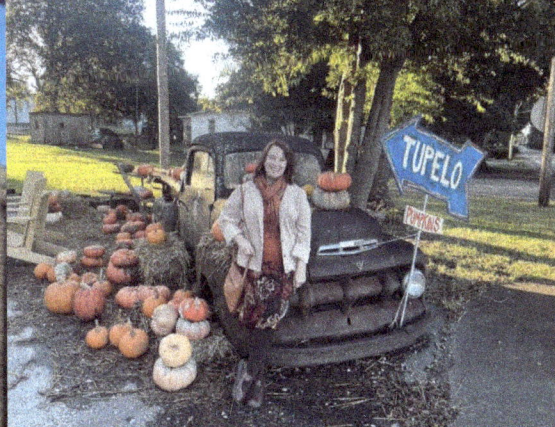

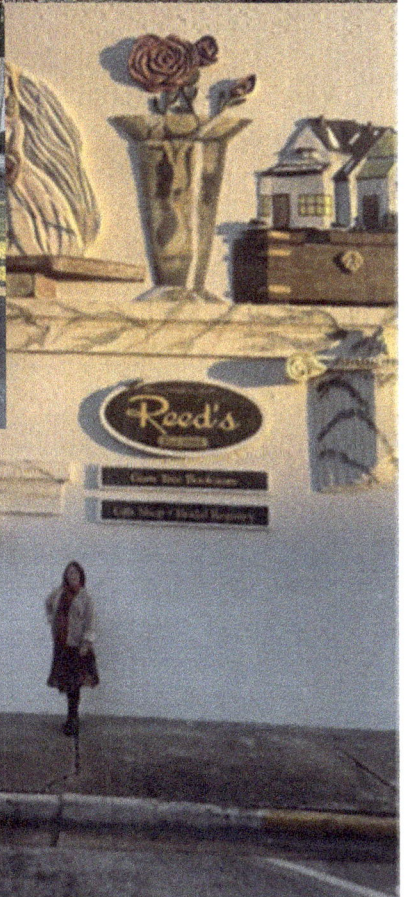

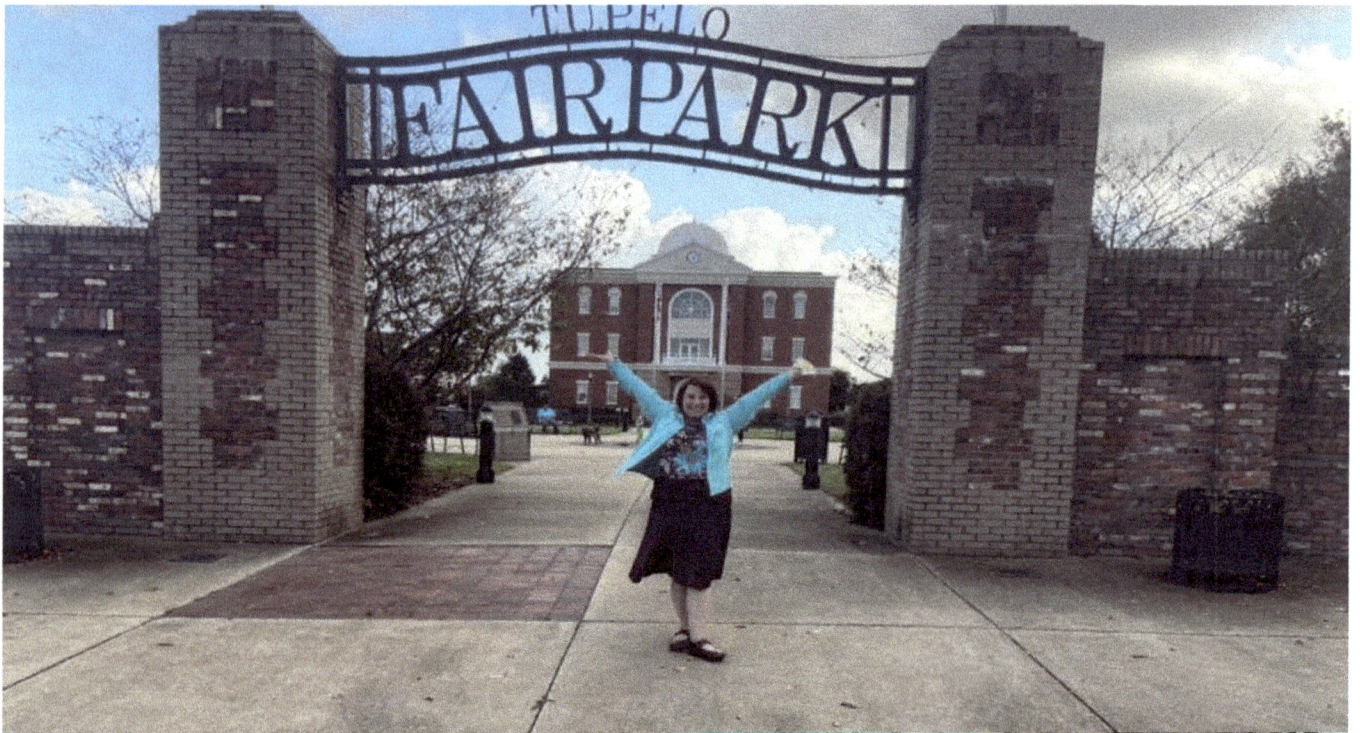

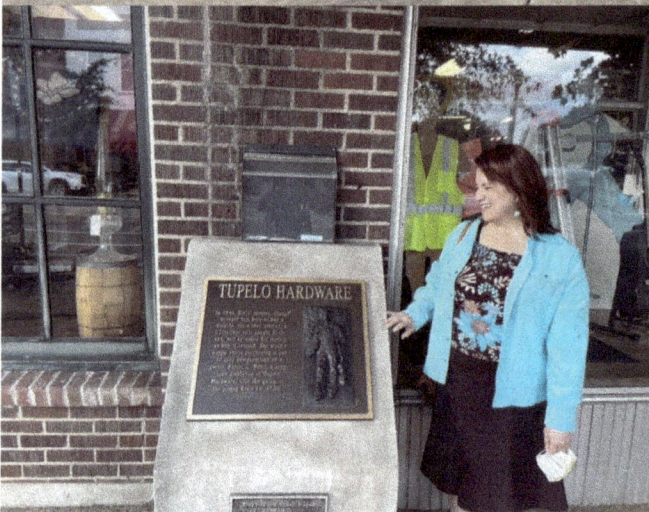

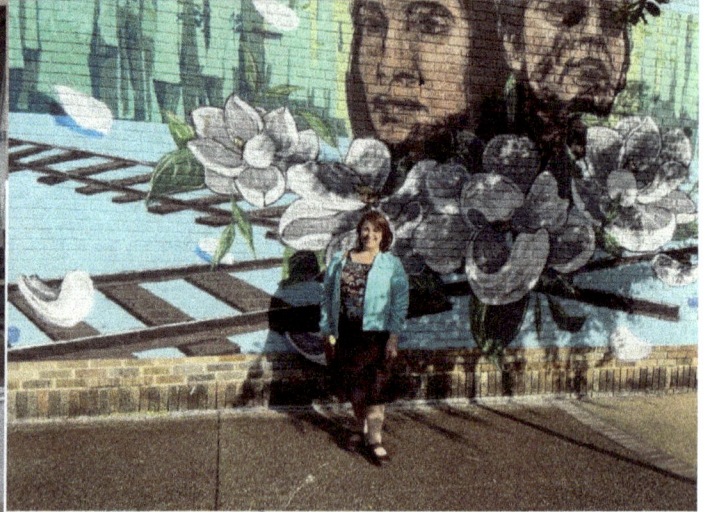

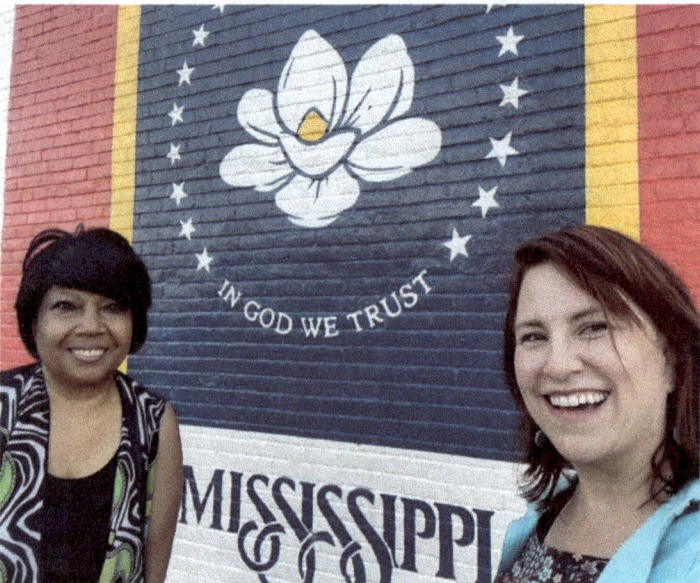

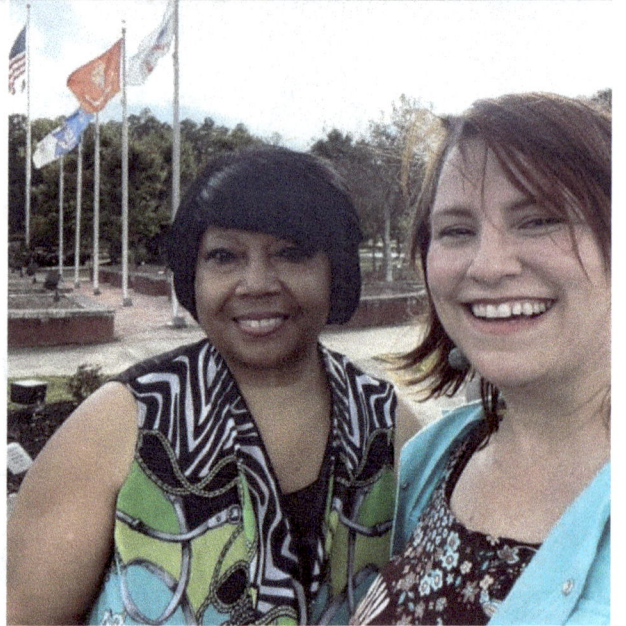

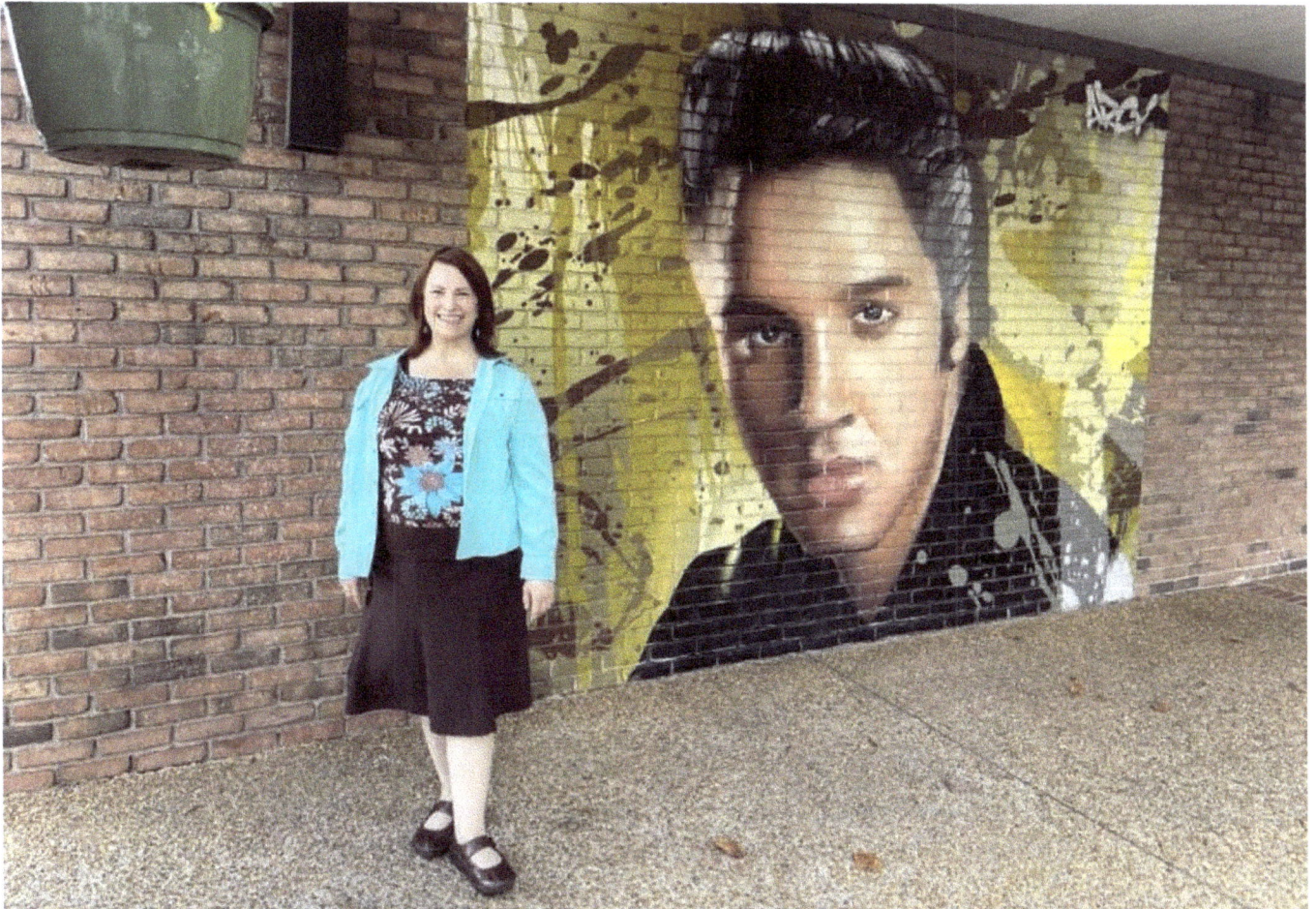

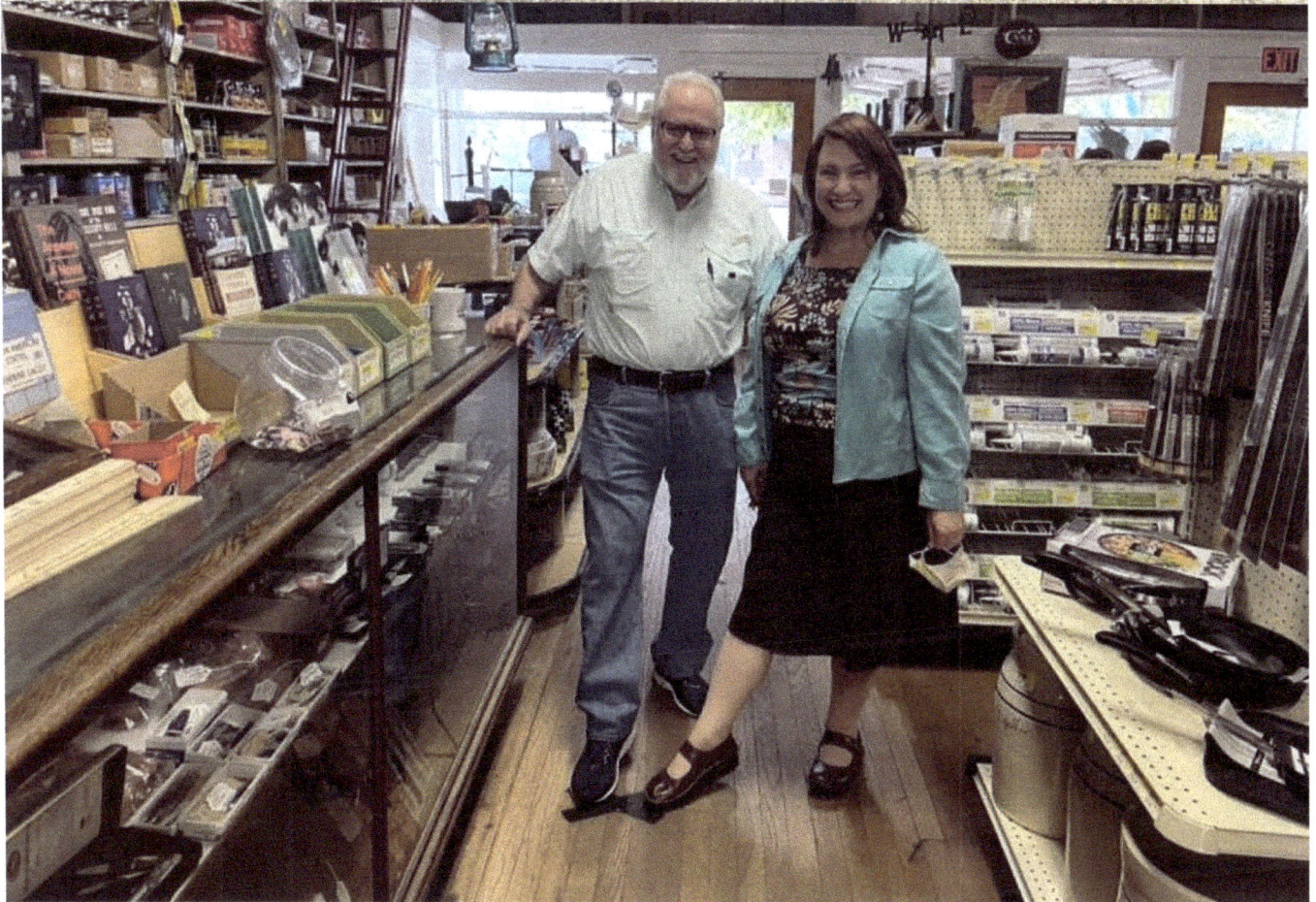

WELCOME TO TUPELO

We welcome you to Tupelo
With wide open arms
Here, we Let Our Hospitality Show
And exude southern charm
We invite you to the Birthplace of Elvis
And the headquarters of the Natchez Trace
Discover the history and heritage
In abundance, in this place;
Learn all about Mill Village and Chief Piomingo
Shakerag, The National Fish Hatchery and more
Find the place where "The King" got his first
guitar
At our own Tupelo Hardware Store
Visit the Oren Dunn City Museum
With our proud past displayed at it's best;
Sample a true southern delicacy
At the annual Dudie Burger Fest.

Explore this First TVA City
Nestled in the Mississippi Hills;
Those looking for fine dining and shopping,
Can certainly get their fill.
Take in a show at the Lyric Theater
Or try the yearly Gumtree Run
Tour our All -America City
And find all kinds of fun
You can visit our local art museum
Or see exotic animals at the Buffalo Park
You'll discover that there are endless
adventures
On which anyone can embark
Let us show you the Tupelo Spirit
Forever shining bright;
Streaming out from Northeast Mississippi
As a true beacon light
Patricia Neely-Dorsey.

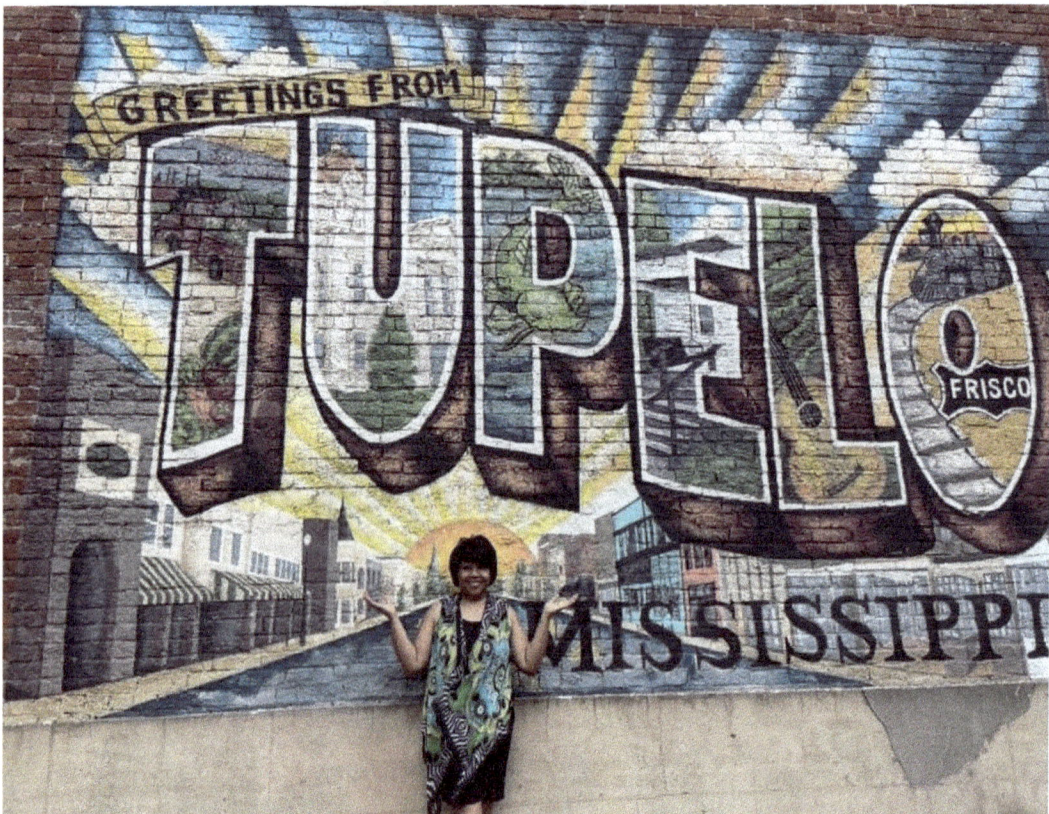

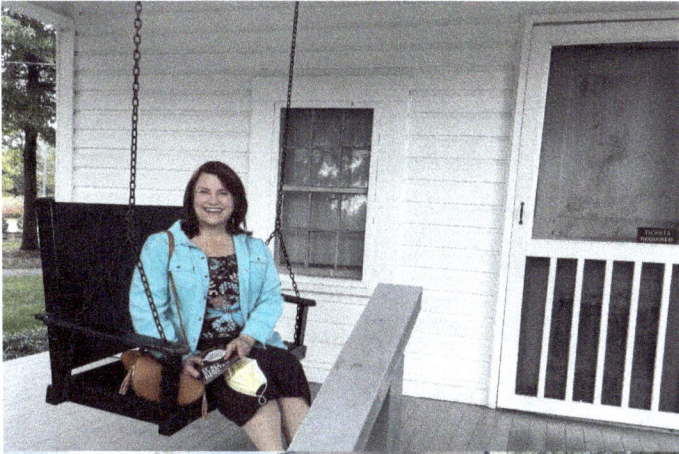
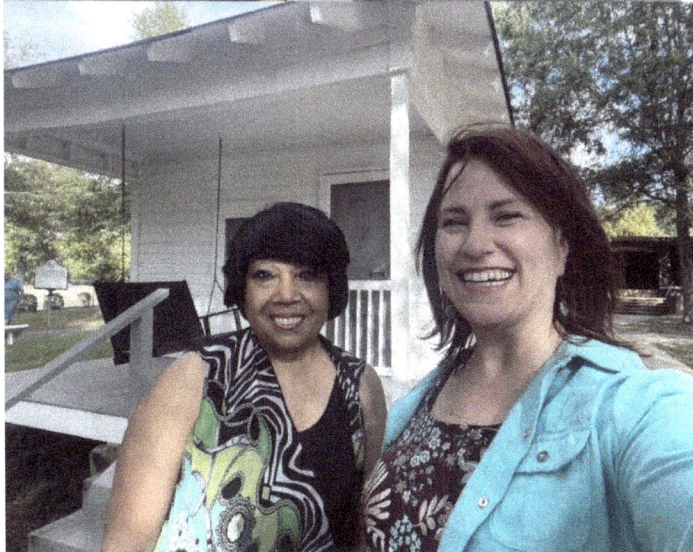
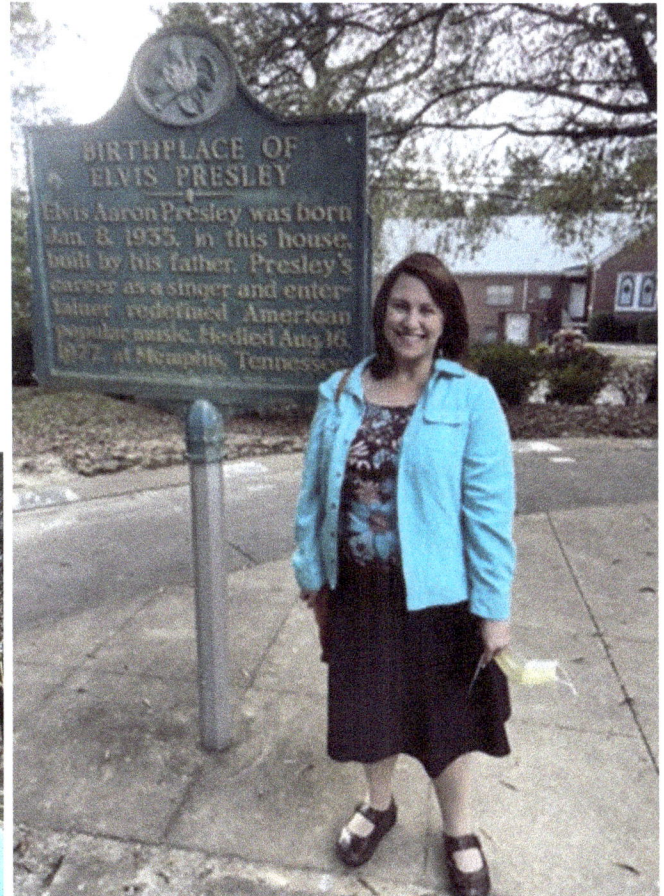

THE KING

(Elvis A. Presley)

born :January 8, 1935- Tupelo,MS

From poor and meager beginnings,
A young man began to sing;
From the small town of Tupelo,
A voice began to ring.
As surely as it's been said,
A man's gifts make a way for him;
This humble diamond in the rough,
Became a sparkling gem.
Velvet melodies and explosive rock,
Were the gifts he'd bring;
The world responded with resounding praise,
And pronounced this man "The King".
2012 Patricia Neely-Dorsey

THE BIRTHPLACE

Would anyone have suspected
The stories that these walls held
Of a mother working fingers to the bone
And a father who was jailed?
All the secrets that lived inside,
The world would not have known;
If the young man with the old guitar
Had not ascended to his throne.
Would anyone have wanted to know
About the family from "across the tracks,"
Who could hardly keep food on the table
Or clothing on their backs?
Would anyone have even cared,
About the heartaches, pain and scorn
If this tiny frame house hadn't found acclaim
As the place where "The King" was born.
2012 Patricia Neely-Dorsey

ELAINE

On July 26th, 1935, twin daughters Elaine and Elois were born to Alton Odessa Kilgore and Julia Buckingham Kilgore in Mantee, Mississippi. We were the third and fourth of eight children. The family lived in Mantee until we twins were five years old. I remember those years as being very happy ones. My father was a principal and teacher of a one-room school in Woodland Mississippi. My mother taught in a one-room school in Mantee.

At the end of the month when my parents received their paychecks the family would pile into Alton's Model T and head to Okolona, Mississippi to shop. After purchasing all the house necessities my mother would buy fabric. She would make beautiful dresses for the girls and shirts for the two boys who were born in Mantee. Two boys were later born in West Point, Mississippi. She used newspapers from the Commercial Appeal of Memphis, Tennessee to cut patterns. When I was five the family moved to West Point. All of the children, with the exception of Julia Olexine were enrolled in the elementary department of Ministerial Institute and College. After five years the family moved to the west side of town. The children, with the exception of James, enrolled in the elementary demonstration school of Mary Holmes Junior College West Point. James continued his studies at MI College and received a scholarship to Morehouse College in Atlanta, Georgia. He received a Bachelor of Science degree and pledged Kappa Alpha Psi fraternity. It was the family's introduction to Black Greek letter fraternities.

When I was in the eighth grade, I met a brilliant student: James Henry Neely, president of the student council. He was born August 8th, 1932, to Robert and Missouri Neely. He took note that I was a brilliant student as well and also a talented actress who was always assured of lead roles in the school's drama productions. James wanted to ask me for steady dates, but he had a problem. He could not accurately identify the twin of his choice. Elois and I were identical twins. The school newspaper, The Mirror, stated: James Neely will ask Elaine Kilgore for steady dates when he can tell her from her twin sister Elois. He did not communicate with me until he could accurately identify us. James discovered that I had a double tooth. He also noticed that I was a consistent honor roll student. Elois participated in pageants and was on the homecoming court.

Once we began dating it lasted until we were married in 1954. The marriage lasted sixty-six years. Then The first five years of my life, I lived in Mantee Mississippi. These were some of my happiest days. I have many, vivid memories of my life in Mantee. The family lived on a 100 acre farm with my paternal grandparents Henry and Mariah Kilgore. That land is still in the family as heir property. My immediate family members did not farm for a living. They chose teaching for their careers. My grandmother was a teacher. My father and mother were teachers. The small children received pre-school education because, we accompanied my mother to school each day. My parents and siblings were always well dressed. My father had a car that he loved and maintained very well. He knew everything about taking care of that car. I believe that he learned it from auto mechanic classes that he took at Tuskegee Institute. He would drop my mother off at the one room school where she taught and go to another school where he taught.

Five generations of the family have produced teachers My mother was an excellent cook. We had a very large stove that was somewhat of a status symbol at that time. The stove had an oven , a warming unit and a unit to hold hot water. For some reason, I am not exactly sure why, my father never allowed us to have eggs for breakfast. But, Raisin Bran was always in the house . Raisin Bran remained one of my favorite cereals through my adult life. During my childhood, I remember that ambrosia was always a staple at Christ-mas dinner. Oranges were plentiful in the home during Christmas. They were used in the ambrosia and put in the Christmas stockings ,along with nuts and other treats. One Christ-mas I received a toy washing machine that you could put water in and swish the clothes around. It was one of my favorite Christmas gifts that I received as a child. To this day, washing is one of my favorite household chores. It's really not like a chore for me. It is more like therapy.

Elaine Left, Elois Right with neighbor

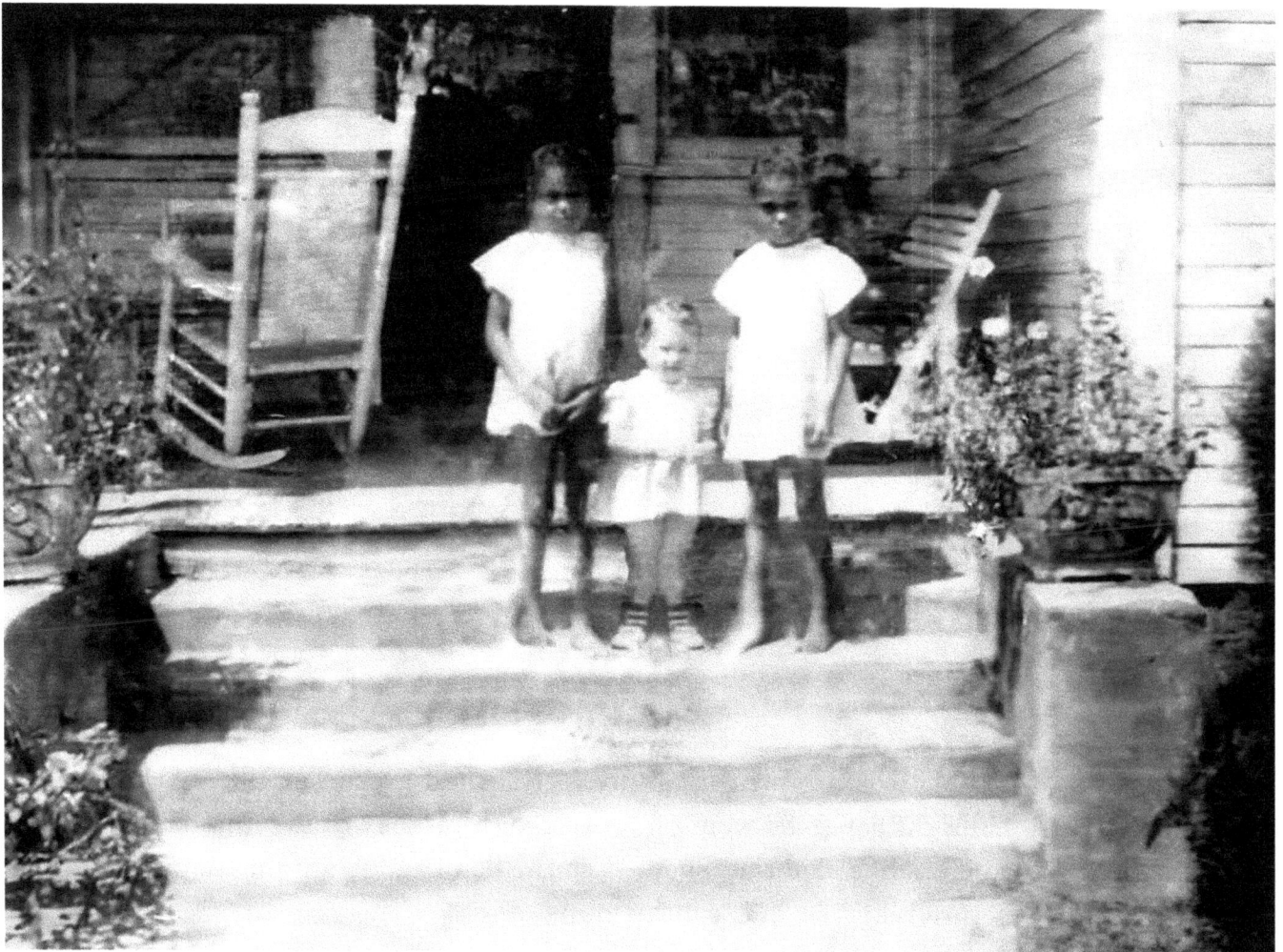

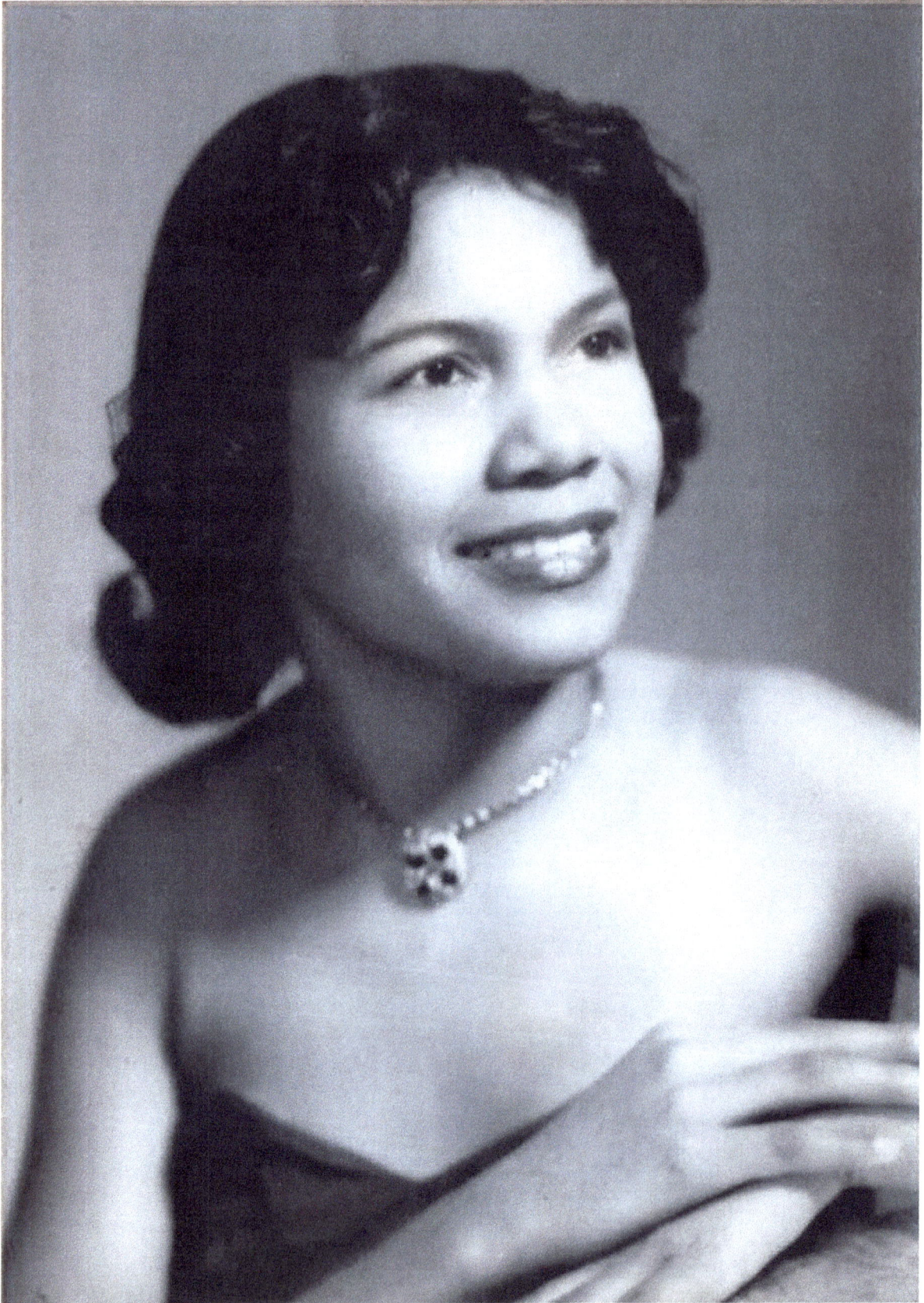

Mom said that this was a brown linen dress. Dad had given her that necklace with rubies (her birthstone) right before he went off to college (Kentucky State) and had asked her to take a picture with it on. She said that she was so thrilled to go to a professional photographer to have her a picture taken for her "college man.

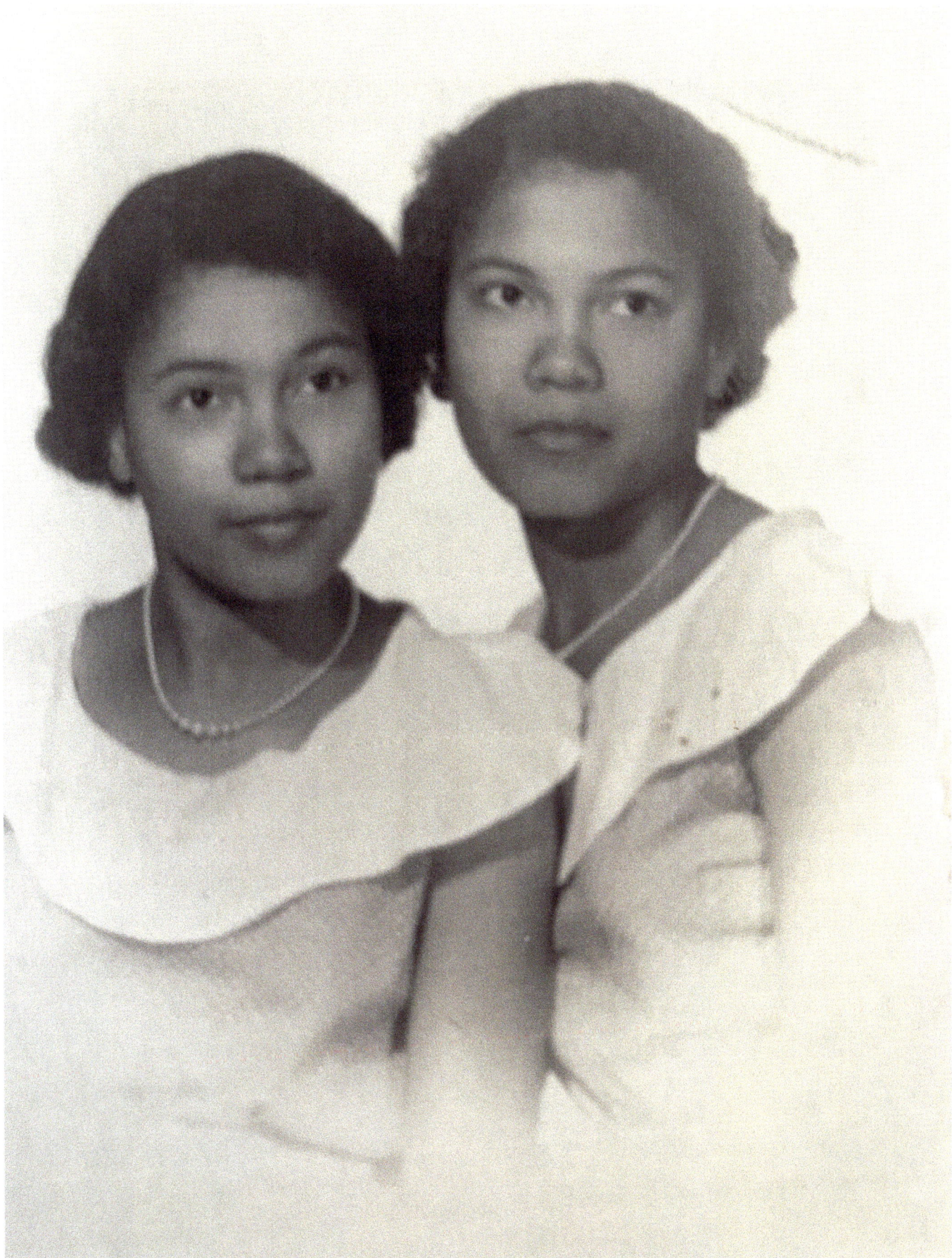

Elaine Left Elois Right

Elaine at Mary Holmes

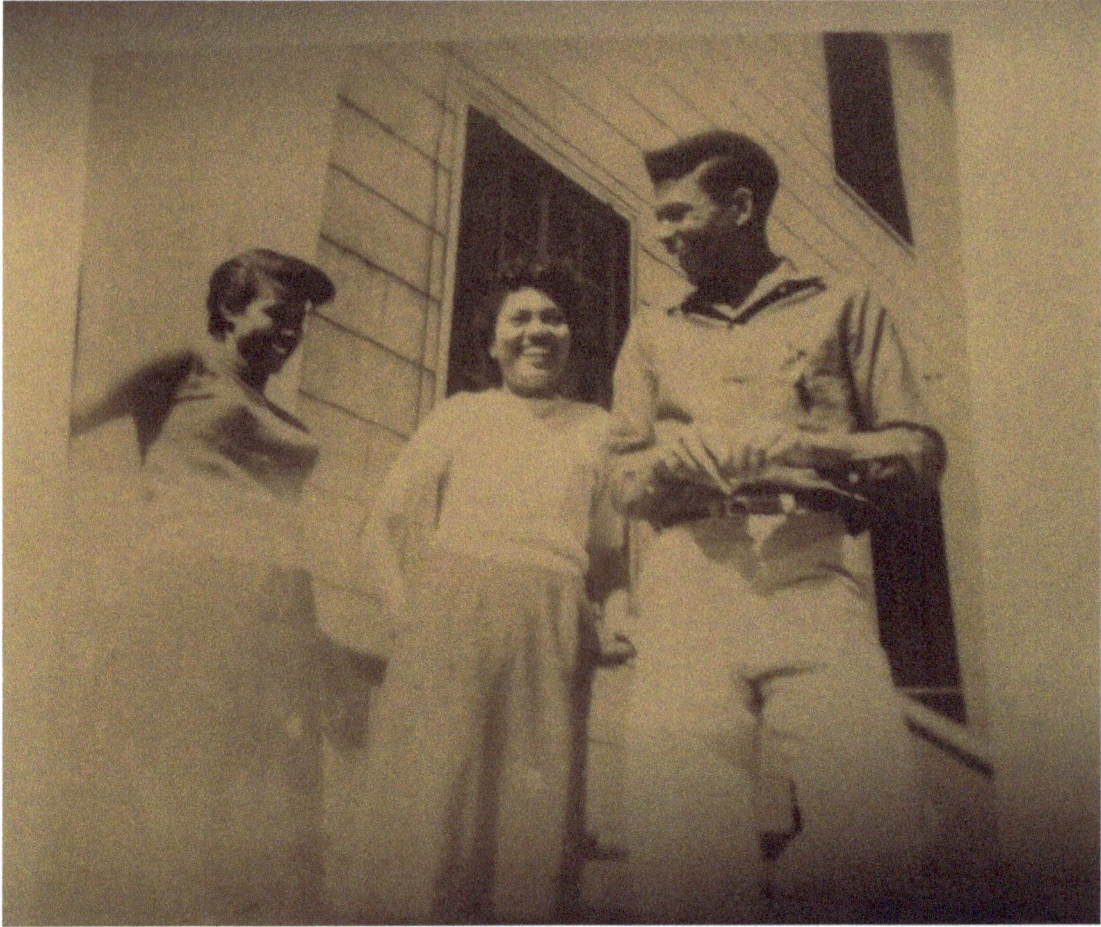

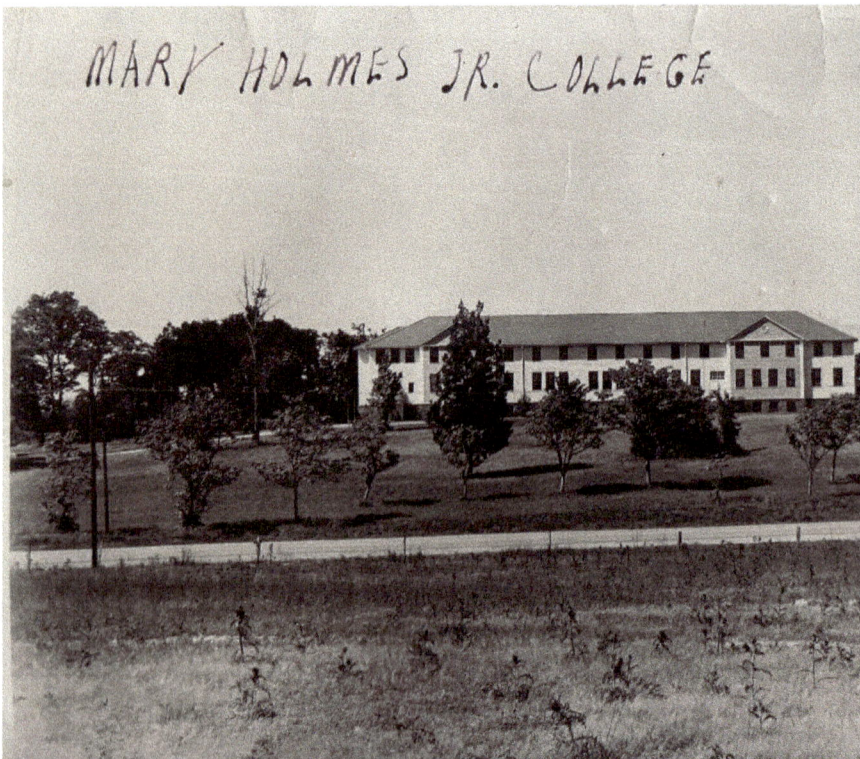

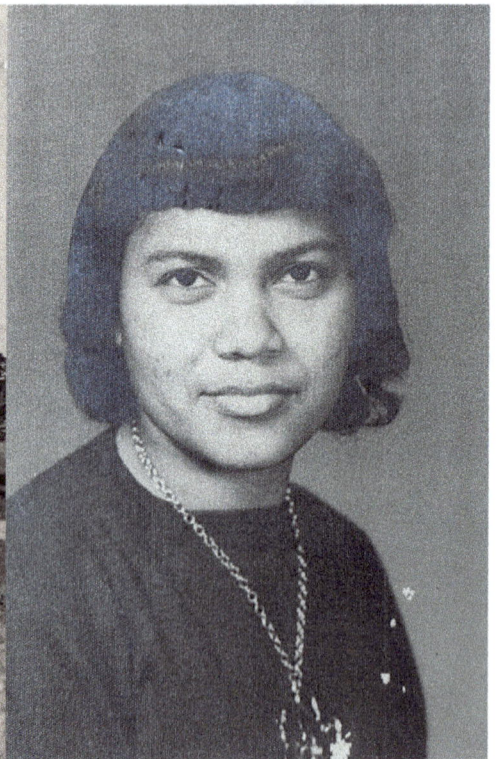

ALTON ODESSA KILGORE

I never knew my grandfather Alton,
But I'm told he was a very smart
man.
Everyone called him professor;
And of learning, he was quite
a big fan.
His parents sent him off to college,
And he was the principal of a one
room school,
He taught the children lovingly,
As he laid down all the rules.
He was my mother's father,
And the father of seven more;
He produced a family of very bright
kids,
All with the name Kilgore.

Patricia Neely-Dorsey

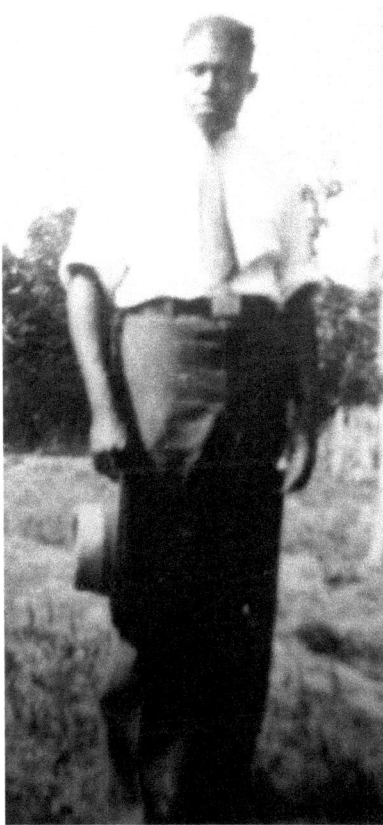

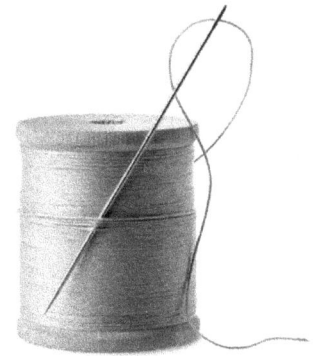

ONE ROOM SCHOOL

My mother told me stories,
Of the one room school;
Where all the grades were taught
together ,
As they went by the same rules.
To this school is where she would
go,
With other children from all
around;
Traveling there in rain, sleet or
snow,
These children could be found.
Each grade had their own lessons,
That they were all to learn;
While keeping warm by an old black
stove,
That in the corner burned.
My mother has high praises
For the teacher who taught them
there,
Because, it was her own dear
mother ,
Who gave them special care.
My mother said that in this place,
She learned so very much;
Like arithmetic and writing,
Basic reading skills and such.
I love to hear these stories,
Over and over again,
For, in passing them on down the
line,
Our legacy never ends.

Patricia Neely-Dorsey

HOMEMADE

Her mother made dresses for them
Old newspapers her patterns
Stitched with lots of love
And worn with pride

Patricia Neely-Dorsey

PND: My mother often tells me
fondly about how her mother would
make such pretty little dresses for
her and her sisters .
She made her own patterns from
newspapers .
Facebook friend Sarah Shelton
wrote:
I would look in the (Sears Roebuck)
catalog, pick out a dress, my mother
would cut the pattern and make the
dress

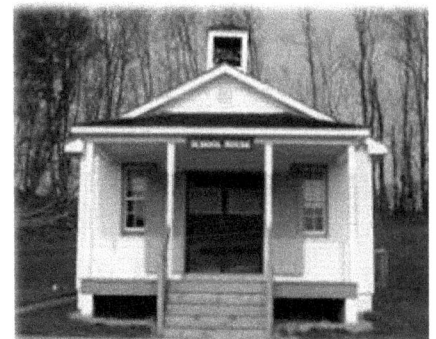

BOOKWORM

My mother, Julia Kilgore, was an avid reader. She had subscriptions to various newspapers and magazines, including The Chicago Defender , The Commercial Appeal, The Progressive Farmer and The Saturday Evening Post. One day as I was reading an article in the Saturday Evening Post, it seemed that the author and I were having a conversation. I thoroughly enjoyed the conversation. Since then, I too became an avid reader. As I mentioned earlier my mother was a teacher in a one-room schoolhouse. I learned to read in that one-room schoolhouse.

—Elaine K. Neely

Reading is fundamental,
That's what they always say;
Without it, I couldn't even imagine,
Wanting to start the day.
My mother's love of reading,
Was passed down straight to me,
And wherever it is that I am,
Some book with me, you'll see.
In my purse, under my arm,
Or maybe in my car;
I'm not so sure where the book would be,
But it couldn't be very far.
My mother says she remembers,
Books and papers 'round her mother's bed;
Where she would spend the whole long day,
With knowledge being fed.
I love to read all kinds of things,
I never get enough;
I guess, I could love without my books,
But, boy, it would be tough.

2008 Patricia Neely-Dorsey

LOOK YOUR BEST

Some of the best advice my mother gave me was to always be well groomed. She said: "Always look your best ". This advice was very valuable to me , because my late husband mentioned how he took note of the devotion I took to my personal appearance. Even in our early years at Mary Holmes, he took note of this. During my years as an elementary school teacher, one principal gave an evaluation of each teacher on personal appearance. I always received a very high rating. People, in general, over the years , have often commented on how well-groomed I look. I have passed my mother's advice on to Patricia. I have always emphasized to her to always look her best when she leaves the house.

—Elaine K. Neely

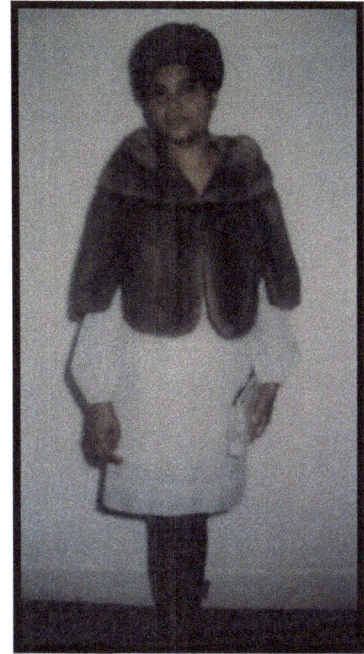

My Mom has always emphasized to me to always look my best when I leave the house. When I was growing up, Mom almost ways wore dresses and was always immaculately dressed. She also had a lot of formal dresses and always had lots of dressy events to attend. I think that this is a huge reason why I love fashion , I love wearing dresses ninety perfect of the time and I love dressing up in fancy gowns, even when I have nowhere to wear them, like during the pandemic! I would dress up in them and Hubby would take pictures "just because"! People think it's interesting (and sweet) that Hubby loves to take fashion pictures of me, almost like a hobby. He. has been doing it for many years. It's definitely not a foreign concept for me, at all. My Dad took pictures of my Mom's wardrobe all of the time, especially of her selections when going on a special trip like the medical conventions. There are dozens and dozens of pictures that he took of her posing in her outfits, in the hotel on their trips. All of them look like outfits that I would definitely wear.

PND

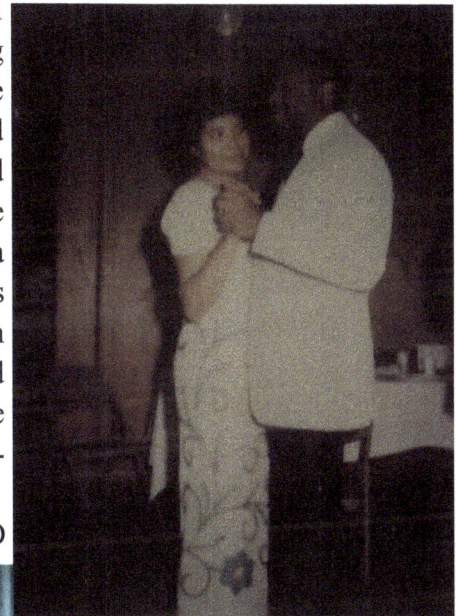

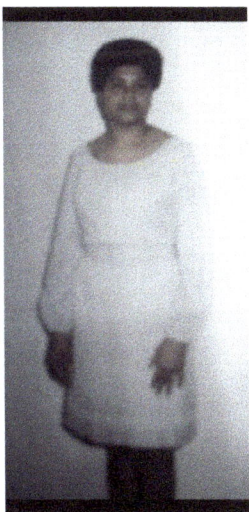
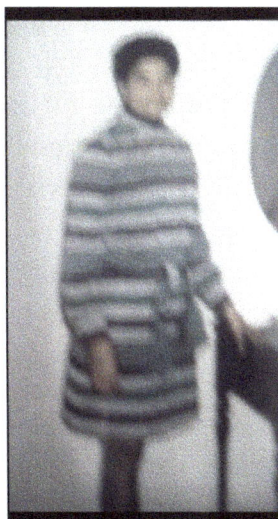
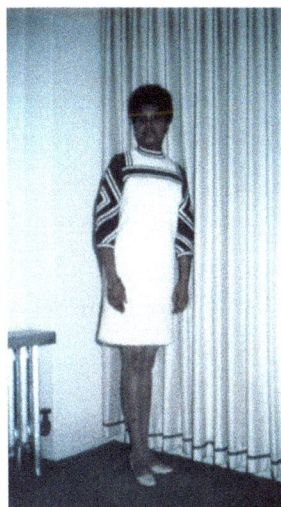

I was six years old when the twins were born. I was the aunt to her and her siblings. But, we were raised more like siblings. I recall Elaine being very reserved and quiet. She was also extremely smart and studious. She always did well in school. As a child, Elaine and her twin Elois would follow along with our group of friends, mostly observing rather than partaking in the activities. I recall times when we would go to the train station to see people boarding a train called The Rebel. This was during the times when people were migrating north. A group of us would go down to the train station to wave goodbye to strangers, then run down the street trying to get into Jip joints.

Jip joints were adult establishments in the alley, behind the stores off the main street that we were not allowed to go to, but we loved trying to sneak in and run away. Other times. we would go to the movies and also have fun times at church on Sundays.

—Pauline Lightfoot

Our friendship goes back decades. I grew up in rural West Point, MS. Elaine, her twin sister and other siblings grew up in town. I stayed with my aunt Minnie and her family in order to go to a good school. My aunt lived on Pee Ridge, a gravel road off of Hwy 45. Elaine lived on the South end of the same street/road. This is where our friendship blossomed , playing with each other up and down this gravel road and at the Presbyterian church/school (next door to her home. Her home sat on the hill next to the church/school. After finishing at the church/school we went on to Mary Holmes. (high school/ jr college)

Mary Holmes was in a beautiful location on a slanting hill where we loved to gather with our boyfriends and girlfriends. We had excellent teachers , commissioned by the Board of National Missions of the National Presbyterian Church. Although we enjoyed the social amenities of the school, we made sure that we excelled academically as well. We finished high school together as Valedictorian and Salutatorian of our class .

After high school we parted ways to some degree. We went on to further our education and married our childhood sweethearts from Mary Holmes, James and Jimmie. Raising children, careers and retirement came along, also. We are separated in distance , with Elaine in Mississippi and me in Washington, D.C. But, we never severed the connection. There are letters, greetings, calls and fond remembrances. We are in our golden years now. From childhood until now, Elaine has always been a gem; easy going, sweet, kind, smart and beautiful-one sophisticated lady.

—Love Your Friend Forever,
Velma Johnson Chandler

I met Elaine when I was about 10 years old. My brother James brought her home to introduce her to the family. When he told us this was his fiancée, it didn't sit well with me. He was my favorite big brother. I made a stink face. Elaine didn't seem to notice. And that was that. My brother was home from school on vacation when we met her. When he left we used to visit her at her family home, maybe two or three times a week- my mom, my dad and my sister. We would visit to check on her and see how she was doing When they married, she moved in with us and got settled. She was very much a student because she studied hard. That's how she spent most of her time. She got really good grades. When she was not focused on her studies, she would spend time with me. I would go in her room and hop up on the bed. We would talk and I would look at her magazines. I remember reading Vogue, Ebony, the Chicago Defender newspaper and all kinds of books with her. She was a great big sister! I developed an interest in what she shared with me like, all about fashion . It was all new to me We would go for walks together around the neighborhood and she would take me to the movies sometimes. My dad wasn't keen on that. Daddy didn't like us going to the movies because of the segregation at the time. She and a couple of other neighbors would sneak me off every now and then to go to the movies.

Elaine opened me up to a lot of new things during that time. She would take me to plays at the college she attended. (Mary Holmes) We would go to the library and to theater events. I enjoyed this very much! Even though I was little and didn't know anything about theater and musicals, I knew that they were really done well! The lighting was beautiful !!! I was totally fascinated. The lighting is what I liked the most. With Elaine, I saw all that the students did and how they enjoyed themselves. It was during this period of time that I decided that I was going to go college, too.

Elaine also belonged to a women's club. When she went to club meetings, she would take me with her. I knew to sit quietly in the corner and listen. I learned that from my mother's women's club meetings , since I was big enough to remember. She would take me with her, and then Elaine. The best part of either one of those events was the food. They would provide really good food , so that was the highlight of the day. Elaine's food was excellent. She made beautiful pies and cakes. My personal favorite was her German Chocolate Cake. The unique part is that Elaine was doing clean cooking and eating before it was popular. She was very careful about the things she put in her food and how it was prepared. We were a family of meat eaters. When she became a vegetarian, Elaine made it work well. She prepared meat for us and she only had vegetables for herself. My favorite dish was her ham. It was so good. Once upon a time we would; have suckling pig for Christmas, until Brian and Pat reached the age of awareness that the pig was once alive. The last year of the pig, there were tears. After that, no more suckling pig . Elaine is my friend, my sister and my mentor. I love her and I would be open to anything she did. I took it all in. She was always there for me. She is always there for me . Always . This is something I knew. This is something I know.

—Erie Jean Neely Wilson

I first met Elaine in 1961, on a bright, sunny day with just a hint of fall in the air. Of my husband's four sisters, I met her last. I remember thinking how much she looked like her identical twin Elois, but minus Elois' shy openness. Elaine was just the opposite; she looked directly at me. I sensed a purposefulness and direction in that first meeting: friendliness but also "I want to know if the dishes have been washed and put away." I read somewhere that often people try to live their lives backward by trying to have money or position to get what they want later. Elaine is not the person who goes rushing through the present to get ready for the future. She lives each day with a sense of purpose for that day. I have always thought that she had, deep inside her, more of what I call the Kilgore mindset: accept, remain calm and don't worry; there is more to life than increasing its speed. Of the eight children, only she is left now and I still see that sense of purposefulness, to live in the present and move with the rhythm of one's own self by embracing life's lessons as they come.

—Naomi S. Kilgore

My Aunt Elaine Neely (Aunt Lane)

How do you begin to talk about someone when there are no words to express the bond that exists between the two of you. There are unspoken words and a spiritual connection. She is the one I could always tell that I had a good childhood but not a happy one. She always let me vent as she listened quietly. My Aunt Elane is a peaceful woman. She is quite; but she talks when she has something to say (and it is always of value and importance). I value her opinion; I look up to her. She is not a judgmental or overly opinionated person; but, if you don't want the truth, don't ask. She is my mentor; she is my friend and she is my aunt and I love her dearly. My Aunt Elaine is classy, eloquent, soft spoken, strong, a peacemaker and a peacekeeper. Her beauty lies inside and out. Her once beautiful glowing black hair now reflects her 80+ years of life and living ,as it is , now, white with wisdom and time. Her face still glows and shines with the good old days ,even when she notes that life was not always a crystal stair. But, she always tries to provide a glass slipper for me. I remember when she would take me by the hand to go over to Miss Lacgie Bug to visit Mrs. Martha Baker. Mrs. Baker had all kinds of fingernail polish and I would be all over the woman's dresser.

I knew better. My Aunt Elaine would sit so patiently and speak to me so softly . Not once would she yell or raise her voice. She would always correct me with such love. My Aunt and Uncle had two children , a boy and a girl, Brian and Pat (to me Sissy Wissy and Brother Ludther)). When I visited, I was always treated like I was one of her children. She taught her children to love. She never made a difference in us, not even to this day. All three of us were Neely children and we could be a bit out of the box (in our own way).

Sixteen is one of my most memorable years. I was turning sixteen, prom bound, sweet sixteen birthday party and all the works. My Aunt Elaine purchased my beautiful ivory and pink prom dress. I was beautiful and my Aunt Elaine surprised me on my birthday with a subscription to Seventeen magazine. At that time, it was the going thing for teenage girls. And my goodness was I happy! My aunt always cooked and prepared my favorite dishes for me. That consisted of green pea salad, fried chicken, salmon croquette, and Russian Tea (Tea and Orange Juice). I remember when I graduated from college and obtain my bachelor's degree, I had married that fall and my Aunt Elaine had a graduation and family dinner for me and my husband and his family. You see, my Aunt Elaine always made sure I felt special and kept me with high self-esteem After graduation, my aunt and uncle provided us with our first home on Hilda Drive in Tupelo, MS.

When my mother passed, my aunt was there for me with open arms. I can remember when I decided to work on my PHD, my aunt encouraged me and gave me great support. As I worked on my PHD, my aunt worked out a situation with my uncle where I could have my own building to build my business. What I enjoy and remember most is every time my aunt and I talk on the phone, our last words are I LOVE YOU. I wish that every person in the world had an aunt like my Aunt Elaine (Aunt Lane) . I Love her to the moon and back.

—Drustella Neely

Mrs. Elaine Neely was more than a landlord to me and my family. My father and mother, former sharecroppers, were finally prepared to move to a better life. Dr. and Mrs. Neely ere instrumental in assisting with this transition. They rented my parents and their 9 kids a house next door. I am still amazed that they were so generous. Most landlords would never have considered having such a large family move next door. My family not only had a doctor near us, but we also had a brilliant educator near us as well. Mrs. Neely coached my siblings and me on the value of striving to do our best in school. She always reminded us of the fact that life in the South didn't mean that using incorrect grammar was okay. Southerners are known to engage in conversations without adherence to rules of grammar. She taught us to learn these standards and apply them to written and verbal expressions. My grades in English Language Arts were always excellent. I later went on to teach Middle School English for several years. Mrs. Neely's inspiration to speak well and read literature helped me develop a love for this subject.

Mrs. Neely also entrusted us with the care of her two children, Brian and Pat. We would spend almost every day with them and would always miss them when their family would leave for summer vacation. The fact that we were poor never concerned Mrs. Neely. She freely shared her kids with my family. She never had a problem with them being around an economically disadvantaged family. No one could have been prouder than she was ,as she followed each of my siblings' careers. I am proud to have had her take such an active interest in the nine of us.

She and her family will always be a part of our lives. I thank God for her believing that we each had the ability to do well in life. She was right. I am happy she and Dr. Neely gave us a home. This enabled my family to leave the never-ending cycle of poverty commonly associated with sharecropping behind.

—Geneva Agnew Matthews

As a little girl, my family was fortunate to move next door to the Neely family. Mrs. Elaine Neely was like a rock. She was always so calm, caring and loving. I always looked forward to sharing my achievements, as well as my siblings' achievements in talks with her. She watched me grow up playing in her house with my best childhood friend, Pat (Patricia) her daughter. When I achieved my goal of becoming an LPN , Mrs. Neely (and the Neely family) was my go to person/family to celebrate my achievement. Once I became an RN , she was one I truly looked forward to again to share this accomplishment. She would look on with a sweet smile and her usual calm manner, but you could see her beaming with joy and pride that another Agnew had done well and beat the odds. You see, my parents were share croppers who later got lower income wages manufacturing jobs. With those low paying jobs they put 8 children through college. As I grew older, I was always glad to share that all 9 of the Agnew children were doing well. Mrs. Neely played an important part in always encouraging and celebrating each of our successes.

—Sharron Agnew Godfrey

It was in the early 2020s at an old Ramada Inn in Tupelo. The hotel did its best to renovate, but the new stuff only covered up the wear and tear from the building's long run. We were there for the Agnew family reunion, where relatives drove from South Bend, Ind., and flew from as far away as California and Arizona. Family reunions in Tupelo for this group were rare to non-existent. But if family came together for a gathering, two people had to be included on the family list: Dr. James Neely and his wife Elaine.

Elaine Neely is the subject of this story. When our sharecropping family moved into a rental home next door to the Neely's, I was only 4. But moving next to Mrs. Neely and her family would prove life changing. Although separated before the move by no more than five miles, our very different lives made the metaphorical gap seem farther. It didn't take long, however, for us to become a blended family that to this day celebrates mutual admiration for each other. The gap that once existed closed quickly. We became family, and remain family, with a history that covers much of the 1960s.

Mrs. Neely was the quiet anchor of her home. She was an educator who, even in her youth, was an avid reader. My interaction with this august person came through her children, who long ago were symbolically adopted as my brother and sister. Mrs. Neely was the one who quietly gave us direction during the day while her physician husband tended to his patients. As long as our requests were reasonable, she rarely told us no. We would go about our business of playing in the unrelenting Mississippi sun only to retreat to the Neely home, where she would look at Brian, Pat, and me and let us have run of restricted parts of the house, even though our clothes had to be dirty and the smell from playing in 100-degree weather unbearable.

The years quickly flew by and before we knew it, we were in middle school. It was at that time that my mom and dad built a house about two miles from our dear Neely family. Back in those days, two miles seemed more like 20. We didn't see our family as much, but bonds like ours are never broken. Mrs. Neely exuded class when we were in her presence. She spoke softly, but her words were meaningful. There was so much to learn from her, and we soaked in as much as we could.

Circling back to that family reunion of years ago, our lives had changed dramatically. Brian and Pat had entered the professional world. And the Agnew children, born on a sharecropper's farm, had beaten the odds and also enjoyed professional success. One of the stories I remember from the reunion was an emotional encounter with Mrs. Neely. I was in my early years of being editor of The (Jackson) Clarion-Ledger, a statewide newspaper with a sizable staff at the time. She approached me, her lips quivering and said: "And that little boy, that little boy, is now the editor of the biggest paper in the state." I knew what she meant. I knew how proud she was. With every obstacle against me and my siblings, we persevered. She was not only celebrating me, but also my siblings. It was a proud moment for us both.

I'd like Elaine Neely to know of her influence in making "me" happen, in making me strive for success. With her home, I saw that one day I'd like a nice home, too. With her elegance, I saw that there was a way to carry myself in the presence of others. With her civic involvement, I saw what it means to give back to my community. With her tenderness, I saw how she loved her children. With her kindness, I saw her treat others as she would want to be treated. The lessons learned from this s Ship. They came from observation. I watched how she lived. And I tried to incorporate as much as I could comprehend into my own life. That's what Elaine Neely did for me. She showed me by example that has been my constant guide

—Ronnie Agnew

Mrs. Neely was the classiest and most elegant woman I knew as a child growing up in the Tupelo/Saltillo Mississippi area. She could have easily been royalty like the Queen of England. She would walk upright and elegantly into a room commanding the respect of those around her. She had a great role to play in our small town, being the wife of the only black medical doctor in the area.

I don't know the story about how they decided to make their home in the Tupelo/Saltillo area. Mississippi is a beautiful state to call home and I am happy they made the decision to live there. I had a wonderful childhood growing up and I believe Mrs. Neely played a role in my child rearing. Mrs. Neely allowed us to play on their land. The front of our yard was so massive, we called it the field. My siblings and I along the Neely's children Pat and Brian would play baseball, basketball and ride our bikes on the land. We didn't have to find a park, there was enough for us to do on Neely's land. We didn't have other friends come over because we had each other. I will forever cherish those days.

On the side of our home, we had a huge garden. We grew all of our vegetables and some fruits in this garden. I remember Mrs. Neely loved to eat egg plants and my dad grew them for her. My family didn't know too much about eating egg plants so my dad would grow them only for Mrs. Neely. The garden was such an important part of our growing up in Mississippi. We would eat from it during the hot summer days especially the tomatoes sprinkling them with salt.

Mrs. Neely could have had a long successful career as a teacher, but instead she chose to stay home and take care of her family. Pat and Brian grew up wanting for nothing. Pat would take ballot lessons looking like a beautiful ballerina. There were times I would be invited by Mrs. Neely to stay for dinner. She made the most delicious meals always healthy.

Mrs. Neely always had a close relationship with my mom. When my mother passed away Mrs. Neely was right there checking on us every day and bringing food to our family. I will never forget how kind and loving she was helping us through those difficult days. I appreciated it so much having her there to watch over us.

I am sure things have calmed down a little for her since raising a family. I am sure that she is enjoying the fruits of her labor and the grandkids. She is a woman of grace which I have had the pleasure to admire for many years. I am happy that Mrs. Neely has been a part of my life.

—Darlene Agnew Sueing

It was in the 1950's in West Point, Mississippi at Mary Holmes Jr. College/ (High School, when I met members of the Kilgore family, Gladys, my classmate, her older brother James and the twins, Elaine and Elois. After graduation, we all went our separate ways. As I remember, my next time seeing Elaine was when she and her husband moved to Tupelo, as Dr. and Mrs. Neely. I had a little meet and greet gathering for Elaine to introduce her to some of the local ladies that I had met. We became friends, again, and visited each other occasionally. Our children formed friendships, although my children were older. We became AKA sorority sisters and have kept in touch with each other and remained friends over the years. Elaine has always been one of the smartest and nicest people that I have ever met .

—Bernice Long

Being raised most of my life at 216 East Barnes Street in Tupelo, imagine being told that we had to move because the house had been sold from under us. The owners of the property lived in California. It had been said that Daddy and MaDear would be considered first, if the owner ever decided to sell. Well, the person sold the house to someone else and we had to move as soon as possible. We ended up on Old Saltillo Road. This area was not strange to me, because several of my classmates who attended Carver High School lived on that road. I used to spend nights with one of my classmates, Clara Mae and her family. I attended their church, Red Oak Grove, also, which was in the community, just up the road. I knew Mr. Johnny Johnson and his family. Mr .Johnson was the Sunday School Superintendent and he worked with my Daddy.

Jimmy Stubbs and other cousins lived on that road, plus a whole lot more. I was aware of the new African -American (Black) doctor in town, Dr. James Neely. Well, his family lived on this road, too, and I got to meet them. Brian and Pat became friends with my brother Woody and sister Andromeda (Meda). Mrs. Neely regularly taught as a substitute teacher at Carver, so I saw her frequently. I am not sure when I became close with Mrs Neely, but I did. She was to me my secret Jackie Kennedy- first lady -first class all the way. I admired her , greatly, and still do. There was one special occasion involving Mrs. Neely that meant/means so much to me. The first was on August 28, 1971, the day of my wedding. Mrs. Neely was the coordinator/ director I was late-real late-getting to Spring Hill Church (Tupelo).

I was at the Bel Air Center , which was the reception venue. I was nervous , sweating and totally stressed out , when I arrived. Mrs. Neely with her calming voice and sweet smile pulled me aside and as I was dressing she said "Betty , settle down. This is your day." It was all that I needed to hear. I felt much better. I did , however know that I should have not been late. I knew better. Mrs. Ratliff taught us and would have others come in her class to teach us about manners, etiquette, etc. I have said for years , "Carver taught us how to live, survive, succeed." My husband is a minister, Dr. Walker PHD By her example, Mrs Neely helped me to be able to adjust to being married to a professional , public man. By listening to her and watching her I learned so much about how to conduct myself and take care of my family and home. On one of my summer vacation visits from South Carolina back to Tupelo in recent years, I went to visit Mrs. Neely at her home.

I asked Meda to take me. Pat came to the door , welcomed us and led us to her mother in the living room. I got a chance to speak with Dr. Neely as well. Mrs. Neely and I had a wonderful conversation, especially when Meda and Pat left the room for a while. I was able to tell her that I owed her many thanks and tell her how much she has meant to me and helped me over the years. In these words, I want to thank her again. Fabulous does not fully describe Mrs. Elaine Neely. She is so much more!

—Betty M. Walker (Betty Lou)
(George Washington Carver Class of '67)

I have fond memories of my Aunt Elaine.

When we were children, we would come to visit, spend the night, and enjoy wonderful meals my aunt would prepare.

I loved her string bean casserole. I remember her giving me some advice on life as a young lady. She was always pleasant, loving, and very understanding. I enjoyed her conversations with my mom, Gladys. They would talk about many things and many people, especially from Mary Holmes College. She was very concerned about my education. She called and told my mother she saw my name in the Tupelo Journal for making the President's List at Mississippi State. She never had any negative thing to say about anyone. When I became a mother, she showed my children the same love. My Aunt Elaine is a beautiful person inside and out, and that is why I love her so much.

—With Sincere love,
Camille Kilgore Lenoir

Mrs. Neely was the coolest mother ever!

I remember the Neely family living across from me when the children were very young. I lived at 432 North Spring Street in Tupelo. When her son Brian , as a small child , would have a temper tantrum she would just say, "Now Brian" over and over again. She would never raised her voice or get upset. (I would get upset just looking on!) Actually, I have never heard her raise her voice, not once! Since the time I have known her, she has always been prim and proper, a real jewel!

—Margaret Baker

Elaine K. Neely

If there is such a thing as a perfect mother-in-law, it has to be Elaine K. Neely. She has always told Patricia how important I am to the family and what a blessing I have been. I think my wife is a little jealous of our relationship, because her mother always takes my side. Patricia has often said , on many occasion, that I should have married her mother. Of course, it is tongue-in-cheek. But, she says that we would make the perfect couple. We have never had an argument or cross words in the 31 years that I've known her. She has always been supportive of our marriage. She is not a drama queen. (She doesn't "do" drama)

She minds her own business. My mother in law exemplifies class. She is very soft -spoken . But, don't be fooled . She wields a lot of power. She strives for excellency and will not settle for mediocrity. If it's not first class, she will not cosign, agree or go along with it . I don't know anyone else that reads as much as she does. She is more than an avid reader. Amazingly, she reads a minimum of 100 books a year. She has always promoted higher education and the arts. She is very loyal.

She faithfully visited Dr. Neely during his extended hospital stay and rehab, after a stroke in1999 and during frequent hospitalization in his last year of life. She never complained. I remember her walking through the hospital better than individuals much younger than her. Her dry sense of humor is on a different level. She keeps us laughing . She says things with a straight face that make us crack up. Most of all, I'm very appreciative of the fact that she is authentic . She doesn't try to put on airs. She is who she is . Elaine K, Neely is just Elaine K. Neely, all of the time. And, there is no one else like her.

—James Dorsey

"She walks in beauty, like the night of cloudless chimes and starry skies,
And all that's best of dark and bright, meet in her aspect and her eyes."
Lord George Gordon Byron, 1814

Whenever I think of Mrs. Elaine Neely, the lines of this poem automatically come to mind for it is a most fitting description of her. She is truly a woman of beauty – both outside and inside. Her eloquence, grace, kindness and true humanity are unparalleled and I am so grateful to know her.

My entire family shared this perception of her once they met her. When Dr. Neely first came to Tupelo, my grandparents, Luvert and Virgie Spearman, were among his first patients. Actually, the night he began his practice, Dr. Zuber brought Dr. Neely to their home and immediately transferred them to his care. Soon thereafter, they met Mrs. Neely and their love affair began. Often they did not have money to pay for their visits, either in the office or on his house calls. My grandparents were farmers with very little income so many times, when Dr. Neely, provided care – most of which were house calls for my grandfather, they did not have the funds to pay him. Because, my grandmother always had a large garden which produced a magnificent harvest, Dr. Neely usually left with large quantities of fresh vegetables and eggs as his payment, rather than cash. I recently learned that Mrs. Neely is vegetarian, so although my grandparent's form of payment did little to increase their financial status, I take pleasure in hoping that the many vegetables were of value to Mrs. Neely.

My brother, Frank, became especially close to the Neely's during his formative years. Because of his interest in the medical profession, Dr. Neely became a mentor and advisor to him during his college years and during the years he was in medical school. He paved the way for him to gain practical experience in both his office and the office of other local physicians. Frank spent a lot of time in their home and became a true "Elaine Neely fan". He would always talk about how thoughtful and intuitive she was, and in fact, while Dr. Neely provided wise and sound professional advice, Mrs. Neely became his "de facto" life coach. He never failed to seek her guidance, direction and advice on personal issues and always found comfort in her positive and analytical responses. When he made the decision to marry, there was no doubt as to who would be responsible for the wedding. He immediately asked Mrs. Neely to be the wedding planner and coordinator. The wedding was eloquent, classy, and one of the most beautiful ceremonies I have witnessed. Mrs. Neely would not have it any other way!

If I was in town when he visited, I would accompany Frank to their home and it was there that I got a chance to meet Mrs. Neely. I quickly discovered that she was all of the wonderful things he had described and more. As a "country girl", I was overwhelmed with her and her surroundings. The elegance of her home, her charm and grace as a host, and her ability to make people feel comfortable (in spite of their economic status) really resonated with me. I could easily understand why my family admired her so much. I always looked forward to those rare, but significant, visits to her home.

Thank you Mrs. Elaine Neely for being who you are and for showing me, and others, how to live with grace and humility, and, more importantly, to always treat people with kindness.

—Virginia Dowsing Toliver

Mom & Dad (Dr. and Mrs. James Neely)

Historically, speaking, parents, family, community, church, civic organizations and academic associations make up the institutions that affect and reflect the core values of a person's ethical frame. We , often, read in books about great families of African-American heritage. I feel comfortable in suggesting that I've seldom met, in-person, families that reflect the grade that we read about in history books. Some families that we see in documentaries have literally changed the landscape of particular communities and organizations, while leaving a larger and lasting impression even on our global world.

The Neely family is one such family. Basically, everything that has been identified as key organizations or first attempts, Dr. Neely had already been successful in accomplishing them all. My first interaction with Mom was a quiet but informative passing conversation. She said just enough to allow me the benefits of becoming acquainted with the Neely legacy. After my continued efforts as a newcomer to Tupelo, Mississippi , Mom would open up to me and my wife more about her variety of life experiences, that would provide much beneficial knowledge. All of this confirmed the fact that , as an emerging leader, the family felt that I had something to offer. As our relationship continued to blossom, Mom began sharing leadership tips concerning the landscape of our community's demographics in an effort to help me avoid unnecessary friction. So well-informed and absolutely aware of the landmines and pot holes of life she refused to let me fall. Dr. Neely offered an equal amount of influence and support. When people take outsiders like my family in as their own, who moved from one of the most prolific African-American communities in the nation, located in one of the greatest cities in the world, New York, NY, it says something big. But it , especially, spoke volumes to me when I was asked by Mom, and the family at large to perform the funeral rites for Dr. Neely. I remember asking myself how I was going to organize my words, and how I could honor the family, particularly Mom, during such a time. I was grateful to have had a mental logbook filled with countless conversations about the family's heart for making a difference and a desire to help future generations realize possibilities and achieve what at times does not seem feasible.

I can honestly say that my family and I are great benefactors of the Neely/Dorsey family value system. We are grateful.

—Dr. Richard Price
Senior Minister -North Green Street Church of Christ

When I recall my memories of time with Mrs. Neely, I think of the time she was my girl scout leader and how she always talked to us about conducting our selves as young ladies and how important it was to use good manners as well as proper etiquette.

—Mrs Virginia Smith

Mrs. Elaine K. Neely. This lady is amazing.

When I think of Mrs. Neely, I feel as though I'm shopping in Neiman-Marcus or Saks Fifth Avenue. Dainty, and the epitome of a woman, Mrs. Neely is a mentor to me, and so many other young women in the community of Parkhill. My first memory of Mrs. Elaine Kilgore Neely was as a little girl. She was a member of the Waymaker's Club. Through the numerous, and various activities that this civic club became fond of her. I'm sure that Ms. Neely has known me since I was born though. When I started the second grade, again I saw this gorgeous woman on a daily basis. I was a little busybody, but Mrs. Neely always was nice to me when I passed her in the halls. She was a special kind of teacher, and I couldn't understand WHY I wasn't I in her class, after all I knew her! When I was told by my teacher that I couldn't go.... me being a third grader, I became angry, and I wanted to know WHY! Instead, my home room teacher only kept saying "now Tally, you know you can't go". She offered me very little explanation! So, what did Natalia do? I got "smart" (so I thought), and started acting like the usual mischievous and hyper little kid. All my other classmates who acted out in class got to go to Ms.Neely ALL DAY!! It didn't work. Sad for me though, all I got was a paddling....ANOTHER whipping, an aggravated Mama and Daddy....and a bruised ego!

It didn't register with me WHY I never had Ms. Elaine Neely as a teacher, until I reached Green Street Elementary School.

I understood finally, but I was angry up until then. Finally, let's fast forward to ADULTHOOD! Ms. Neely is a member of the same church that I attend....St. Paul UMC. As a teen, a young adult I always count on Ms. Neely to be seated on the left hand side of the sanctuary, on that FOURTH pew, by the window. Then, to add icing on the cake, in September of 2000, I became a member of Alpha Kappa Alpha Sorority, Inc. You're talking about a real honor for me, to become my mentor's "little sister". Thank you Ms. Neely for the wonderful example that you set for us little girls.

Thank you mentoring, and cementing a dear friendship between you and I. I love you and appreciate you.

Always and sisterly,

—Natalia A. Davis

Note: Mom taught remedial reading and Natalia did not need to be in her class.

With love and admiration yesterday, today and tomorrow, I will cherish the journey with my friend Elaine.

From the mid-sixties to present, our friendship began with our children who were nursery school classmates and friends. We were also very fortunate to have taught in the great   Tupelo Public School District for many years. Our relationship grew and was solidified as line sisters and travel buddies in Alpha Kappa Alpha Sorority, Inc., by attending meetings, conferences, church services and social events. Elaine is my mentor, my sister, my friend...a beautiful creation God placed in my life. I thank God for Elaine, one of my blessings!

"From the fullness of His grace, we have all received one blessing after another." John 1:16 NIV

Lovingly,

—Christine Partlow

I've had the pleasure of knowing Mrs. Neely for almost 50 years. She did an amazing job being my wedding coordinator. (December 21, 1974) Being Alpha Kappa Alpha Sorority sisters for 30 years, I've learned a plethora of knowledge about our illustrious sisterhood from her both on the chapter and international levels. She is a beautiful and respectable lady in every way. One of her graceful characteristics that I admire is her ability to be honest yet sincere with you about anything. For many years, we have sent each other Christmas cards. I am grateful for the opportunity to share these expressions.

—Roxie Smith

Remembering some of my fondest. memories of my friend Elaine Neely. Elaine has been a member of St. Paul united methodist church for many years. I can recall when Elaine held the office as Superintendent of Sunday school. She took on this position after my husband William Smith sr. retired as the superintendent Elaine did a great job until she retired from this position as well. Dressed in her white attire every first Sunday, Elaine served as a communion steward for a year. Elaine was always eager to serve where needed. Elaine volunteered and helped with vacation bible school for numerous years faithfully in June after the annual conference. Faithful, hard working ,dependable are just a few of the words that come to mind when I think of Elaine Neely.

—Mrs, Catherine Powell Smith

Mrs. Elaine Neely was a fabulous substitute teacher and woman of wisdom. One particular year she was our substitute for the entire semester of fifth grade. She was the kindest, sweetest, most humble, soft-hearted person, with a love for children.

She was an extra-ordinary person. She always surprised us with treats, not just for one, but for all of the children. One side joke was that "she has lots of money" to be able buy all of us Christmas gifts. Her focus was always on the children making the best progress and excelling in their subjects. She worked extra hard and encouraged me while being there, that school year. It gave me the momentum to set my goals high and become the best teacher to my students one day. She left a great impression on me, even to this day. I still cherish and reflect on those memories over 50 years later. I am now a retired teacher and I want to thank Mrs. Neely for the foundation that she laid for me.

—Deloris Fields-Jenkins

I've always admired the way she dressed and always soft-spoken.

—Rochell Harris

I became acquainted with Elaine after becoming a Tupelo Public School educator. Elaine is a very unique lady. She is very intelligent, kind and soft spoken. But, when she speaks, I would advise you to listen. She is the kind of person that you just don't meet every day. And, her company is most enjoyable. She is now my sister for life and an angel of a friend.

—Mary A. Cleveland

I Have Not Forgotten

I have not forgotten.

Your laugh.

Your Grace.

You.

I remember staying with you as a little child. Visits and holidays. The extended stay when my mom was sick and you cared for me. As Uncle Jim watched over Mom's life while she fought to stay with us. I worked my big cousins nerves!

After all, they were six and nine years older than me. I was three. One particular day, a Saturday I believe, we had one too many tea parties, changed into one too many dance outfits, read one too many books. My cousins were at their wits end! Patti, with Brian's support, drew up the indictment- a pictorial letter outlining my offenses. I was brought before the judge a jury- the high bed where you and my uncle were resting and Pat presented my charges. In writing. I'm not sure if I cried but I know I felt bad. There were no raised voices. No scorn. I was sentenced to getting in bed. With you guys.

Snuggled between you and Uncle Jim to watch whatever you were watching on TV, which I probably was not interested in at all! I knew not to whine or complain. Gentle parenting at it's best. You two knew I wasn't being intentional in my actions. I simply wanted attention and my mom. You did the best you could to give me the love she would have. That was intentional. And I received. This is the only memory I have of that time without picture reminders. Pat and Brian's exasperation, no malaise. Your lovingkindness and gentle scolding meant to keep me safe. Comforted, not punished. As the years seemed to fly by there were beautiful holiday dinners. Special birthdays. One on one time with you for almost a year when my grandmother was sick. The epic win in your sorority's fundraising pageant. Of course we won-you could do anything you put your mind to and you taught me the same thing too! I have not forgotten. All the things you taught me. The melody of your voice. Your patience. Your love. I could never forget. I am so blessed to call you my aunt. Family. You are simply unforgettable.

—Tracey Bowen Bell

Having a friend like you in my life has been one of the best things that ever happened to me. I will forever cherish every moment that we spend as sisters. Your loyalty has been unshakable. You are one of the most creative, kind and level-headed persons that I know. You are a true friend that accepts who you are , but also helps you become who you should be .

You are a person with grace and poise. You are never arrogant. I've never known you to boast about your success to make yourself look good. You would always rather bring people up than bring them down. You have a great degree of self-awareness. Your social etiquette is always on point. You are a person who is always prepared. Thank you for all of the positive traits that you exemplify. Because of all of these qualities , I am so very proud to call you my friend. You are indeed the best among the rest and I will always strive to live up to your expectations. Thank You for being a part of my life and letting me be a part of yours.

—Pamela Coleman

As a child I remember Mrs. Neely visiting my Mom (Shirley M. Armstrong) house on Saturdays with her daughter Patricia. I would always stare at her because she reminded me of one of my dolls, but she was a real person. She is a very soft spoken woman with an inviting smile. I have always admired her and the presence she brings in any room. She enters with her style, beauty and grace. Mrs. Neely is the epitome of a lady and I am so proud to call her my Friend and My Soror.

—Rhonda Armstrong Gibson

It is with pleasure for me to write these few paragraphs about Elaine which could be many more paragraphs because of her involvement in the community. I became familiar with Elaine when she was teaching third grade at Pierce Street Elementary School. She was a quiet-spoken person. I had heard about Elaine way before we met because she was the wife of the new black doctor that moved to town. We were so proud to have them in town. I don't remember if they came to town before integration of the schools. Our rooms were on the same hall at Pierce Street Elementary. I remember we were in the teacher's lounge and we introduced ourselves to each other. This is how we became acquainted. We enjoyed talking to each other. Those were some days that you would want to hurry up and forget because of the pressure from parents, students, and administration. When we had our break together, that was the sunshine on a cloudy day, and we encouraged each other. Still today I am thankful because God took care of us, so today we still give him the glory.

Elaine was the wedding planner for several weddings in the city, and I was the musician who played at the weddings. We often worked on several occasions. Her planning was very thorough. Everyone in the wedding party knew what to do and where to be. Most of them, as I can recall, started on time.

I can't remember when Elaine became a soror, but during our local meetings we used to sit together and enjoy each other's company. I remember when I went to the first regional conference which was in Jackson, Mississippi. We were so proud to be apart of such a prestigious group. To see beautiful black women dressed for business and just looking good. As years passed I had to drop out, but I continued to see the continued progress AKA was making. The sorors implemented progress in the city and the county, and I wanted to be apart of it. So I reinstated and was very happy to know that Elaine had reinstated as well. For two years we didn't get a chance to see each other because of COVID, but I am always happy to see sorors, Especially Elaine.

—Ollie Scales

Magnolia Mornings

Eight a.m. my eyes were opened by the flooding of light through the antiquated windows of my grandmother's bed and bathroom. I lifted my body from the fresh floral printed duvet that I had been nestled into the night before. Turning sideways I gazed directly into the mirror formally ,attached to a large dresser. I could smell breakfast, and I knew that my grandmother's daily routine had already begun. I remember the long walk down the hallway to the kitchen, where strawberries and green stripes encompassed the walls. I walked past paintings of copper skinned sorority women draped in pink gowns and pearls and the parlor where I was instructed not to enter. I greeted my grandmother and in her southern drawl she would politely respond, "Good morning, Ivy". I usually declined everything that she prepared .Her own personal breakfast of choice was raisin bran. After breakfast, I would watch her clean. Her kitchen was immaculate, as if it was from a magazine. She would then continue her daily schedule which included lessons.

She taught us writing, social studies, and culture. So, well that I can remember winning my fourth-grade geography competition without even trying, for which she attended. The best part of the day would be the few hours we were allowed to play outside. We were granted acreage in which we were permitted to explore. My sister and I particularly enjoyed rolling down steep hills lined by azaleas. The azaleas made Easter our favorite holiday.

Grandmother would prepare the best Easter dinner served at the same time every year, around noon. She had so many eggs, that we would help dye beautiful colors. She would combine the eggs with plastic ones and scatter them for acres. My strategy was to check the lawn mower first, and then to the yard. She completes the entire event dressed to the nines. She was the epitome of womanhood, grace, and class. One thing that I remember for certain is that every morning at grandmother's house smelled like magnolia.

—Ivy Elainea

More than likely my first opportunity to meet Elaine was at my sister Delores's beauty shop, in Tupelo, long before we became sorority sisters in the mid 80's. She visited my home in Pontotoc, on one occasion with Delores and then my husband, James, at the time, and I visited her home in Saltillo on another occasion. I think we attempted opportunities to socialize.

My most lasting memory of being in her presence came when I was invited to join the Nu Sigma Omega Chapter of Alpha Kappa Alpha Sorority. During that time we met at various venues to accomplish the desired goals and on most of those occasions food would be served. There was an occasion when we had met at a gathering and I was served a drink in a Styrofoam cup, whereupon Elaine had the drink returned and I was served in a proper container, a glass. The incident was a clear indication of Elaine's proper upbringing and social graces, as she is the epitome of Southern grace and charm in matters of etiquette.

One might go as far as to say she is a modern day portrayal of the woman mentioned in Proverbs 31: One who is of noble character, full of confidence and lacks nothing of value. She is clothed with strength and dignity, speaks with wisdom and gives faithful instruction. It is an honor and a pleasure to be an affiliate and a member of some of the organizations of which she is also a member.

Best regards,
—Cora A. Givhan Ford-Ingram

Elaine and I are sister in-laws. We were married to two brothers who are now deceased. I first met Elaine when my husband brought me to Mississippi to meet his family(or should I say "my new family"). Elaine welcomed me to the family, and she was very supportive, She made me feel real proud to be part of The Neely Family. Her positivity, wit, laughter, and love were infectious. She was a school teacher and believed that every child should have the best education possible, and she did her best for all her students, and her own children Brian and Patricia to receive that education. She loved to entertain, and whenever we came to Mississippi she invited us over for dinner. She also loved to cook and I think she was one of the best cooks I know.

One year her husband called me and said they were in California at a Medical Convention. My husband and I went to L.A. to picked them up and brought them to our home so we could entertain them. We were so happy to have them in our home. I remember the last two times I saw Elaine. One was for our 55th Wedding Anniversary. The year 2014. Everyone was there except Erie Jean and her husband. Her husband was too sick to travel. The next time was the year 2016 and Erie Jean and Her husband were able to come and we were able to meet her husband and we were so happy to meet him.

Elaine, I thank you for allowing me to write something to you. It has brought back a lot of memories of our families. You take care Elaine, and God speed
Your sister in law,

—Mildred Neely

I can't remember exactly when Dr. and Mrs. Neely moved to Tupelo, but I do remember I was in elementary school. It was in the 1960s, because the schools were still segregated. Dr. Zuber had been our physician and his wife, Mrs. Zuber, was our piano teacher. So when the Neelys arrived to town our parents, U.S. and Ruth Mayhorn, were introduced to them by the Zubers and subsequently, the five Mayhorn children met them and we became Dr. Neely's patients, along with our parents and paternal grandmother. Of course, we were in awe of the second Black doctor we had ever met and his young, beautiful wife, Ms Elaine. Over the years, our mother, Mrs. Ruth Staggs Mayhorn, and Mrs. Elaine Neely became good friends. We would visit each other's homes. I remember Mrs. Neely, even trusted my older teen sister, Gloria, to babysit Brain and Pat when the Zuber Reading Club would meet. I was always around and felt as though I was babysitting too. Ms Elaine was doing a great job with the children because they were good children and could hold interesting conversations at a young age. Ms Elaine was quiet and very ladylike. A definition of "ladylike behavior" is she behaves in a polite, dignified and graceful way. Some synonyms of ladylike are refined, cultured, sophisticated, elegant, proper, respectable, polite, genteel and courtly. Ms. Elaine was all of this and more.

What stands out to me the most in referring to Mrs. Neely was her quiet, respectful and elegant manner. Don't get me wrong, she was very friendly and conversant when among her friends. I know that Dr. Neely was a highly intelligent man, however; I do think that it was Mrs. Neely's daily influence on the children that influenced their outgoing personalities. As I grew older and went to high school and college, I didn't visit the Neely home as much as I did in my early years. Needless to say, when it was time for my wedding, the first person that we thought of to assist us was Mrs. Elaine Neely. She in my opinion was the epitome of elegance and I knew that if she directed the wedding, it would be done in the proper manner. My wedding , on December 24, 1975, was all that and more thanks to Ms. Elaine and her kind and gentle manner. Although, I no longer live close to Mrs. Neely or her adult children, I still consider them to be close family friends, who I respect and love.

—Stella Johnson

In the summer of 1965, I returned home from Jackson State to learn we had a new family in Tupelo, MS.

The family was Dr. James H. Neely, his wife Mrs. Elaine Neely, children Brian and Patricia from West Point, MS.

This new family would become family friends to my parents Mr. Luther (L. C.) and my mother the late Mrs. Gloria Sims along with my six younger siblings. Dr. Neely was Tupelo's new local physician replacing the late Dr. W. A. Zuber, Mama's great uncle.

It was clear my family thought a lot of the Neely family with Mama immediately telling me she would be keeping the children whenever needed. Mrs. Neely frequently visited our home. .

She had and has a laugh that no one can repeat. It is just different!

Being new to Tupelo, Mrs. Neely did not hesitate to ask Mama about Tupelo and its people.

Of course, Mama provided her with the latest updates.

When Pat and Brian visited/stayed they were considered a part of the family, eating, sleeping just as one of Mama's children.

I remember Mrs. Neely always saying "act nice and mind". Of course they always did.

I shall never forget when Mama told her I was getting married. Mrs. Neely immediately told me a church wedding would be ideal.

I had been a flower girl, years back in Emogene Ratliff's wedding .

But, my sisters had home weddings and I did not have a clue about how to have a church wedding. Mrs. Neely did !

She reassured me it would be "The Wedding".

For bride maids, etc. I selected my sisters, Gloria Joyce, Gladys, Janet and Wanda .

To complete my wedding Miss Patricia Elaine Neely was the ideal flower girl and she handled being my flower girl perfectly.

Mrs. Neely guided us through the complete wedding planning process, and yes, everything was by the etiquette book, including wedding programs. It was clear she enjoyed what she was doing and that this was one of her "callings".

Being employed part time at Dr. Neely's office during this time, he would often laugh when he asked about how things were coming along.

He would say, "Elaine is enjoying this".

It was obvious Mrs. Neely enjoyed taking the lead and our guests were able to see the results of her appreciation for social graces.

The late Mrs. Lillie M. Lockridge, got right in and made sure all the food related issues were taken care of including the , bride and groom cakes, and rehearsal dinner.

Many years later when we attended Pat's wedding and reception dinner, it was handled with perfection, of course.

Mrs. Elaine K. Neely was and is always a soft spoken, sophisticated, intelligent lady who is very proud of her family.

—Phyllis Sims

My husband Ike passed away at our hospital. I came home that early morning to a big ole empty house, just in a trance! I walked around the house for I don't know how long until I heard a knock at the door. I went to the door, and it was Elaine Neely. I think she said that she was there to be with me for a while. I said, I think because I really don't exactly remember what she said, but she walked in, dressed immaculately, and asked if she needed to get me anything. I remember drinking sprite and lying across my bed. The bed that only the day before, both me and my husband had lain in. I slept, for I had been awake, the night before, waiting in the intensive care waiting room, writing lesson plans.

Elaine stayed with me for hours until my sons came...then she left quietly. I never will forget how kind that was. She showed true sisterly love. Her husband, Dr. Neely, was our physician. Her daughter , Patricia and I pledged Alpha Kappa Sorority, Inc together in 1989

—Ora Baldwin

I have wonderful and glorious memories growing up down the street from The Neely family in Saltillo and having Pat as my lifelong sister· friend. I thoroughly enjoyed every minute. And I will always cherish those glorious years of sisterhood. They will last for a lifetime. We played every day, practically. Pat would come to my house to swim. I remember my worst overnight stay with my sister friend. She had a bed with a canopy. I had never seen anything like that before. It was so beautiful. But, I couldn't figure out that arch over our heads. The only thing I could relate it to was a casket. I was terrified as we laid in it . I cried until midnight. Pat had to wake Mrs. Neely up to try and comfort me. I was so upset that Mrs. Neely had to call my mom in the middle of the night to come and get me. Little did I know that I was privileged with a friend of the upper echelon at an early age. Lol

I often think back to those precious memories and how we used to run and play together without a care in the world. And Oh My, how our once playing ground has drastically changed. (The place where our house stood and the surrounding area is now a huge subdivision) The Neelys are and will always remain as my extended family for life. Hugs, kisses, and much love for life

—Andromeda Hamilton

She's my grandma. The voice and welcoming smile that would let me know I was at home away from home when I was very young. Kind. Caring. Giving.

—James Henry Dorsey

I often say that, if my grandmother had been born in a different generation, she would have been a Senator. She has a brilliant mind for politics, an understated charm, a sharp wit and an inherent and irrepressible curiosity. But having been born in the 1930s, in Mississippi and Black, she became many things- a teacher, a doctor's wife, a mother and a grandmother, all of which were considered a best-case scenario of a life for a woman with her beauty and aptitude.

As a teenager, I spent more time with my grandmother than anyone. She drove me to and from school in her silver Cadillac with butter soft leather seats and a steering mechanism that was so smooth it felt like it drove itself. She drove me to piano lessons and to the hairdresser every Friday, making one stop to allow me to grab a lemon filled donut from Shipley's on the way. She gripped the wheel tightly and drove in silence, except for my youthful chatter that I did not feel obligated in any way to temper or restrain. I talked and talked while she listened without response, until prompted with some open-ended question that was no doubt focused on me. She would take me shopping for clothes of my choosing, parking at the mall and sending me inside with cash while she remained in the car, pulling whatever paperback book she was reading at the time out of her center console. She gave me a weekly allowance and once a week, took me to the grocery store to buy whatever I needed to make my own lunches and dinners, as I- like her- had adopted vegetarianism, a very unpopular thing to be in our town at the time. She would hand me cash but would never traverse the sliding glass threshold of a place that had too many people for her liking. She had her book and I had money and my task. I would need to figure out what to do with both.

Complicit to the deeply engrained norm of remaining in a child's place, I rarely asked her personal questions, only breeching that familiar rule to satiate my fascination with her almost telekinetic relationship with her identical twin. I knew her, but I didn't know her and as an adult, I carry deep regret for not asking more questions, for not pushing the norms, for not learning all that I could from such a complex and multifaceted individual at time in my life when I could have benefitted from it the most.

My grandmother's beloved children and all of her other grandchildren all look like my grandfather. I look like my grandmother. Every year, I look more and more like her. But that, especially as a teenager, I believed was our sole similarity. She was a quiet person, surrounded by gregarious extroverts, all of us having a propensity for laughter, loud talking and intense intellectual debate. Despite this, she would, in her quiet way, always manage to get us all to do exactly what she wanted- whether it was sitting in the formal living room on a hot July day when we would all rather lop around in the cool, casual comfort of her den to our immediate family only dinners that were still hosted at a formally set table with place cards- regardless of how ridiculous we may have pretended her request was.

She loved nothing more than to be lost in a book or surrounded by periodicals of every kind- voraciously absorbing every pop culture factoid or piece of news that she could find. She could hold her own in any conversation, but she often preferred the role of observer. She was known for her elegance and her entertaining. Stories of her dinner parties in the 60s and 70s still rattle around her former social circle and pop up from time to time in conversations with family. I remember sitting in her pantry admiring her sets of special occasion china and the crystal glasses with our family crest and name etched into them, feeling fancy as I studied the patterns on each piece. She set a perfect table. She was an immaculate dresser. She was civically active and exceptionally regarded in our community. She gifted the best books.

I think back to being a trend conscious, people pleasing teenager, annoyed by my grandmother's desire to dress to go into "town." She wore pristine two-piece sets- often jacket and skirt, but sometimes a smart pant suit- with a statement brooch. Her left hand would be adored with the massive diamond solitaire that was given to her by my grandfather- albeit rarely, either because of safety concerns or because she deemed it ostentatious; I don't believe I ever asked. Her shoes were either Ferragamo or white canvas Keds- no exceptions. My Aunt Patricia and I would jokingly tease her about her shoe collection, feigning eye rolls and giggling as we poked fun at her multiple pairs of what were basically the same shoe, varying only slightly by color and even more slightly by heel height. To us, they all looked identical. To us, they were boring. To her, they fit, were well made and were what she liked. And to her, that was being practical.

I now realize that the shoes, the driving in silence, the constant reading, the working when she could have easily and happily subsisted comfortably as a housewife, were all about control- a control that was denied to women of her generation. What I learned is that my grandmother was the first woman I had ever known with true agency. She was empowered by having her own money, a wealth of information and the talent and skill to do things, whether she chose to do them or not. I would come to understand that she was teaching me incredibly valuable lessons that would eventually empower me. She was teaching me that I could make my own choices about what I could wear and what I could learn. She was teaching me that practicality and comfort always trumps trends and status quo. She taught me the beauty that is learning how to do many things well, while having the choice as to what to do with those skills and with whom I share them. She taught me to budget and to be financially independent without ever expressly telling me how to or that I needed to do either.

My grandmother is still with us. I write of her in past tense, because she is a very different person now-no more hosting lavish dinners and parties, no more packed social calendar, no more civic engagements, no more patiently teaching young children experiencing learning challenges the happiness that is reading and the freedom and power that is reading comprehension. She still loves her books, and my greatest joy is to bring her a stack of them when I visit her- still beautiful, still impeccably dressed, still very interested in the "goings on" in Decatur and Atlanta, politically. Her greatest joy these days is to be in her home, surrounded by quiet and books and seemingly neighborless acres of land, living the life that she wants to live for herself, unapologetically and with grace. She has found her peace and I have found myself aspiring for the same.

I admire my grandmother immensely. I am an elected official, an avid reader and a mother, who has been told on more than one occasion that I host a lovely party. And as I sit here, wearing my black t-shirt and jeans combo that has defined my personal style, with a stack of books to my right and within eyeshot of my closet that is lined by simple black dresses with only the slightest of variation among them, I realize that I am so much more like her than teenage me could have ever imagined or understood. Of that, and of her, I am deeply proud.

I love you, Gramma. I am all that I am because of you. Thank you.

-Lesa Neely Mayer

Sometimes home can feel like a person, and it's because of the things they teach you that you carry with you your entire life. Home is not the single mailbox at the end of a long driveway or the crunch of gravel under your tires. It is not a faint but comforting hello from the other end of your knocks at the door or the familiarness of strawberry wallpaper. Some would argue that home is the smell and taste of homemade sun tea, rows of cookbooks, or handwritten recipes. Home could feel like endless birthdays and holiday dinners, meticulously Planned and executed with perfection. Home might feel like a place where you watch the seasons change or watch people change in ways that are almost unrecognizable. But, I don't think home is any of these things. These things are just a result of everything that my grandmother poured into her home because of her love for her family. It is the care and attention she gave to those around her, even at expense of herself. We and everything we had the benefit of all came from her. So for me, home is the gentleness of my grandmother's presence, a softness that is shadowed by more intelligence, strength, and power than ever exuded. Home is her unwavering class, grace and style. Home is the sharing of our experiences, her desire to teach me, and her willingness to learn in the process. I have grown by many years and traveled many miles but I have never left my home or the safety and comfort she provides.

—Julia C. Neely
Brown

As I Know Elaine

A devoted wife and caring mother! Has always been to me a real inspiration , urging me on by faith and friendship. Provided guidance and a listening ear. Possessed dignity, character and strength. Possessed a passion for authentics and books. "A fine Christian woman whose virtues have not enveloped her head in the clouds, but who has ever kept the common touch."

-Rob（Robbie Neely Jones）

"My friendship with Mrs. Elaine Neely has spanned over fifty years. She is a true friend, who is resourceful and has a regal and cooperative spirit. She has great leadership qualities which I have witnessed in various church and community activities. I specifically remember our days in The Ladies Waymakers Auxiliary where she coordinated and compiled our cookbook for sale to fund a summer camp for children. She got the job done in outstanding fashion and style! Elaine has been a gift to me and the entire Tupelo community. I am blessed to be her friend."

-Dorothy Townsend

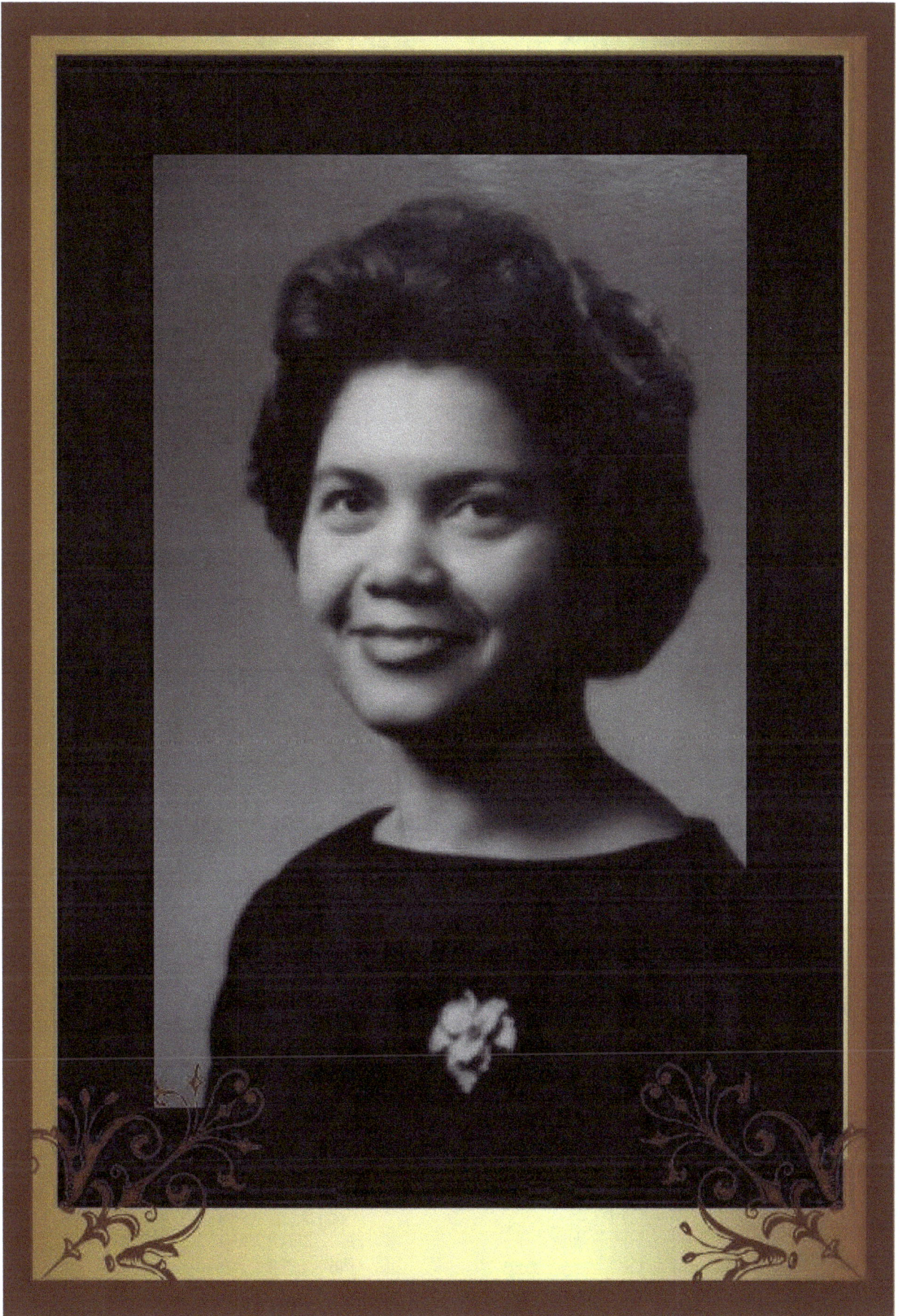

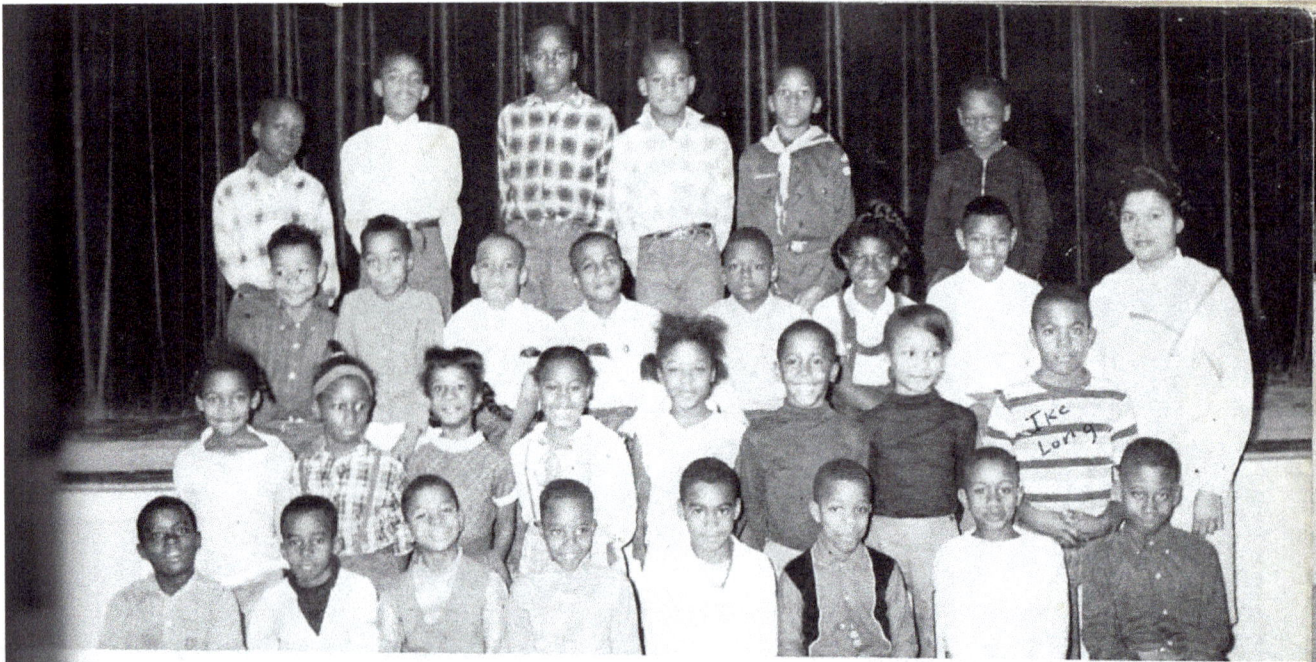

THIRD GRADE DIVISION III   MRS. E. NEELY, Instructor

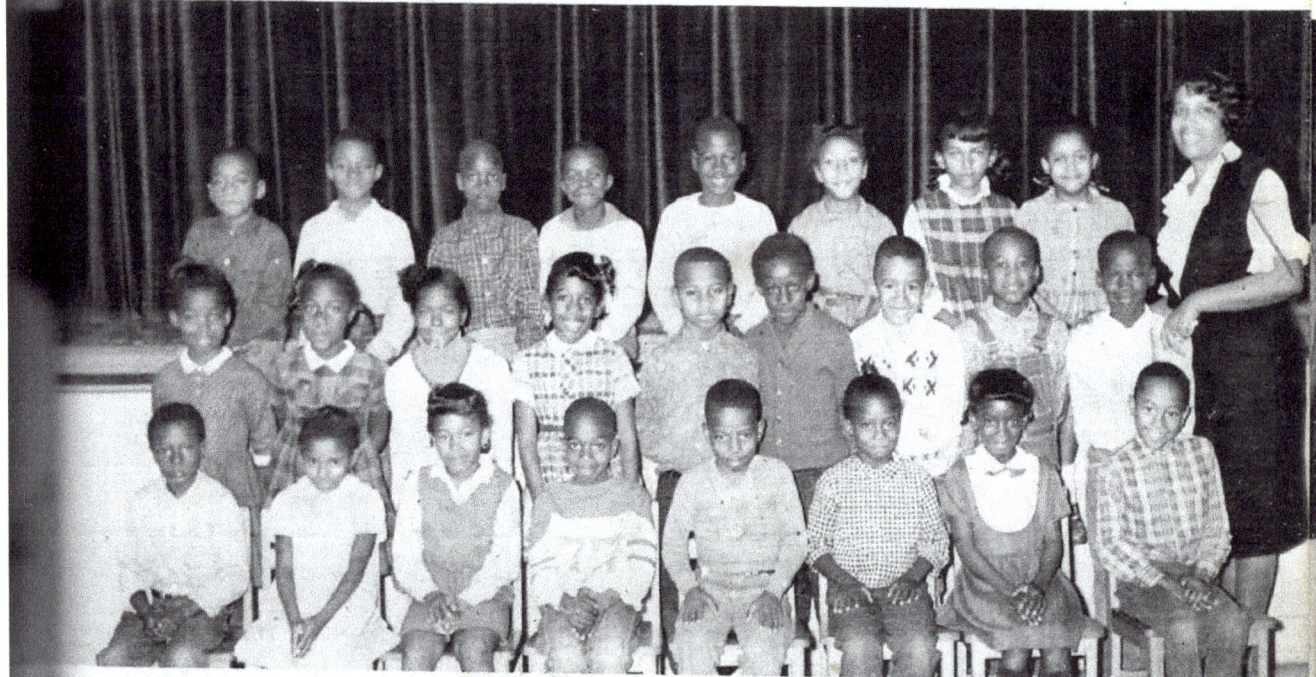

SECOND GRADE DIVISION I   MRS. E. C. FOSTER, Instructor

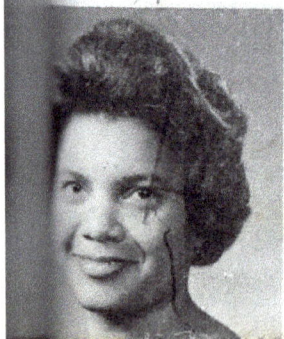

MRS. E. NEELY
B.S., Lane College
Jackson, Tenn.

MRS. F. C. FOSTER
B.S., Rust College
Holly Springs, Miss.

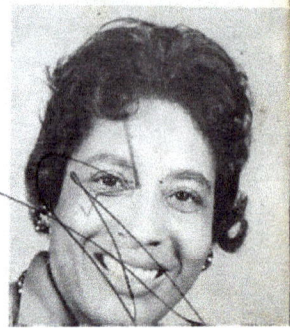

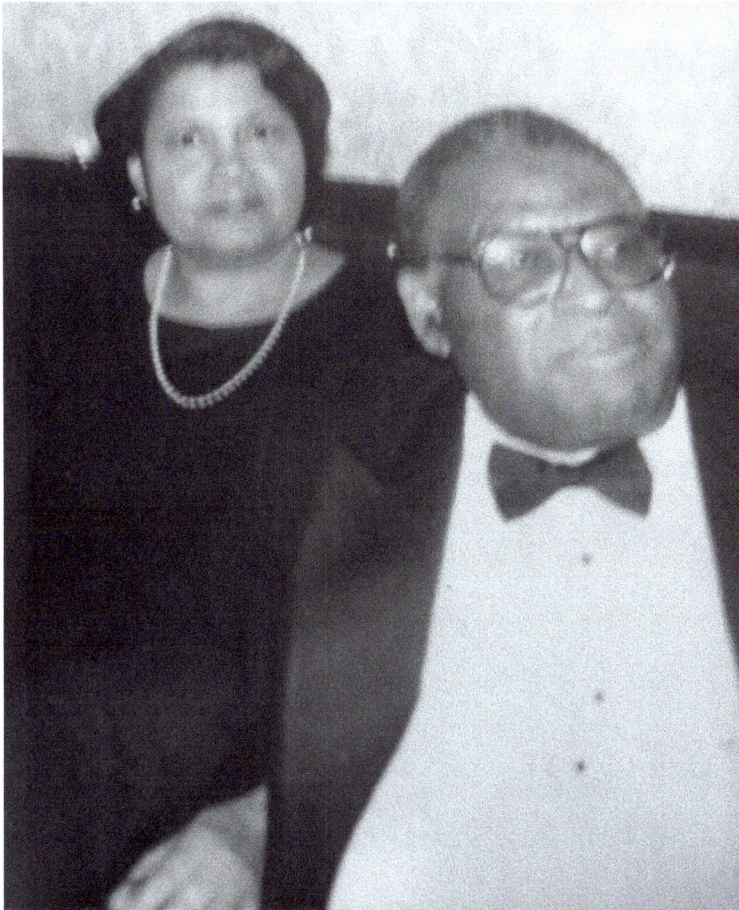
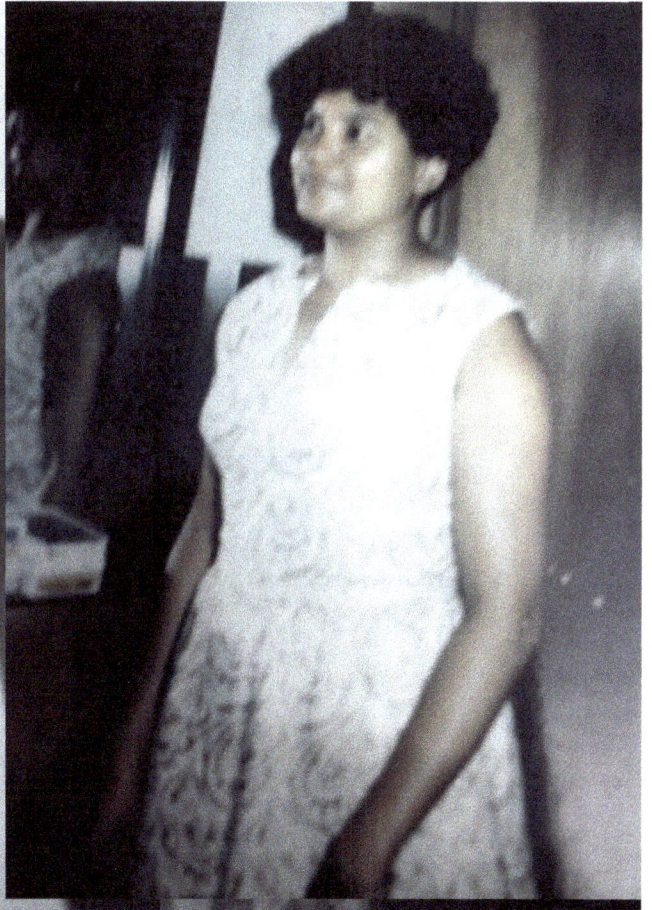
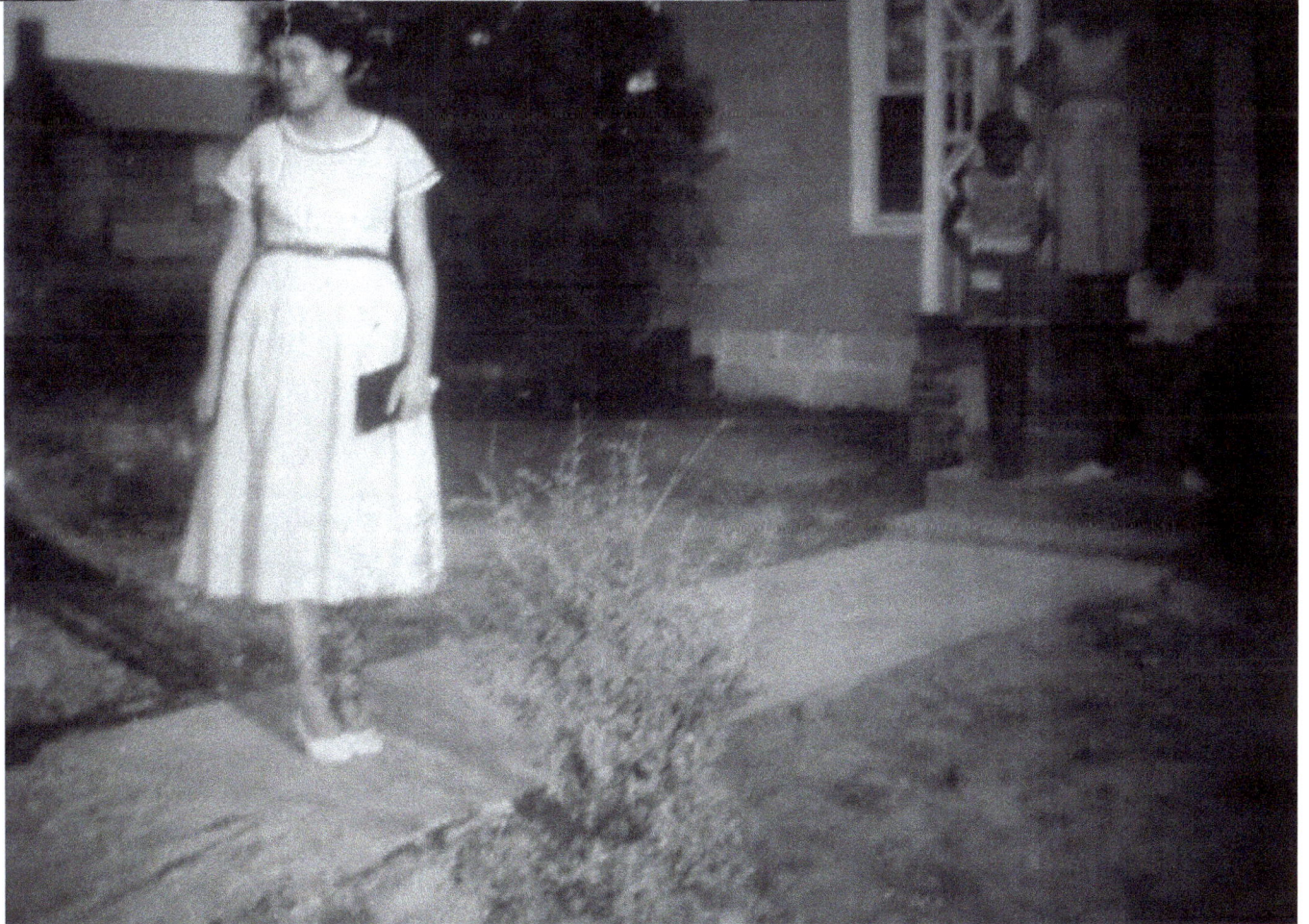

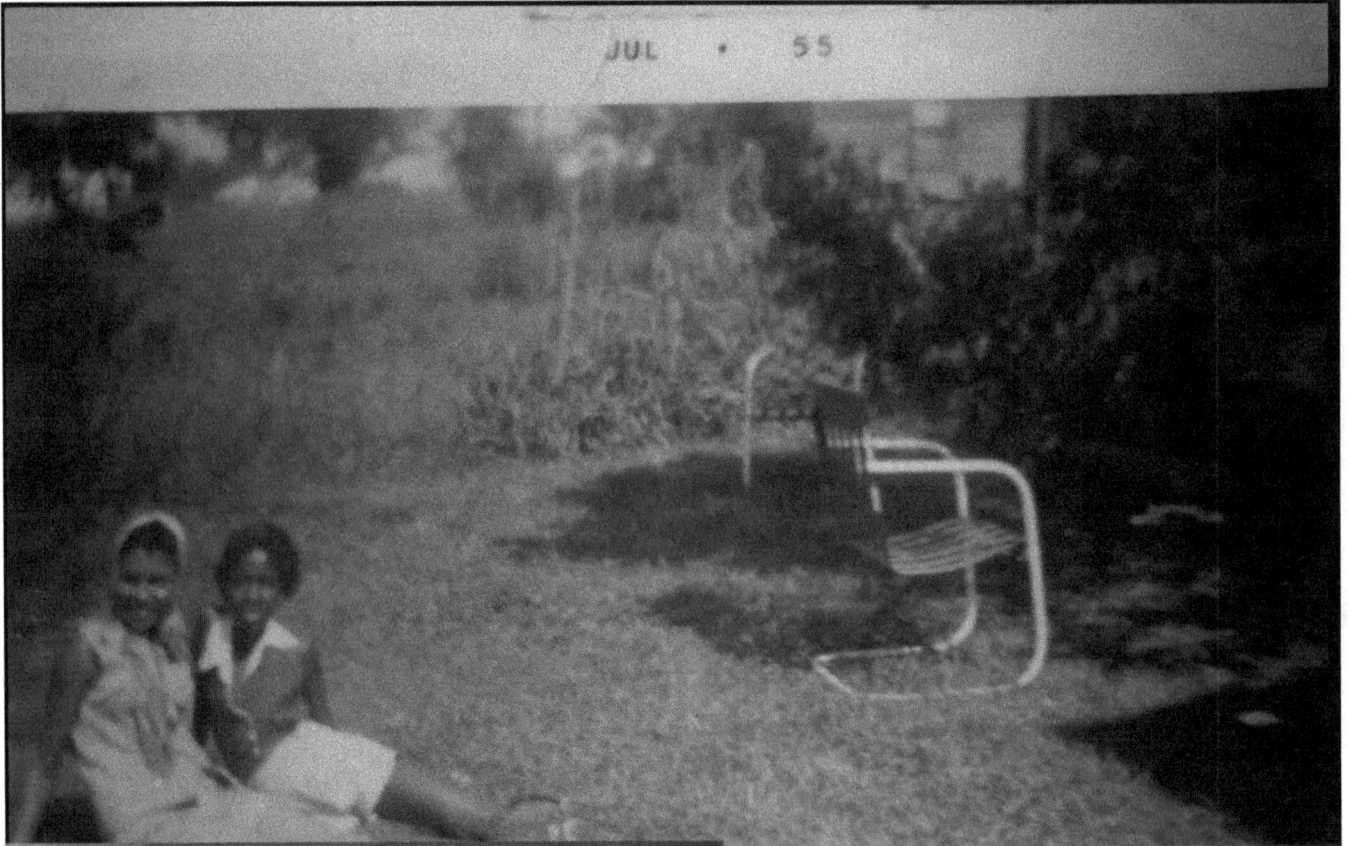

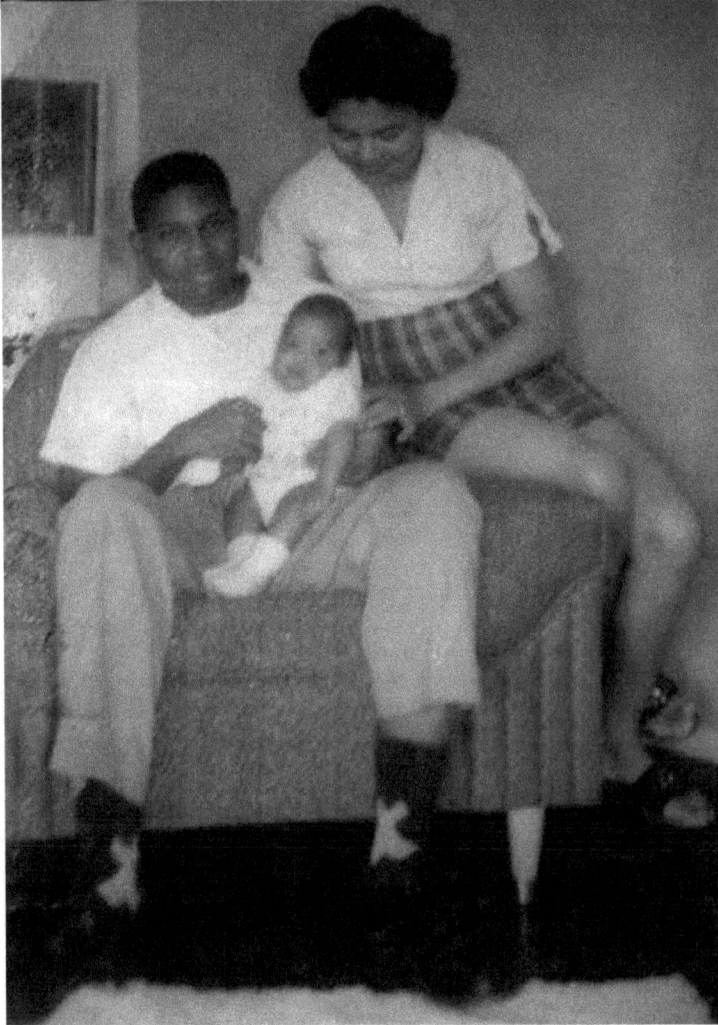

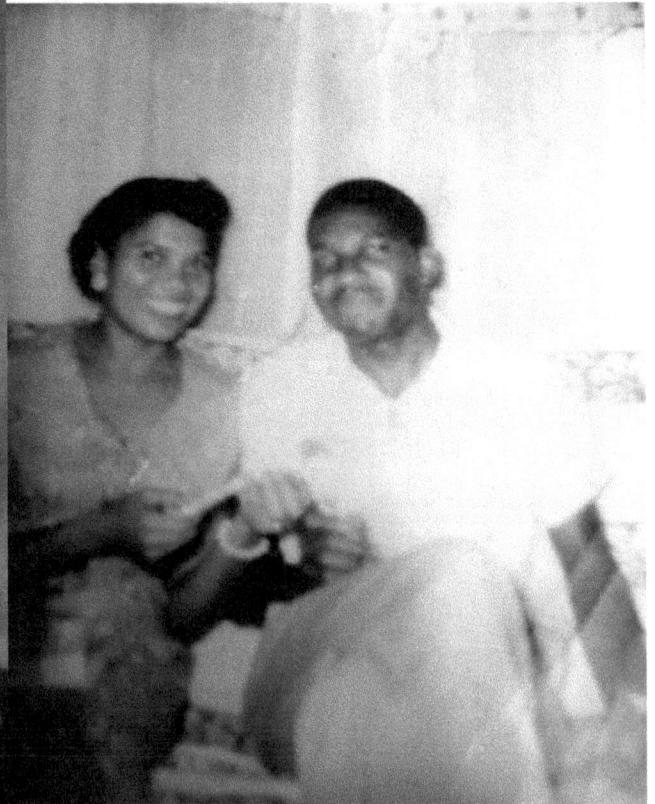

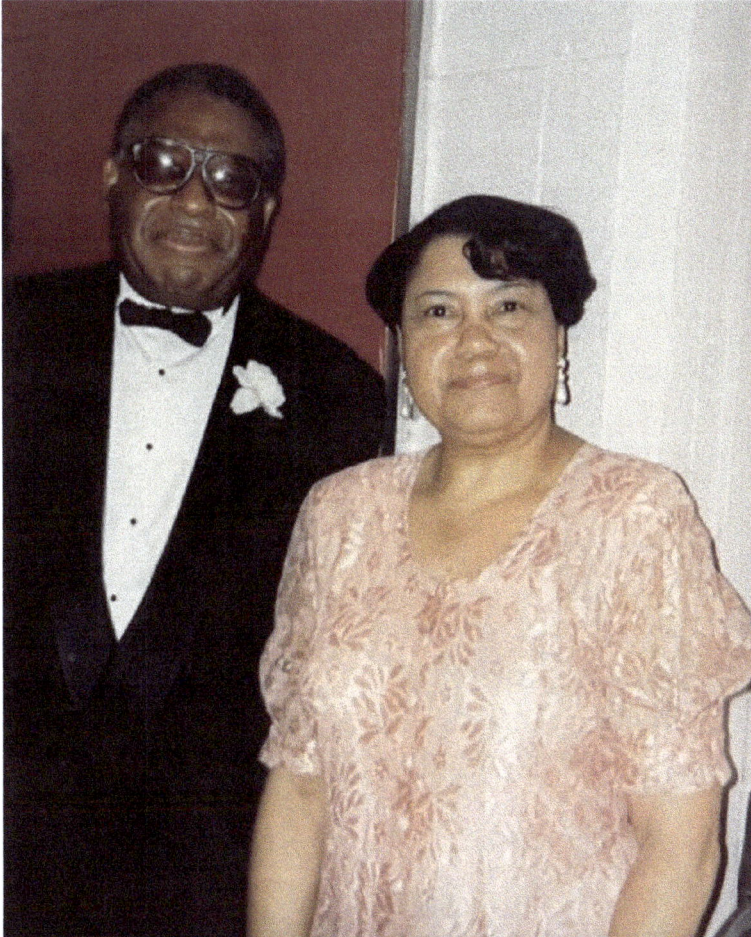
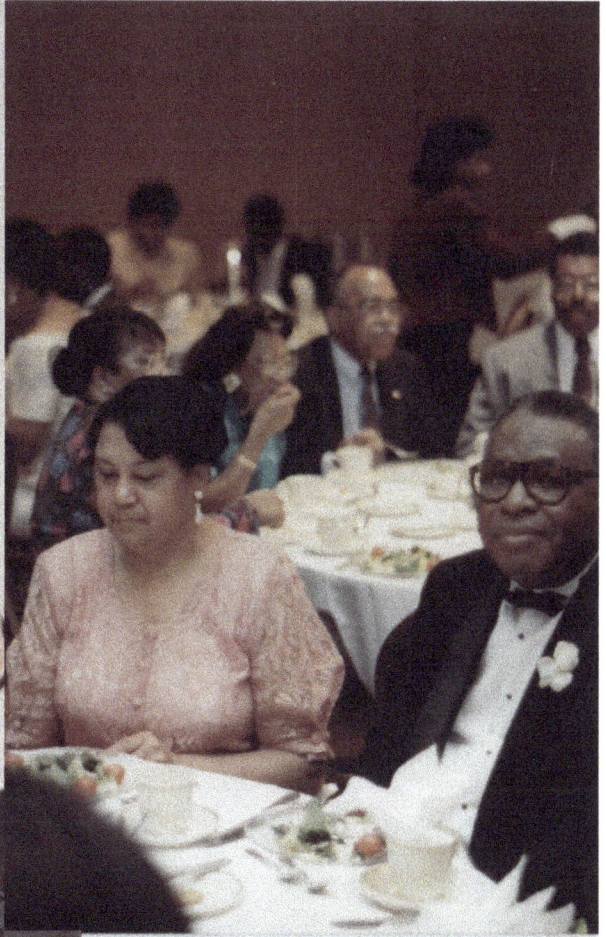
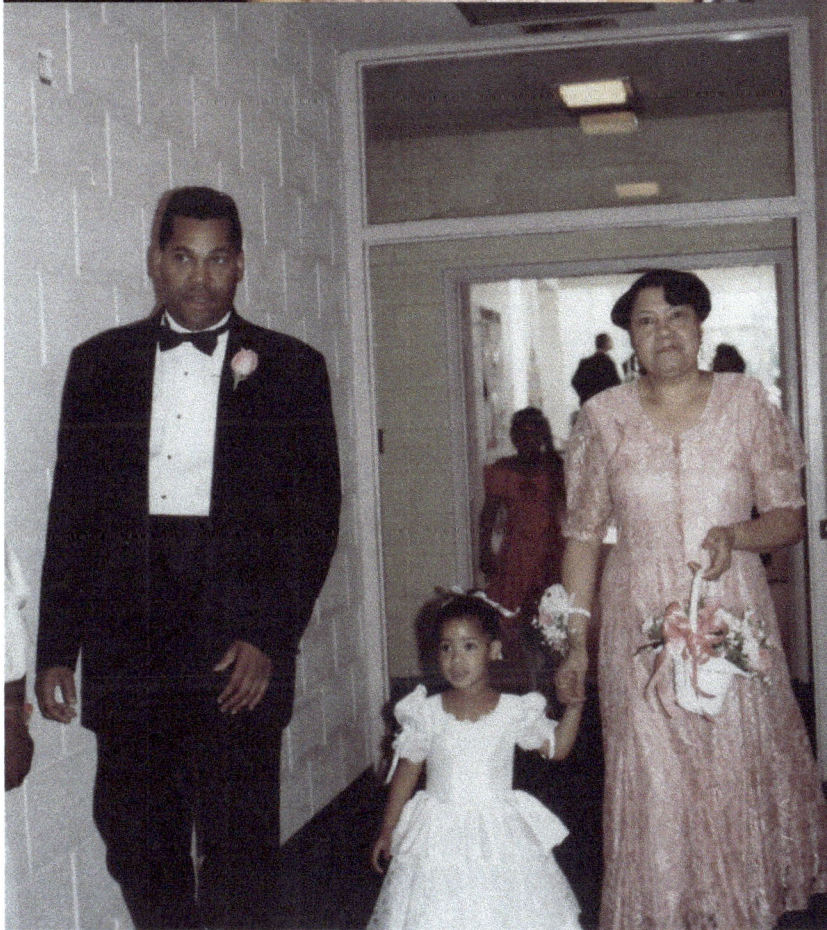
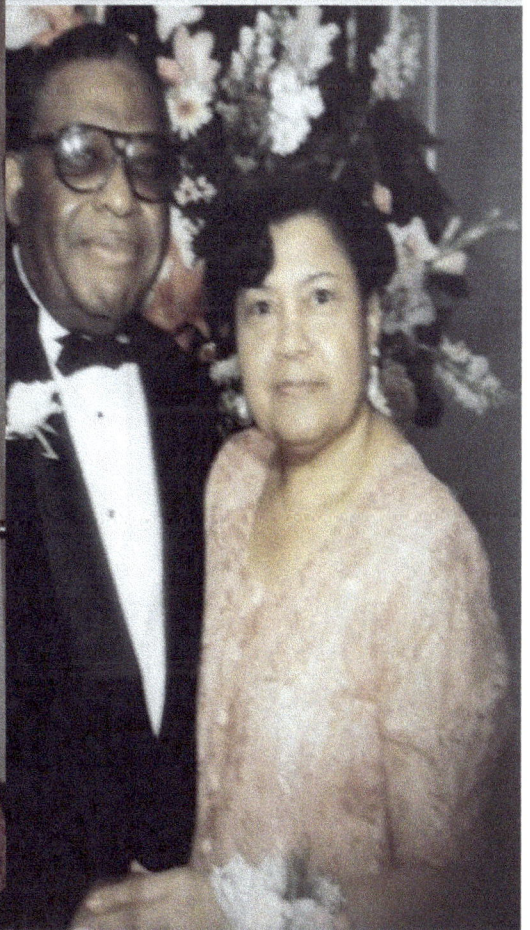

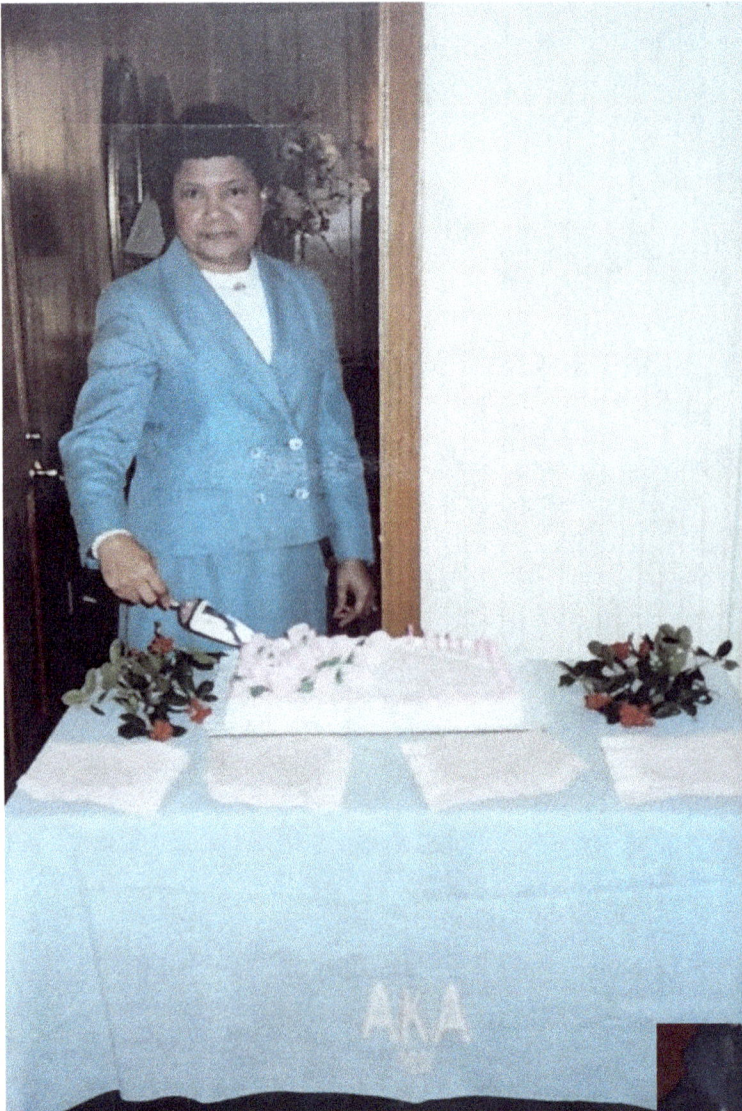

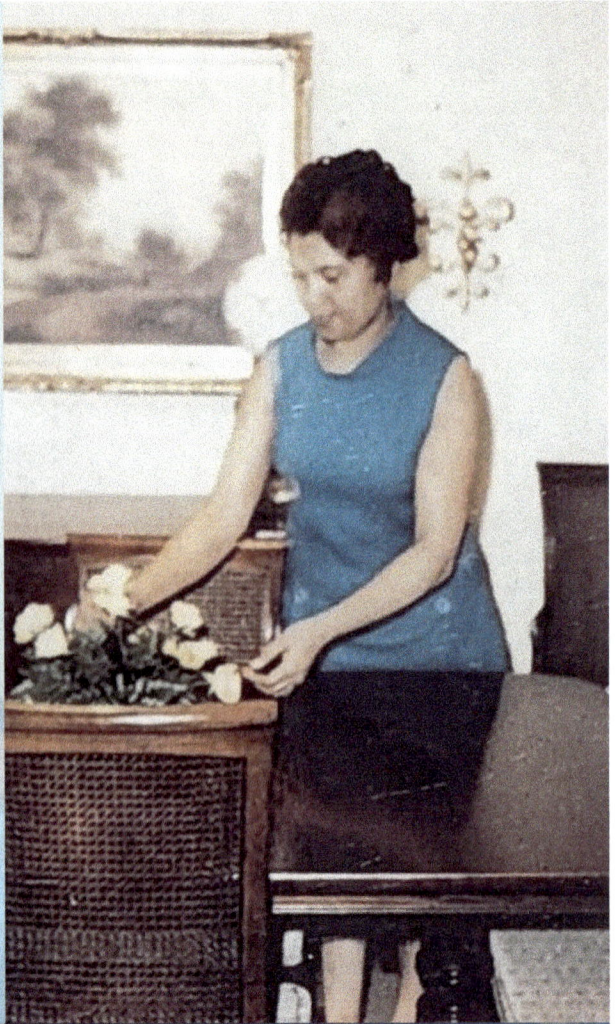

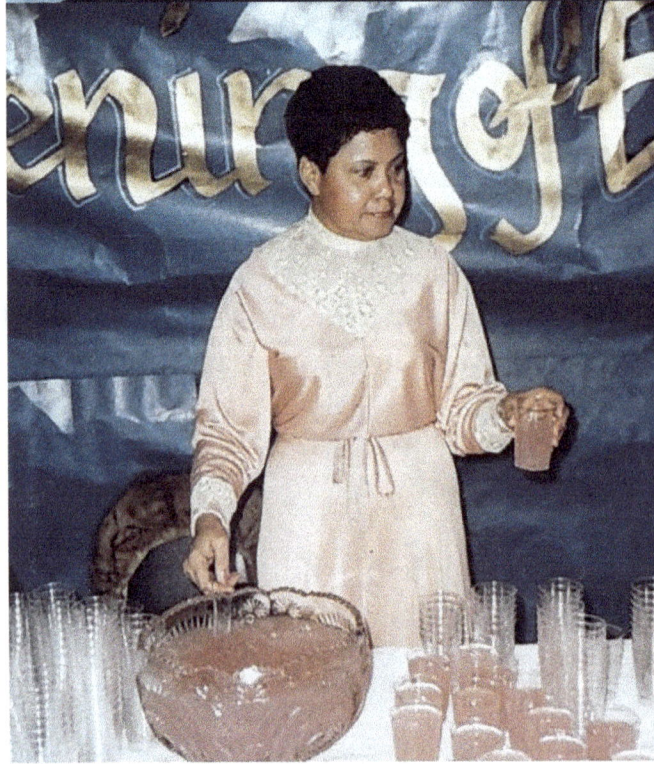

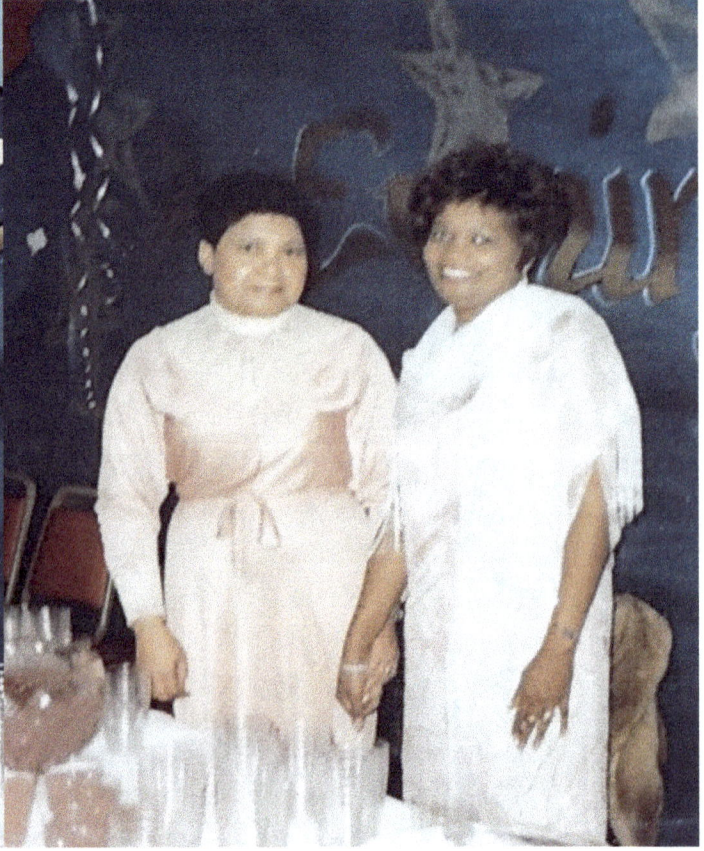

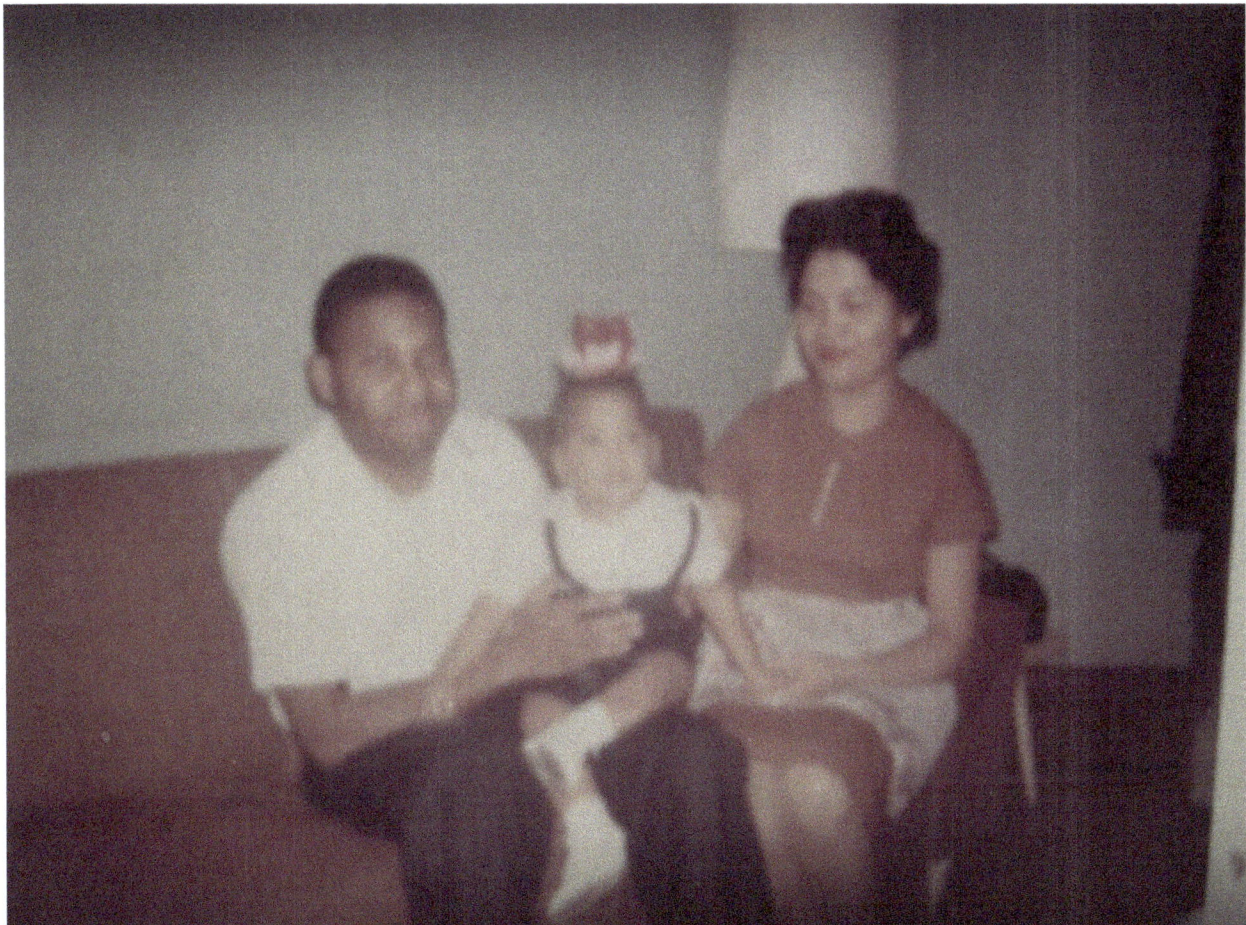

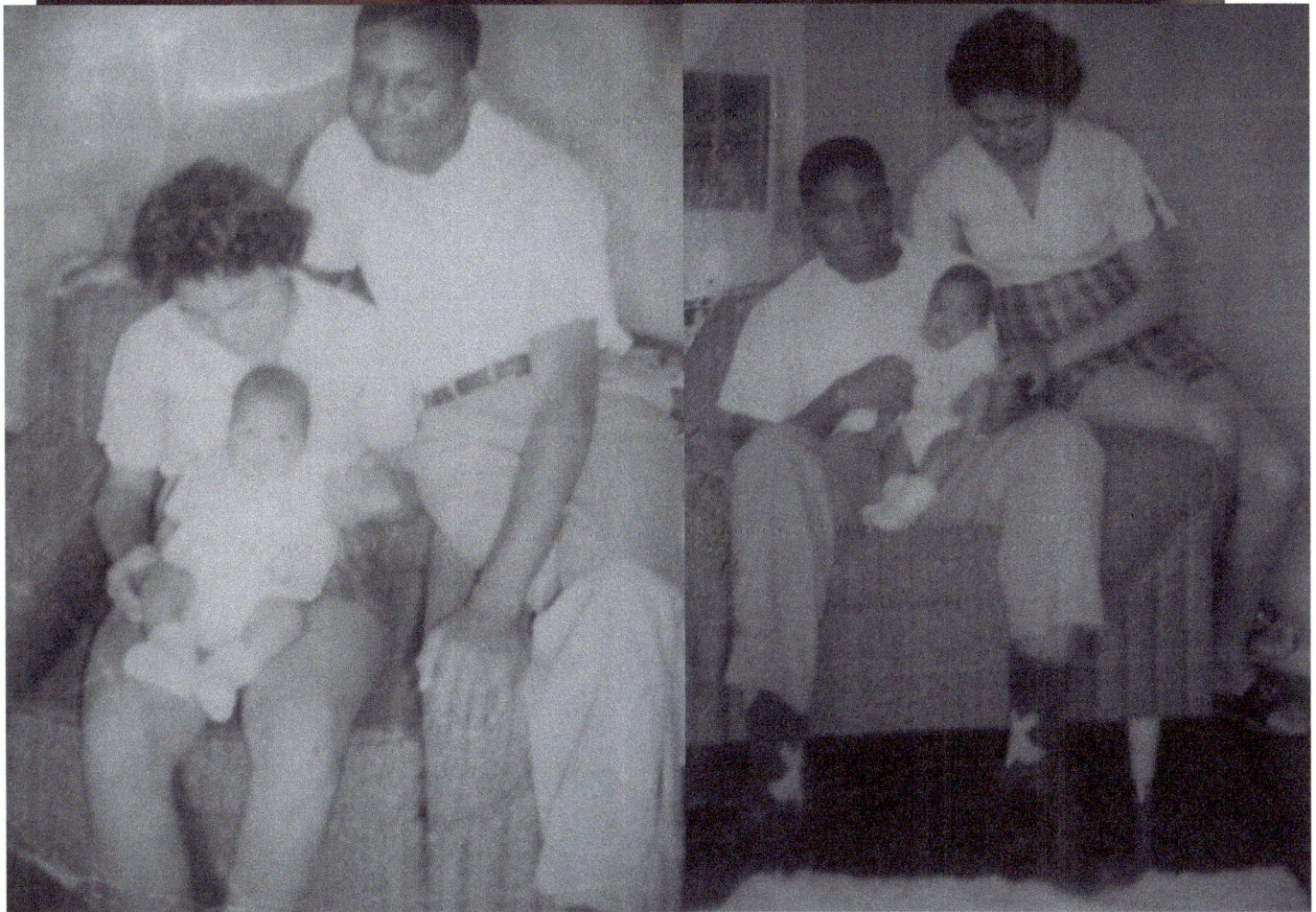

Mom and Dad with Brian

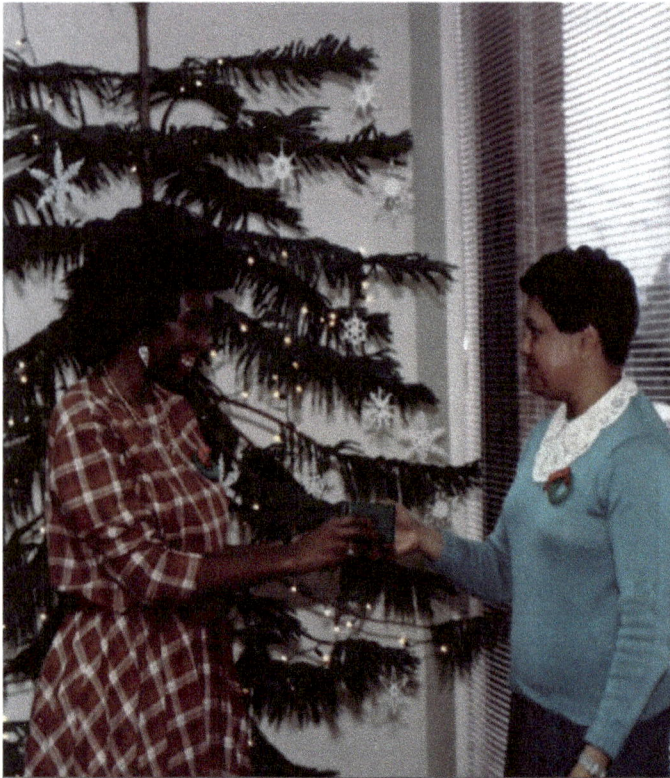

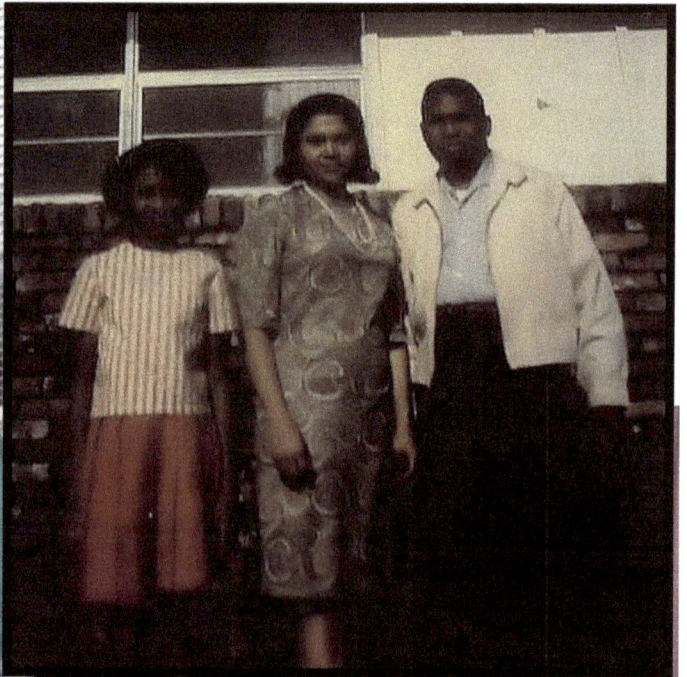

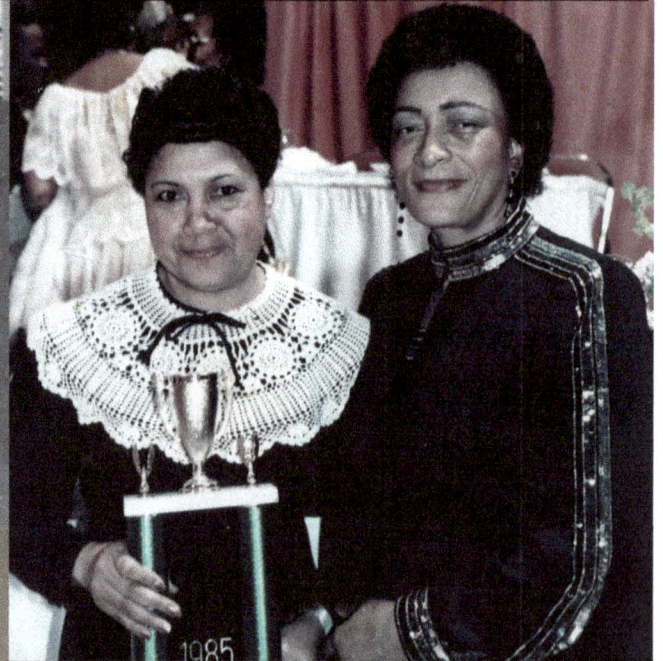

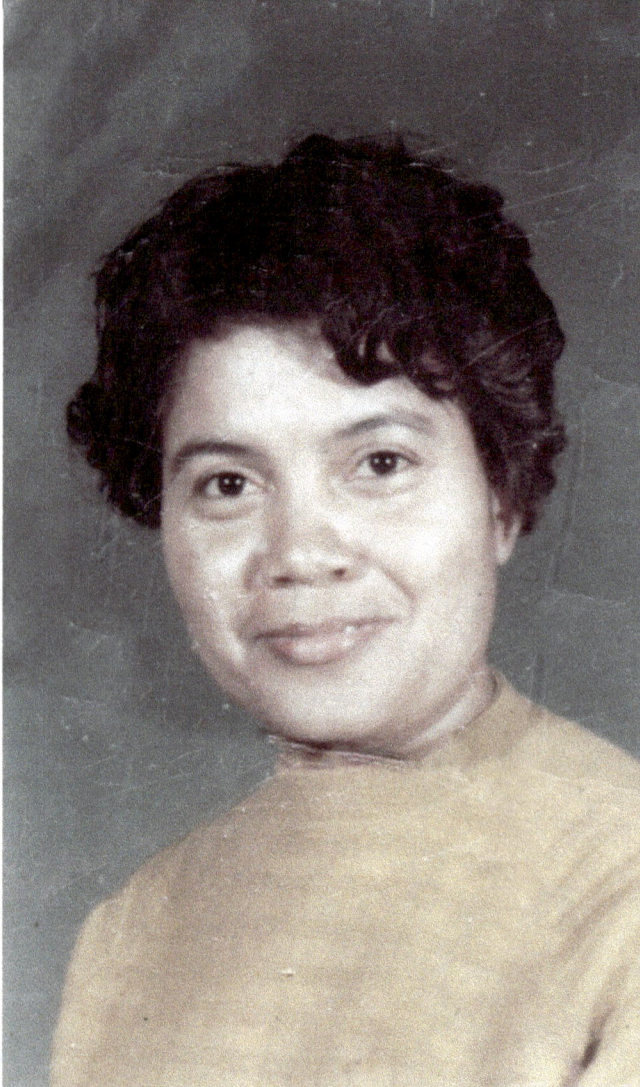

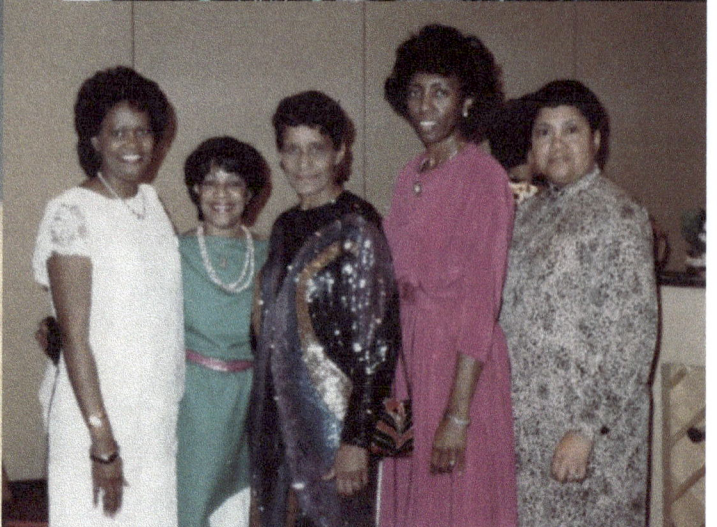

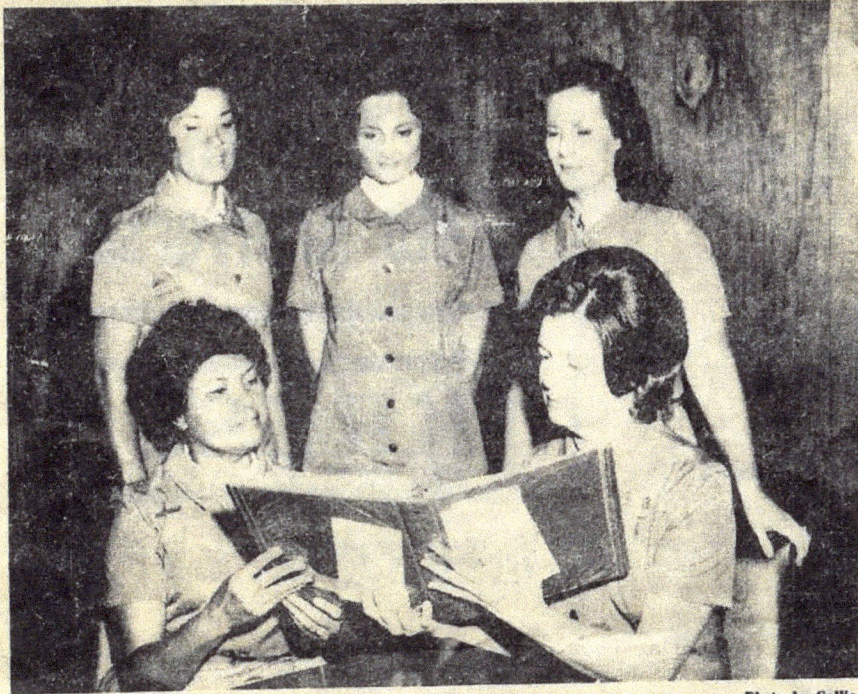

Daily Journal, Tupelo, Mississippi, Thursday Morning, August 15, 1974

Photo by Sallis

SCOUT ORGANIZERS MEET --Organizers for Girl Scout Troops of the Tupelo Neighborhood met Wednesday in the home of Mrs. Charles Moore, chairman, to make plans for the new Scout year. They are, front, from left, Mrs. James Neely, Green Street School; Mrs. James W. McCarty, Thomas Street; back, from left, Mrs. Ralph Holland, Church Street; Mrs. Wayne Washington, Lawhon; Mrs. Charles Moore, Milam Cadettes. The organizers recruit new leaders and place girls in troops. Other organizers not in picture are Mrs. James McKinney, Joyner; Mrs. Donald Green, Rankin; Mrs. Lea Pasley, Pierce Street.

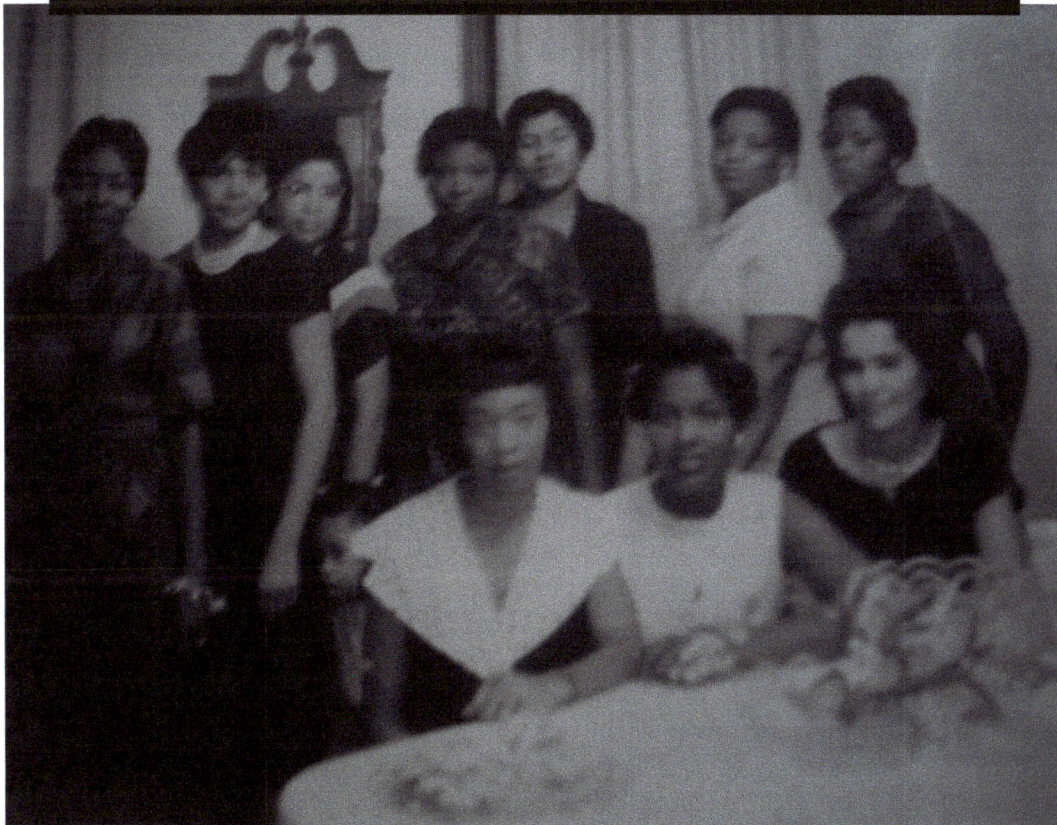

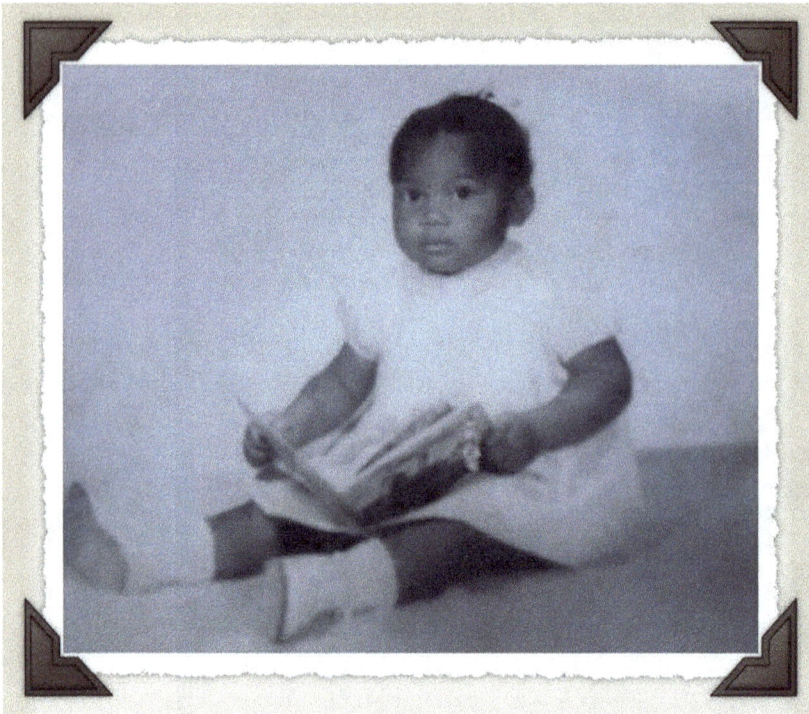

Always a reader!!! My mom said the book was one of the photographer's props and I started crying because I didn't want to give it back!! I also took a picture with a ball and some other things that day. But of course I was obsessed with the book !!!! Mom had a portrait of my brother done in a little blue shorts jumper when he was about the same age. I had on a pink dress and she had the photographer colorize it to have me in a blur dress that matched my brother's picture .

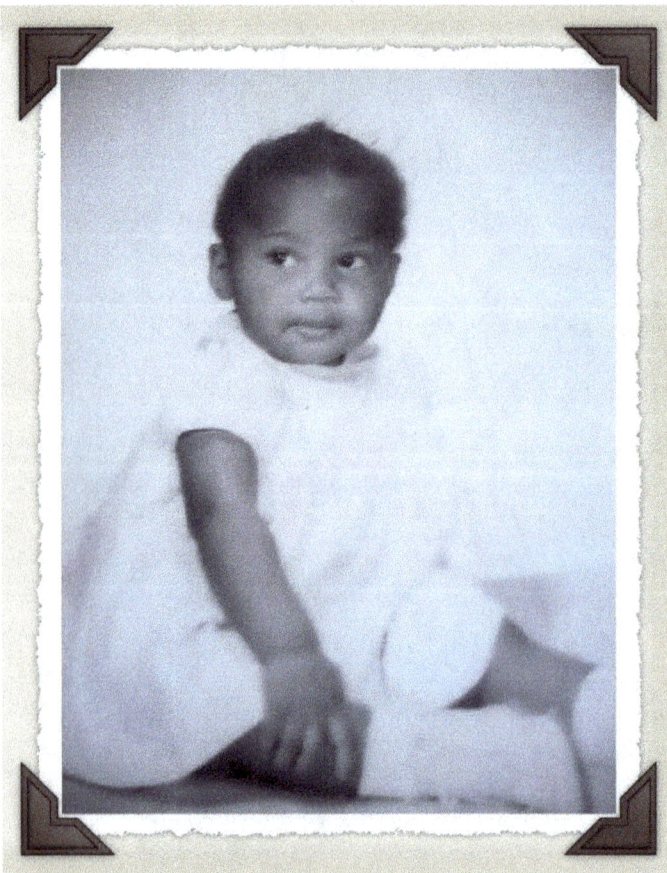

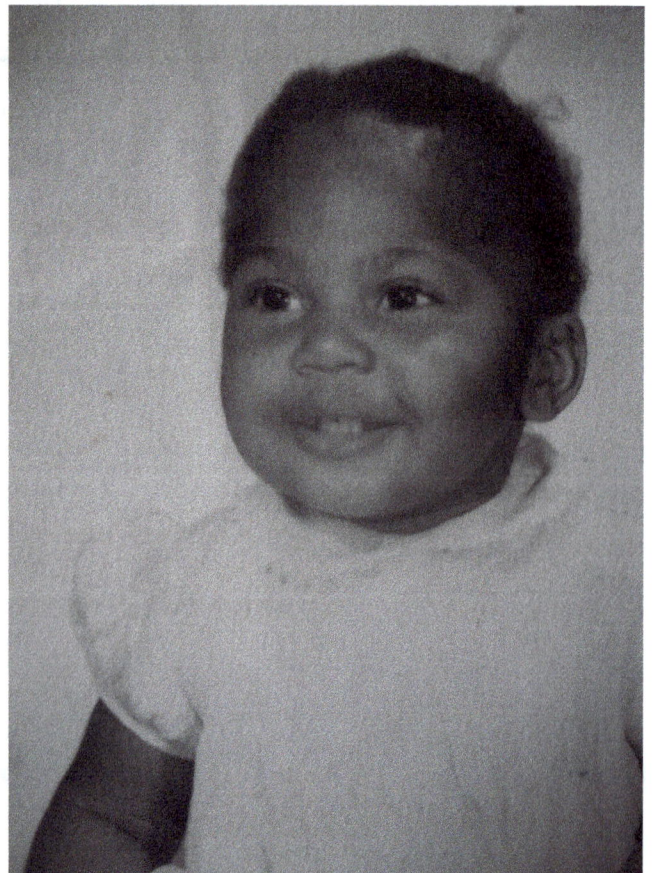

My mother often talks about how her fondest childhood memories were before the age of six. (pre-school years) She also comments on how vivid these memories are. She says that she remembers them like they were yesterday. This is the same for me. So many of the poems about childhood in my first book of poems, Reflections of Mississippi Magnolia-A Life In Poems, were memories from my pre-school years. All of the sights and sounds, conversations and activities flood my memories, almost as though they are not distant memories at all, but rather recollections of things that might have taken place only days ago. I don't think that I have a photographic memory in the truest scientific sense of the word, But, I must say that I know it comes very , very close. I once wrote that the poems were snapshots (pictures in poems) of my daily life growing up. I see every details of those days in bright , vivid detail and easily able to transfer them to paper. In fact, my subconscious mind did all of that for me .

As I wrote in the foreword of my first book, I never intentionally sat down to write any of the poems. They basically came to me totally packaged (fully formed) like a gift, with title and all. I would just write them down. I woke up on February 14, 2007 with a poem swirling around in my head. I woke up and scribbled it down. After that that the poems started to flow and flow.

In a few months, I had hundreds of poems. One of my most vivid childhood memories was of Carver band marching down Green Street on game days , just to give the community " a show". We would hear the drums beating, almost like a bell signaling everyone to gather , because gather they did. The shop owners would basically shut down their businesses (there were many all along Green Street) and everyone congregated on the sidewalks and all along the street to watch Carver march through. I always had one of the best seats. My lifelong friend, Verner Parlow (Wilson) lived on Green Street and there were steps in front of her house, coming up from the sidewalk. We were able to comfortably sit and have a wonderful view perched on those steps. This memory is probably is so vivid because there was so much fanfare associated with it. Before integration so many of the activities in the black community, in Tupelo, centered around Carver. So, whenever they did something (anything), the whole community basically participated and celebrated.

Partlow's Band

Though technically
It was Carver High School Band,
To one man it belonged;
If you thought that there was any other rule
They you'd be sorely wrong.
On game days we all knew
The band would give a show
From the school, they'd make their start
And down Green Street They would go.
First we'd hear those mighty drums,
And then the marching feet;
The anticipation was so great,
As crowds lined along the street.
The majorettes were a sight to see
In glittering and gold;
And little Gwen who led the say was maybe 9 years old

With batons twirling in the air,
And tassels wagging on their feet;
There was always a special show
For each corner crowd they'd meet
Each girl was stacked and built
Not a one of was boney
They'd twist and turn and prance about,
And Gwen would do "The Pony."
Mr. Partlow with head held high,
Would walk along the side;
He'd strut like some male peacock,
With confidence and pride.
Mr. Partlow has passed away,
But history does repeat;
His son's Partlow's Drummers carry the torch
With each resounding beat.

Another very vivid memory that I have is all of the programs and activities that we had in "our" little library, A M Strange Library on North Green Street. I recall so many fun days in that place. Of course, there was just the simple joy of visiting the library, reading and checking out books. There were cub scout meetings there , which I often tagged along, because mom was a Cub Scout leader for a while. There were girl scout meeting there, and mom was also a Girl Scout leader for a while. There were summer reading programs , of course. The main librarian during my childhood was Mrs. Vaughn. She was the sweetest person that you could ever want to meet. She was also one of Mom's very close friends and we spent many days at her home. They talked and visited and I would read or watch tv. I always remember that.

AM STRANGE LIBRARY (picture below) · North Green Street Cub Scout Meeting Bursting the Pinata (I was between 5-6 years old) Pictures always bring back SO many memories!!! One of them was that I was ALWAYS hanging with the fellows ! My mother was the cub scout leader and I was always at their activities ! When I got older and my bother was driving, Mama always made him pick me up from night time events and activities. He hated it !! LOL!! Of course he had his whole crew with him ...and again..hanging with the guys !

Every time we pass the little (once) AM Strange Library building on Green Street , Hubby always says, that building is so small, it couldn't have had a full library in it or many books. I am always telling him. It was ! It did! It was all of that for us! He is amazed (or befuddled) when I so excitedly tell him how there were hundreds of books lining every wall , tables and chairs in the middle and in the left corner was the children's section, librarians' desk and bathroom I have SUCH fond memories of this place! Years later, my love for reading and this little library came full circle when I was asked by Orlando Purnell to coordinate a summer reading program through CDF. It was a tremendous success!

I wrote about is having a "Double Life" growing up. Like the story of the city mouse and country mouse , I had two very distinct set of experiences. I had a set of "city friends" and activities and a set of "country" friends. and activities. Dad had his office in "town" (Dr. Neely's Office North Spring Street) and Mom had many associations and activities in" town". Mom would mostly purchase her groceries at Cherry Street Grocery off of Barnes Street and often at Asby's Grocery. I loved the big bin of penny cookies and all of the candy behind the counter. Apple sticks were my favorite! Some-times Mr Burress would deliver the groceries to the house. I remember being in the sand-box playing and seeing his truck come up the long driveway. I would get super excited be-cause I knew that he would have a little brown bag folded and stapled oh so neat-ly,filled with candy, for me and Brian. Anoth-er person who always brought us a little treat was Mr. Bo Traylor. He kept our yard oh so meticulously! He would often come twice a week in the summertime. Every week he would always bring a pack of Wrigley's gum for me and for Brian. Brian got Juicy Fruit and I loved Doublemint.

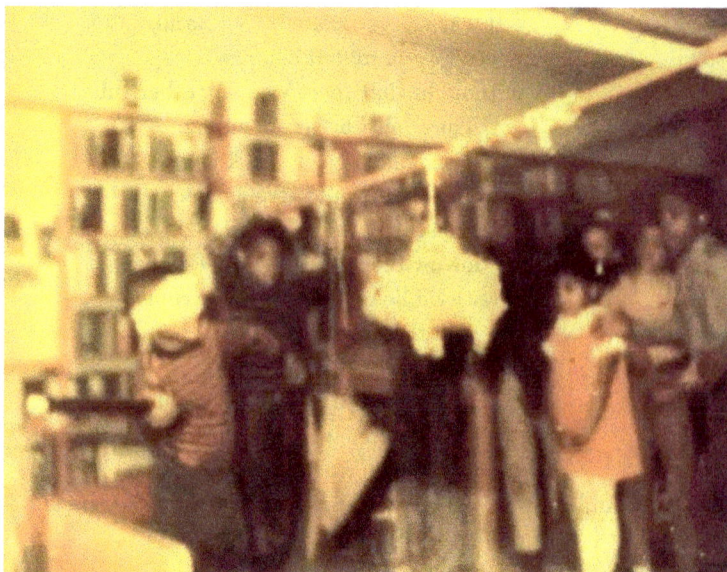

DOUBLE LIFE

I grew up as a country girl.
But, I had my city friends;
The activities of my daily life,
On which side it would depend.
With the country crew, I was a no shoe girl,
With hair wild upon my head;
I'd run and play and make mud pies,
Until I went to bed.
There were chickens and cows, goats and pigs,
Animals all around;
And somehow, everything we did ,
Was connected with the ground.
We'd root around in the garden,
And go fishing in the pond;
We'd pick wild berries on the path ,
And have all kinds of fun.
We'd walk along the dusty roads,
And eat the red clay dirt;
In the country , we always knew,
A little dirt could never hurt.
But, then, on the city side
We'd mostly do house things;
We'd play with Barbies and paper dolls,
Or try on sparkly rings.
We'd play games or watch t.v.
Or walk along the street;
We might go to the corner store
To find some sugary treats .
I truly had a double life,
That's plain for all to see;
It was a unique way of life,
But one so right for me.

2008 Patricia Neely-Dorsey

SHELLING PEAS

It's summertime in the country,
And the kids buzz around like bees;
But, when that silver tub is placed on the porch,
It's time for shelling peas.
From the smallest to the oldest,
It's something we'd all do;
At first, of course, the little ones,
Didn't have a clue.
They'd watch to see just how it went,
And soon , they'd give a try;
Then look amazed as fingers stained,
As though dipped in purple dye.
When we'd first get started,
It seemed an insurmountable chore;
There looked like half a million peas,
Or maybe even more.
But, after we all got the flow,
We'd turn it into fun;
We'd have a race to see just who
Would be the first one done.
We'd each one have our own bowl,
and a paper sack;
We's slip our fingers through the hull,
Then throw it empty back.
At last, when all the shells lay empty,
And a tub of peas was done;
We'd let the grownups take the haul,
Then look for some new fun.

2008 Patricia Neely-Dorsey

NEIGHBORHOOD GROCERIES

Asby's Mayhorn's Cherry Street
Pickled Souse
Rag Bologna
Liver Cheese
Dill Pickles In A Jar
Penny Cookies
Coconut
Chocolate Chip
And Butter
Stage Planks
Moon Pies
Apple Sticks
Tootsie Rolls
Point out what you want
Behind the glass.
Service with a smile.
Home folks you know.

Patricia Neely-Dorsey

GOING TO TOWN

Making the rounds
And stopping in
Or Passing by
Marlin Cook
Ben Franklin
Kuhn's "Kent's
Kermit's Bakery
Pryor's
McGaughy's and Scheinbergs
Reed's , Westbrook's Black's
Two Sisters
And of course
The Corner Shoe Store
We'd always make a day of it
Going to town.

2012 Patricia Neely-Dorsey

A.M. STRANGE LIBRARY

That little one room library
On North Green Street
Held a special place in our hearts.
It was our neighborhood place to go
For story hours , book reviews
And exposure to the arts.
We'd sit at the little tables
Or form circles on the floor
Mrs Vaughn , our wonderful librarian
Was so soft-spoken , kind and sweet;
With a warm smile and welcoming voice
Each child there she would greet.
To many of us bookworms,
It's where we got our start;
And to my childhood loving of reading,
It played an integral part .

2012 Patricia Neely-Dorsey

LANDMARKS
"Can you tell me how to get to..."
Yeah you know...
You go past the bridge and Lockridge store
Henderson's Cleaners, Carver School, The Daily
Bar,
Asby's Mayhorn's Debro's,
Tolbert's Funeral Home, Springhill Church, The
Graveyard andThe Tank
Turn up there by Lane Chapel and Brown's Cleaners
It's down from Vaughn's Motel, Ms. Herbine's
Nursery,
Dr. Neely's Office and The Dixie Bell Around from
the R.C Plant and Grayson's
Across the tracks
Over by the Packing House
You know....
"Yeah, I know where that is ...
I think. "

Patricia Neely-Dorsey

THE RULES

Most southern folks have rules we're taught ,
From when we're very young;
And most of us throughout our lives
To these rules have clung.
Life can be much easier
When you know what to do or not;
And you're sure to learn a lot of them
If southern parents' you have got .
One of the first rules you come to know is
Children are to be seen and not heard ;
It's best if you sit down somewhere
Quietly as a bird .
You always say "Please " when you're asking ,
And "Thank You" when you receive;
You address all your elders as
"Ma'am" or "Sir",
And if you don't do it you'll grieve.
Don't touch anything in the store,
Keep your hands to yourself; If it's not something
you plan to buy,
Leave it soundly on the shelf .
Always say good morning , Soon after you awake;
And always greet people pleasantly,
If friends you are to make. Don't slam a door as you
walk out,
You don't live in a barn;"
You'd better close it gently.
Is what they's always warn.
If you open a cabinet or anything, Always close it
back; Once you do it repeatedly,
You'll always have the knack.
Don't call someone before 8 a.m.
Of after ten at night :
If it's something you feel you must do ,
It's an urge that you must fight.
Never ask for food when you visit,
Although the host may ask;
Sometimes it's best if you decline , And let the moment pass.
These are just a very few of the things, We Southerners are taught;
Without some rule for every occasion, We are never caught .
2008 Patricia Neely -Dorsey

RIDING THE BUS

One of the fondest memories of our school days
Had to be riding the bus
I'm sure that all of my friends will agree
It was quite fun for all of us
Early every morning
We'd walk out to the road
We'd stand around all chatting
'Til it was time to load
Mr. Townsend our bus driver
Would flash that great big smile
And lovingly talk of his daughter Patrice
Along each and every mile
The ride was often bumpy
And we kids were exceptionally loud
A dozen or so of us together
Sounded like some roaring crowd.
During school elections,
We'd try to solicit votes;
But mostly we just giggled,
And passed our little notes.
When we neared the school house doors
We'd say our quick goodbyes
And gather up all of our things
Then, from our seats all slide

Patricia Neely-Dorsey

UNDERSTOOD
Growing Up...
We all knew
THE Store
THE Corner
THE Shortcut
THE Hiding Place
THE Candy Lady
and ...
The Rules

2012 Patricia Neely-Dorsey

NURSERY SCHOOL

I loved the walks that we took around the neighborhood. We were always greeted with friendly faces and waves from people that we knew and that knew us. That was pretty much everyone. Sometimes , I wished I could just go to my Daddy's office to stay. It was just down the street at 608 North Spring Street. We passed it every time that we went out. One day we walked all the way up to Page's Grocery Store which was outside of our usual parameter. That was a big deal and a huge thrill. One day we took a field trip to the Royal Crown Bottling Company which was at the end of the street across from Grayson's funeral home. We were taken on a tour throughout the plant and received a bottle of soda when we left. The building is now the location of The Mayfield Law Firm and has been for many years.

I loved story time when we were read excerpts from a book each day. The one that I loved the most was a red leather bound book The Little Brown Bear. I looked forward to hearing about the little brown bear every day. I had my mom look everywhere to find it or me. She finally did. I wore tights one day and kept picking at them for some reason and by the middle of the day, I had a big hole in them . I was so upset. and embarrassed. I cried a lot about it that day. Of course at the end of the day when Mom picked me up, she calmed me down and let me know that something like that is no big deal. (I really could have just taken them off,

I loved watching Sesame Street . It was a new show at that time and very exciting! It debuted in 1969. So, we were among the first group of preschoolers to see it. I learned a lot from the show. I think my favorites were Bert and Ernie. Mom would bring me a new book every Friday as my gift for the week. During that time she got me a set of Sesame Street Alphabet books that came out weekly at the grocery store. She gave me a whole set of Sesame Street books one at a time. I was an adult before I knew that a Mississippian , Jim Henson, was the creator of the Sesame Street Muppets. That would have been something amazing to know , a that time.

I remember the presentation by a community group of Patch The Pony. We saw the film and learned the song about staying away from strangers. His name is Patch the Pony . He says Nay, Nay from strangers stay away. We were given little badges and coloring books. One year, probably, 1968 or 1969 ,we were chosen as the photo for the Grayson Funeral Home calendar. (which was located right down the street on the corner) We went outside on the front sidewalk and took the picture. I am still in search of that calendar. It was so exciting for the graduating class each year to get to go upstairs to Ms Herbine's house to practice our parts for graduation. We each had some little line to say at graduation. The ultimate thrill was graduation night when we got to wear our white caps and gowns and receive our diplomas on the stage at the big school, Carver. I loved that diploma SO much ! It was so colorful and had pictures depicting all of the .nursery rhymes all around the border of the diploma. I don't know what happened to it and still long to find it! Mrs Herbine Reese was very sweet and kind. She was all about teaching us to have good manners and knowing "how to act" !

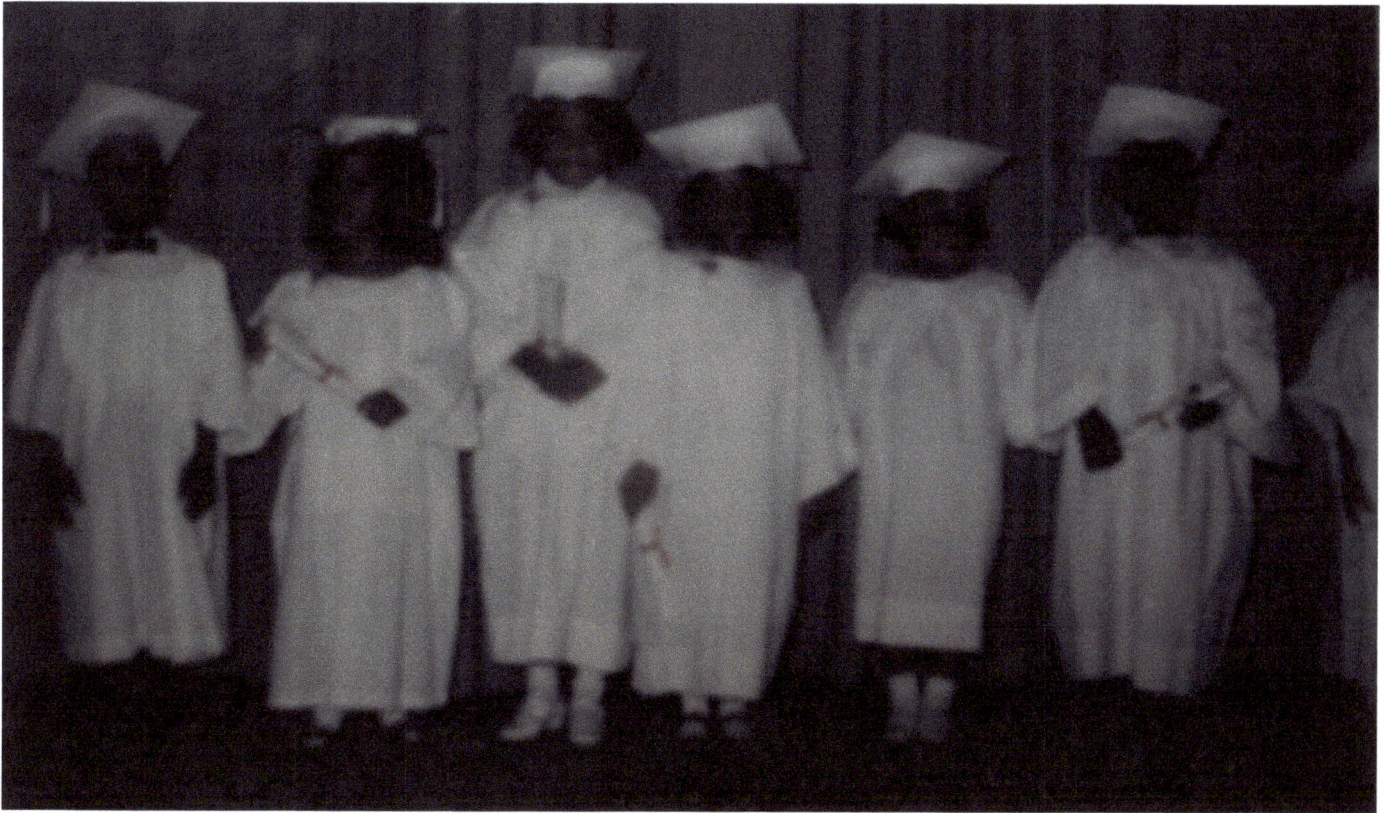

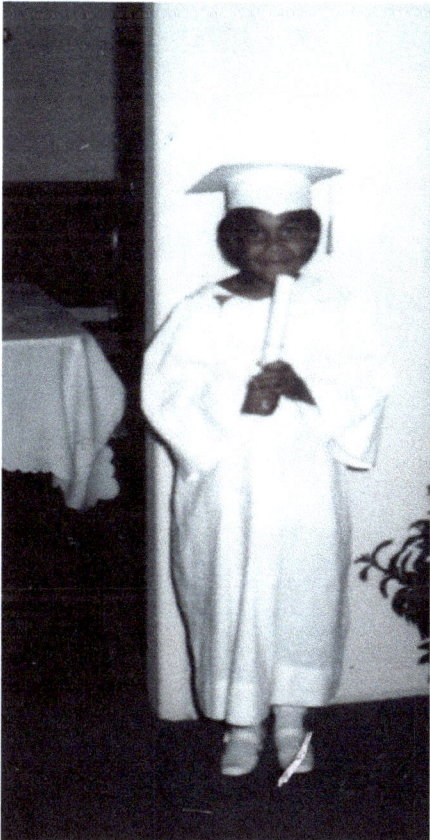
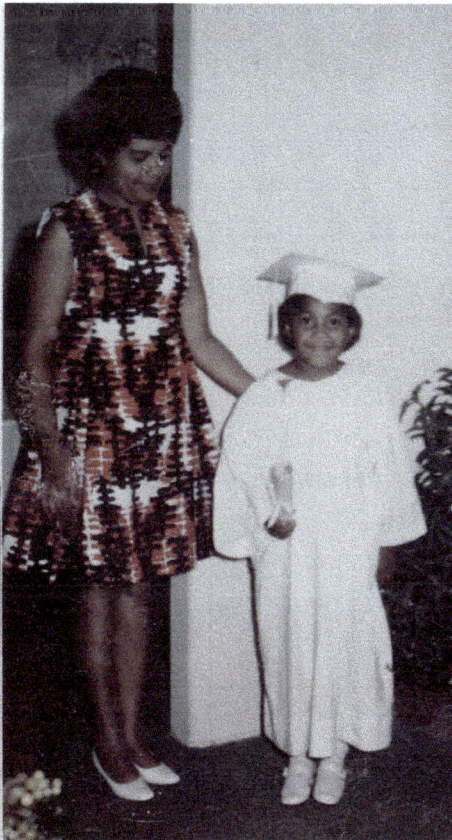
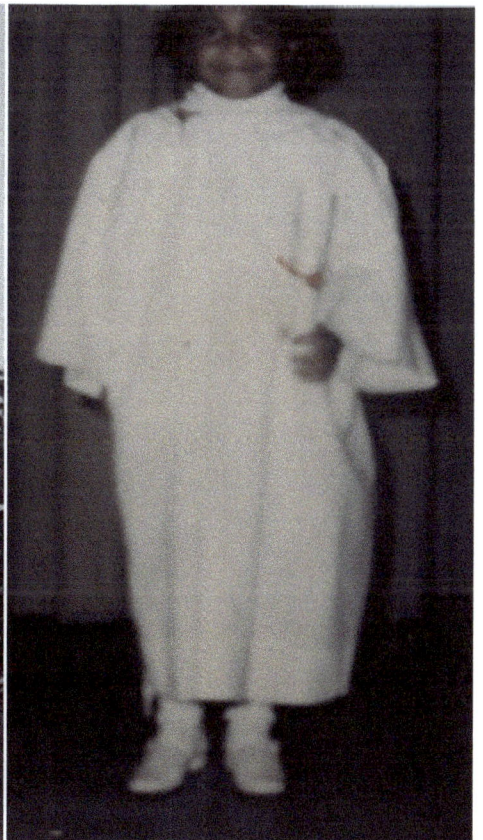

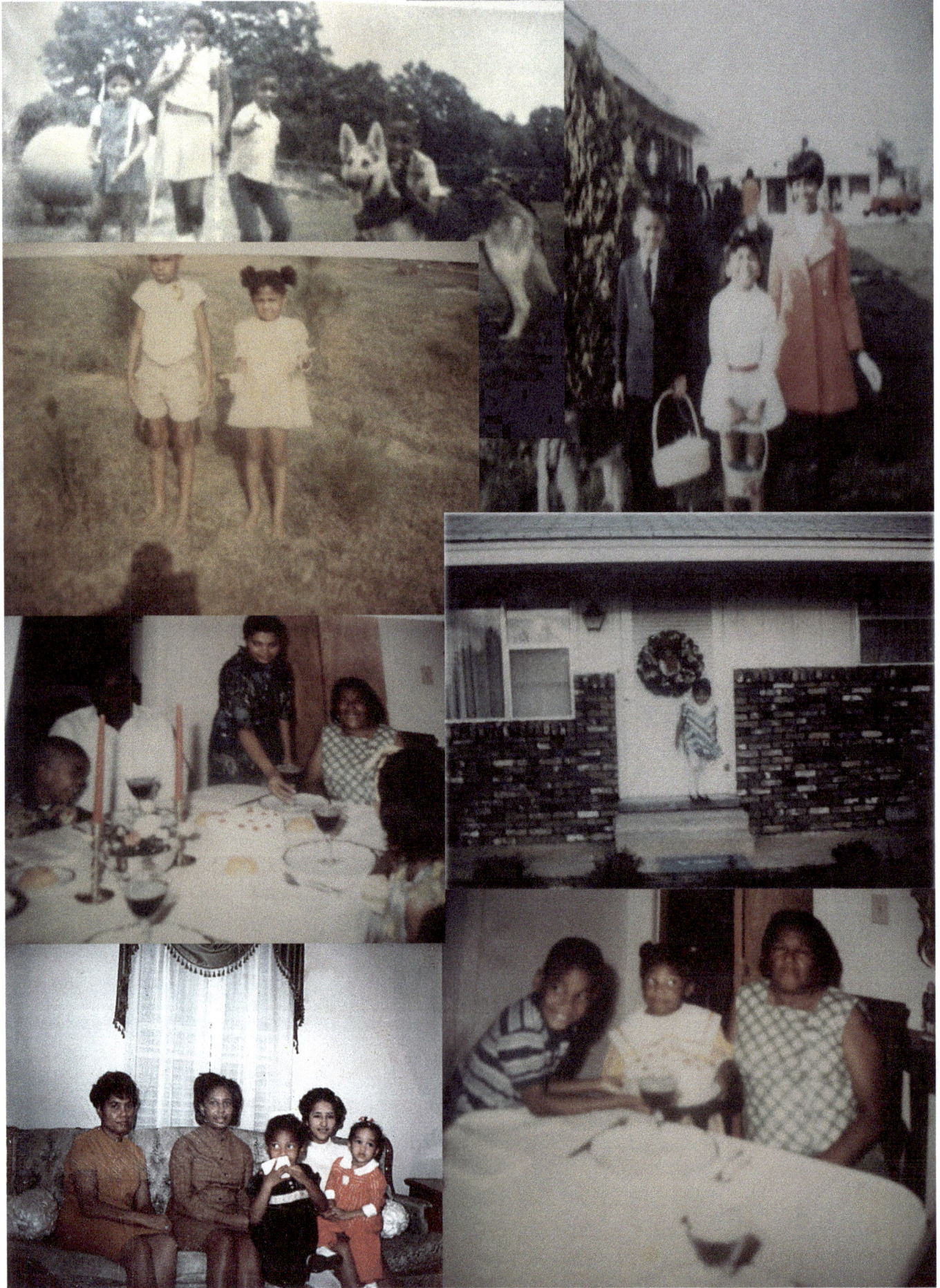

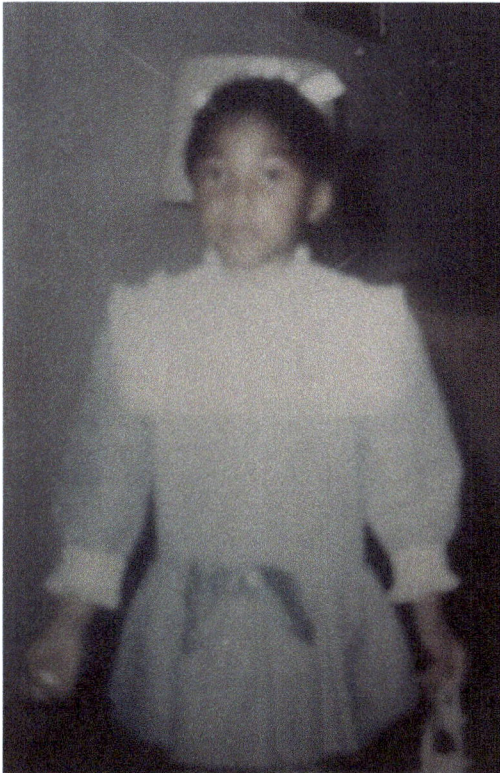
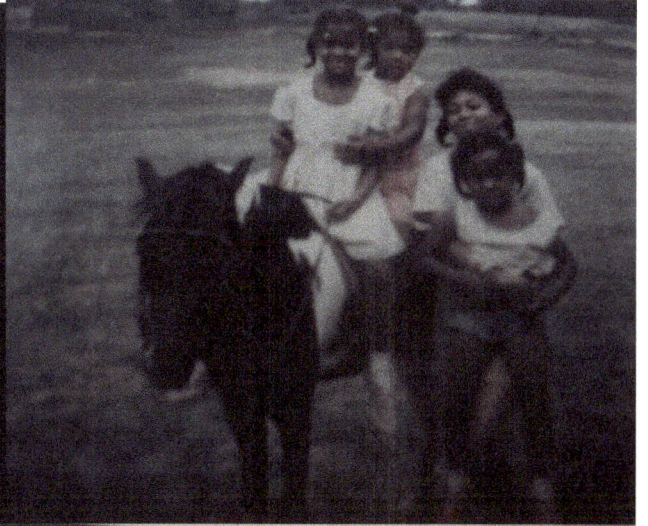
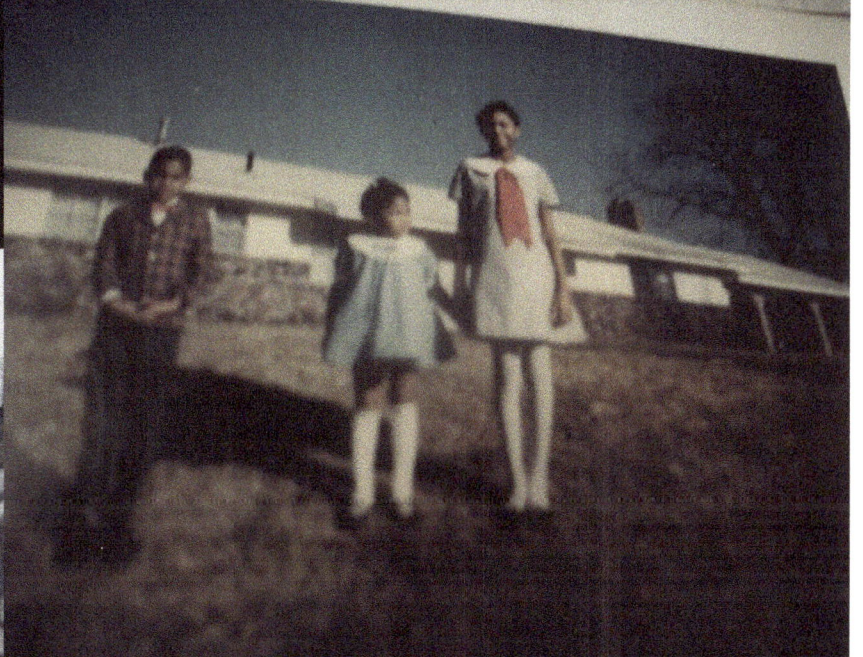
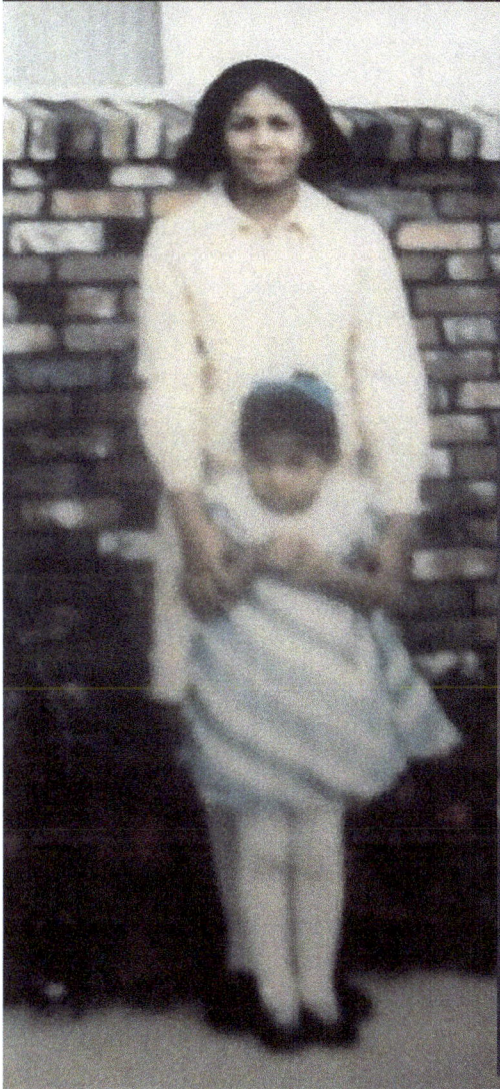
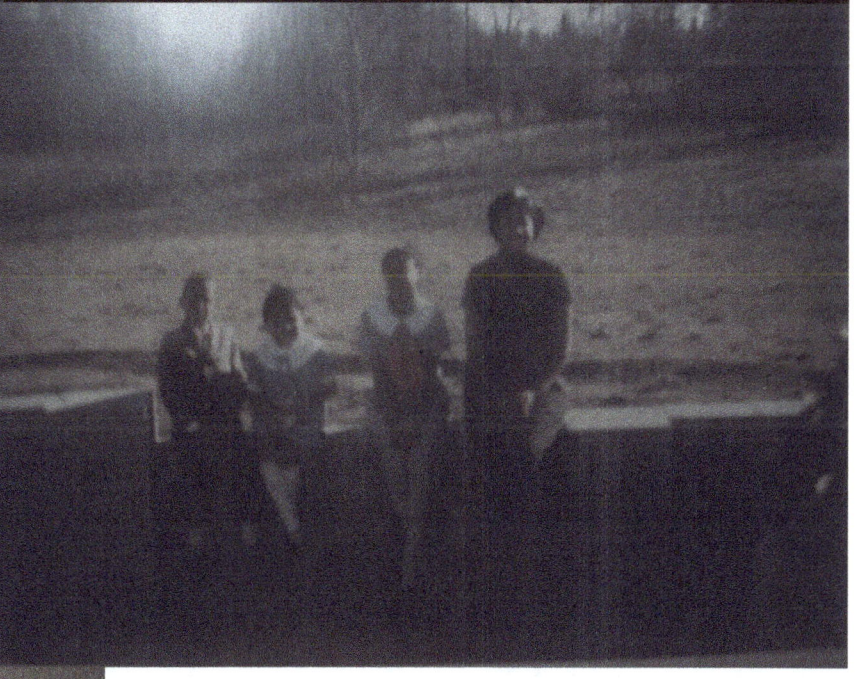

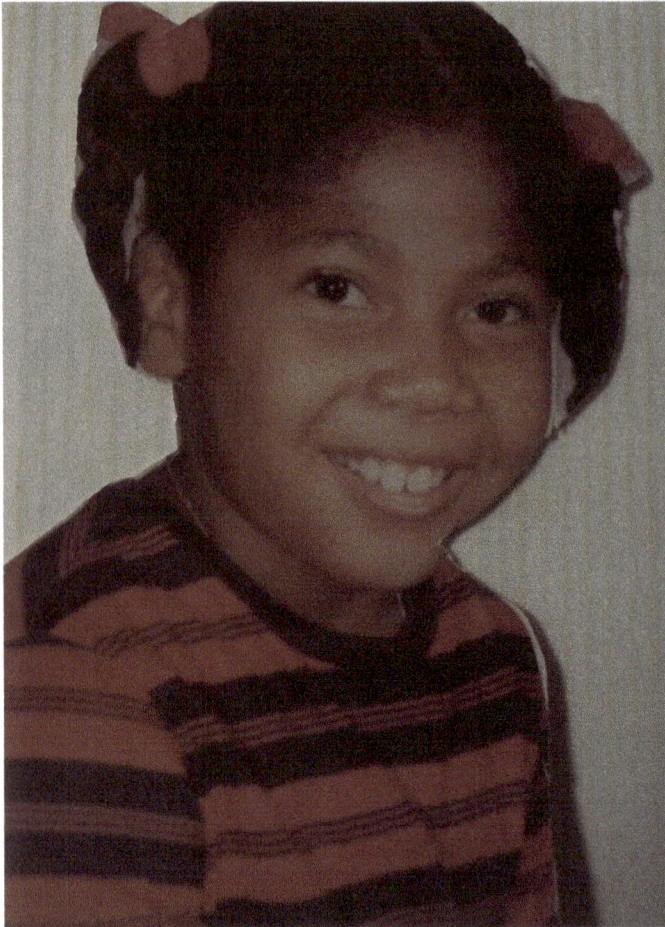
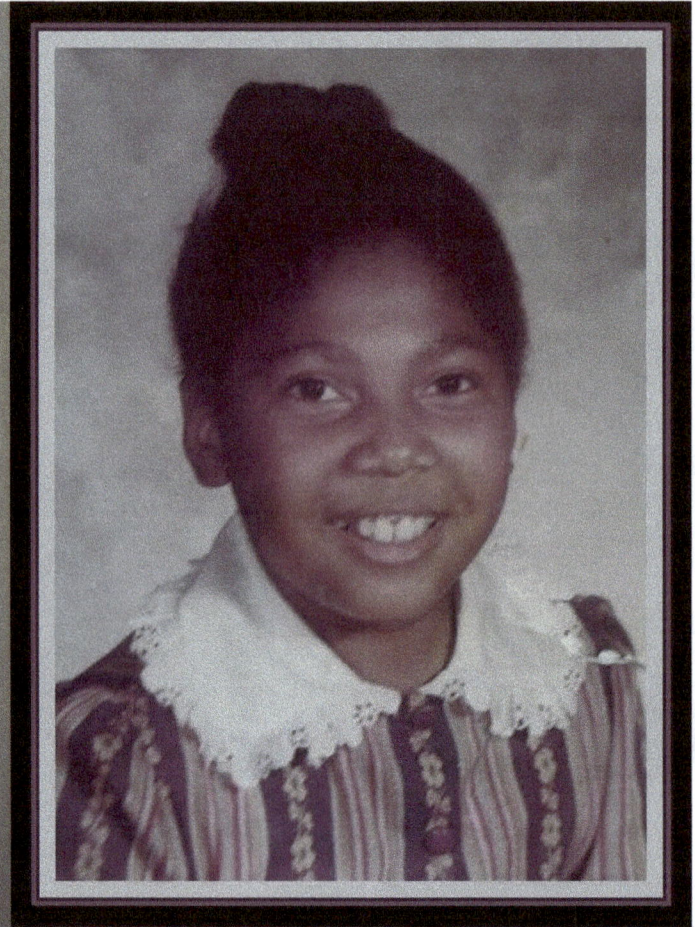
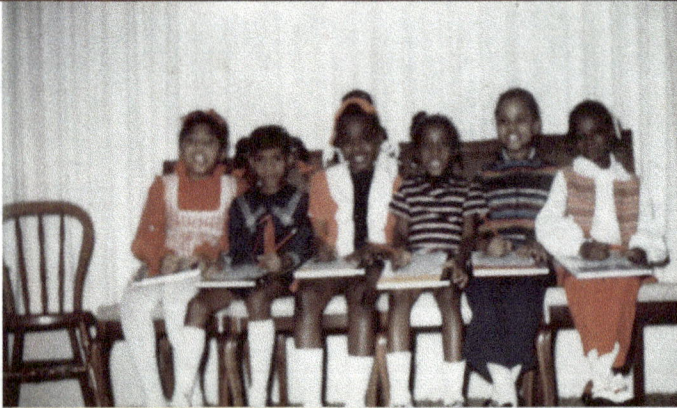
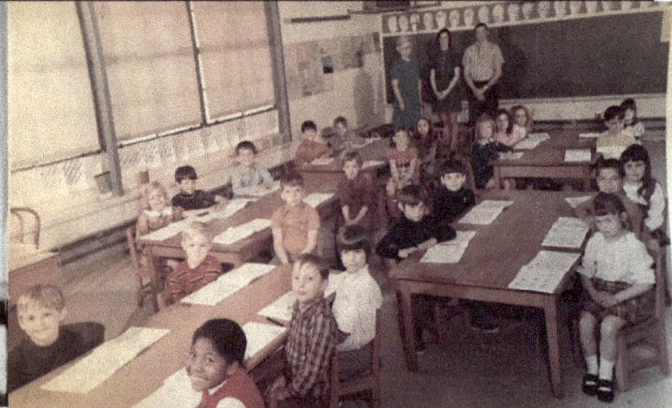
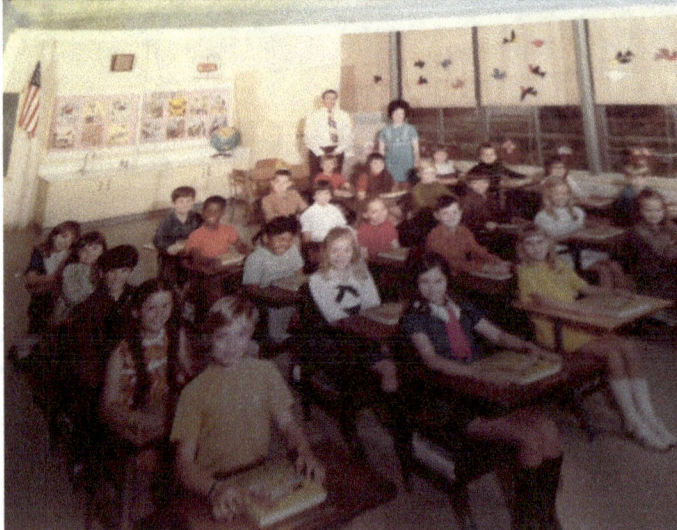
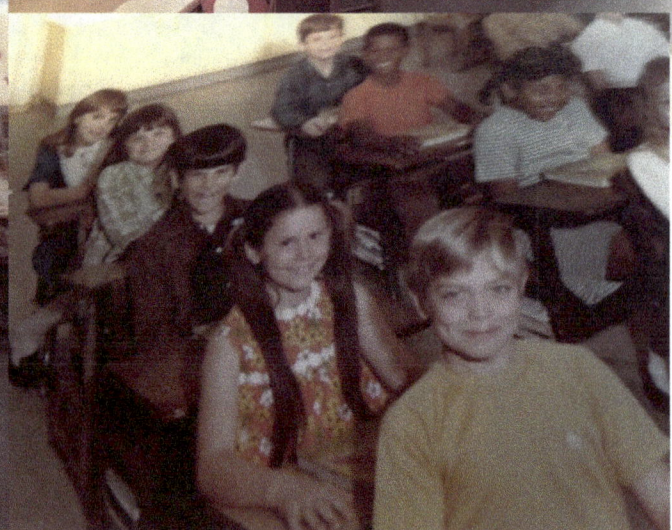

RESULTS OF A SOUTHERN MOTHER

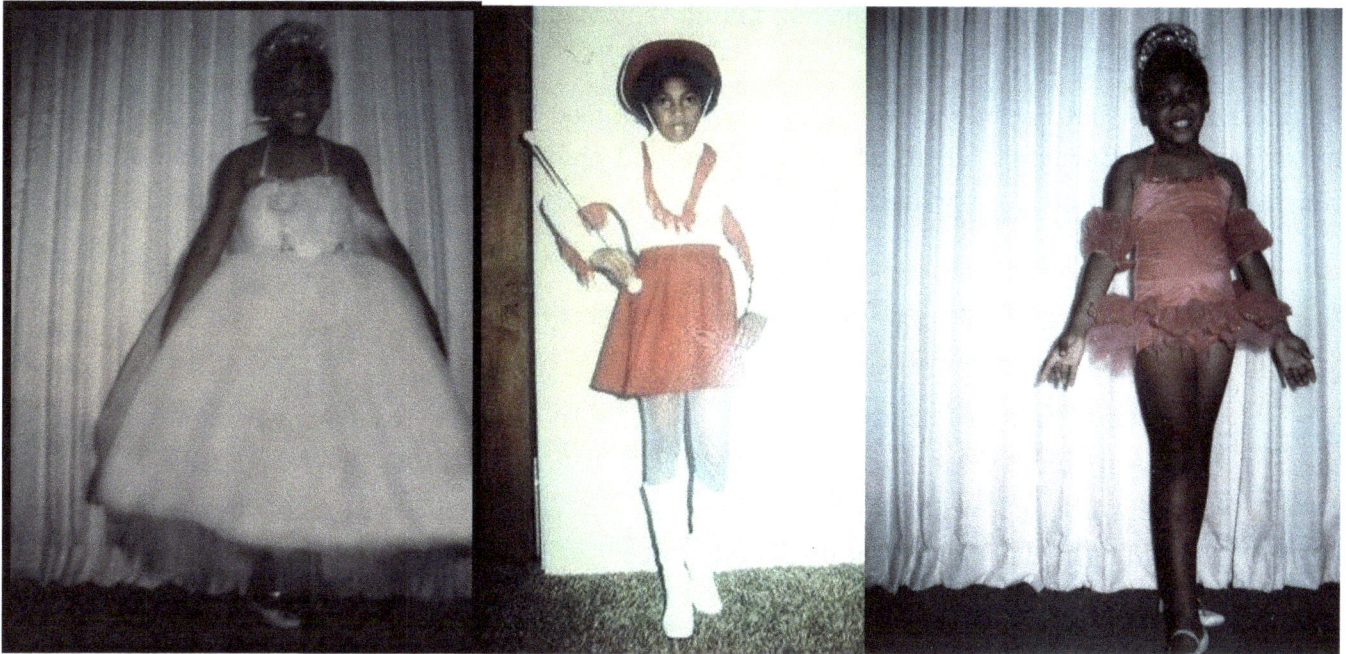

I took violin lessons and every other kind of lesson you could name
(piano, ballet. tap, jazz, baton....the list goes on) And of course , I was in Girl Scouts.

Piano Recital

Patricia Elaine Neely

May 21, 1977

YEAR ALMOST GONE — 1973 is fast drawing to a close and Girl Scouts of Tupelo are currently staging their drive to "keep body up to date" — with a sale of 1974 calendars. The colorful calendars have pictures of Girl Scouts involved in various activi. The group of Scouts here include, from left, front, Resa Randle, Lynn Paslay, Lisa Paslay; back, from left, Marsha Boyd, Paslay, Patricia Neely. Patricia is the daughter of Dr. and Mrs. James Neely. Dr. Neely is a member of the Medical Staff at North ippi Medical Center.

I love to hear the stories of my parents' childhood Christmases.

My father says that during Christmas, when he was growing up, his mother would cook at least seven or eight cakes. One of those, he said, would always be a Jelly Cake. He says that there would always be a lot of meat from the hog killing that his father would perform right before Christmas.

My mother says that her mother would prepare lots of food and always had a Pound Cake and Ambrosia for every Christmas meal. She remembers that the children were always excited about getting lots of fruits and nuts, which they didn't necessarily get regularly throughout the year.

CHILDHOOD CHRISTMAS

Christmastime at our house
Was such a joyous thing;
There was much anticipation
Of what the day would bring
For many months prior,
The list making would begin;
There were so many things I wanted,
On pure memory I couldn't depend.
I carried handy 'round with me
A trusty little list.
There was not one single thing,
I wanted my parents to miss.
And every year, without a doubt,
I couldn't ask for any better,
For I 'd get everything on my list,
Down to the very letter.
The night before, my brother and I,
Would always try our best;
To catch ole Santa in his tracks,
So we'd get little rest.
We'd try to keep ourselves alert,
With a flashlight by our side;
But, every year ole St. Nick
Would cleverly by us slide.
We must have fallen fast asleep,
Before the morning's light;
Because our toys appeared miraculously,
Sometime through the night.

In our den, the floor was covered,
With toys of every kind;
The sheer volume of them all,
Would surely blow your mind.
We'd jump around from here to there,
And squeal with pure delight;
We couldn't have concealed our excitement,
If we tried with all our might.
Later on in the day,
The relatives would pour in;
For the traditional Christmas dinner,
With us and all our kin.
We'd have such an array of food,
Usually, specialties of the South;
One year, we even had a whole roasted pig,
With an apple in his mouth.
We'd exchange gifts and laughter,
And each other's company enjoy ;
The men would often help assemble,
Some child's complicated toy.
Our festivities usually lasted,
Way into the night;
And after all was said and done,
We felt that everything went just right.
from Reflections of a Mississippi Magnolia-A
Life in Poems
by Patricia Neely-Dorsey, Copyright © 2008

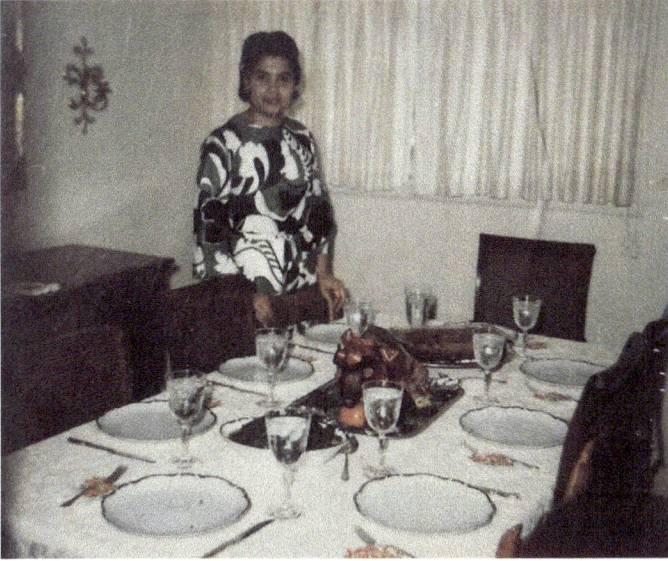

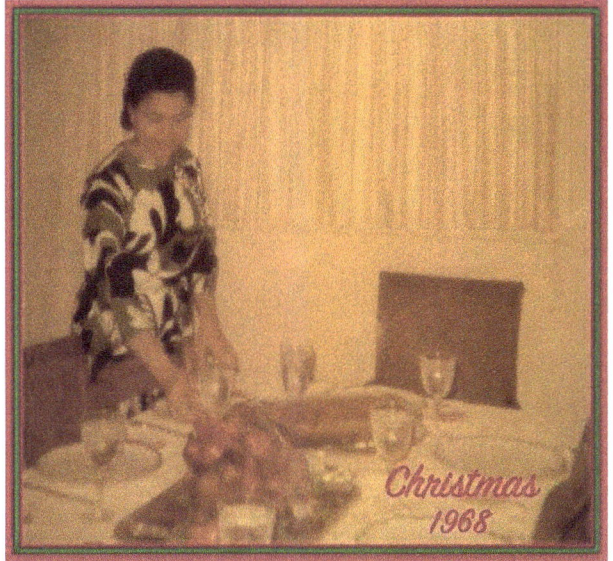

Christmas 1968

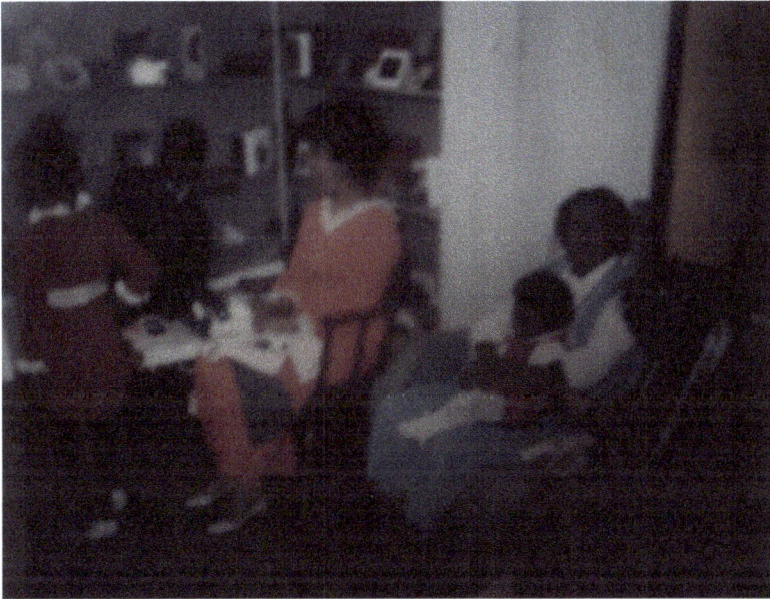

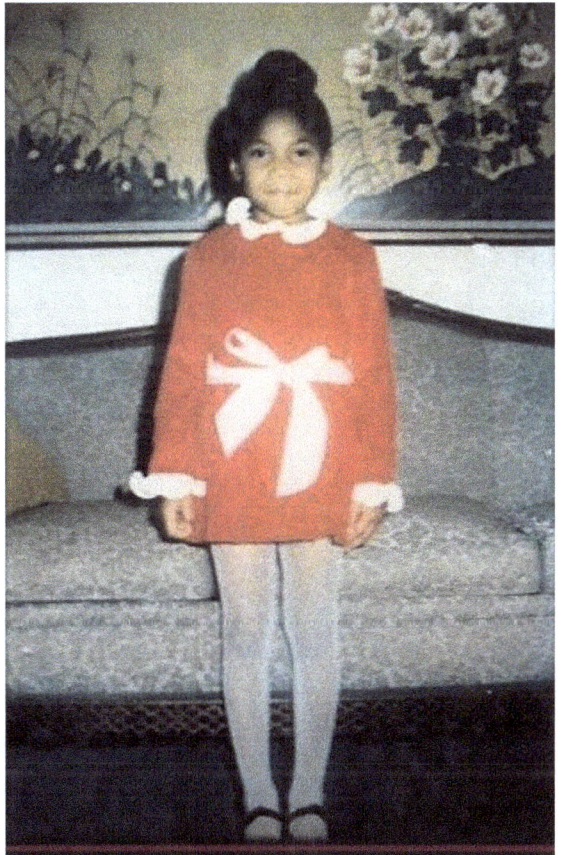

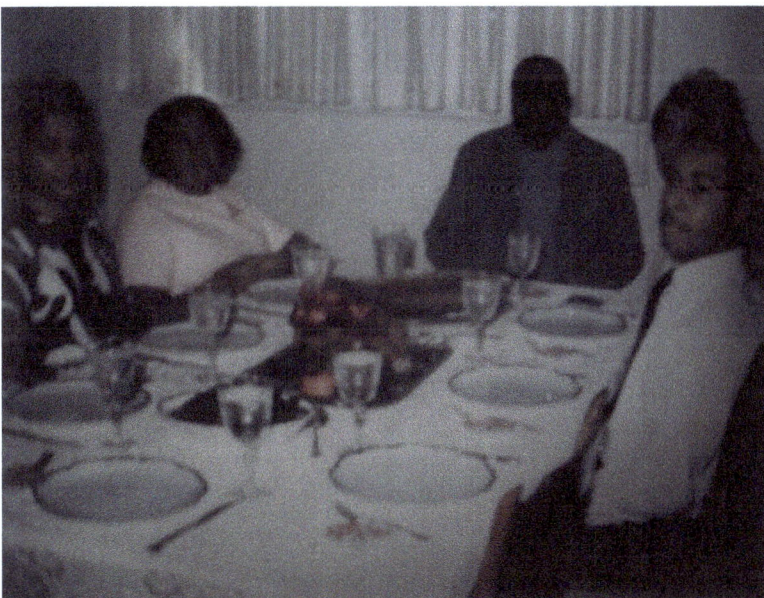

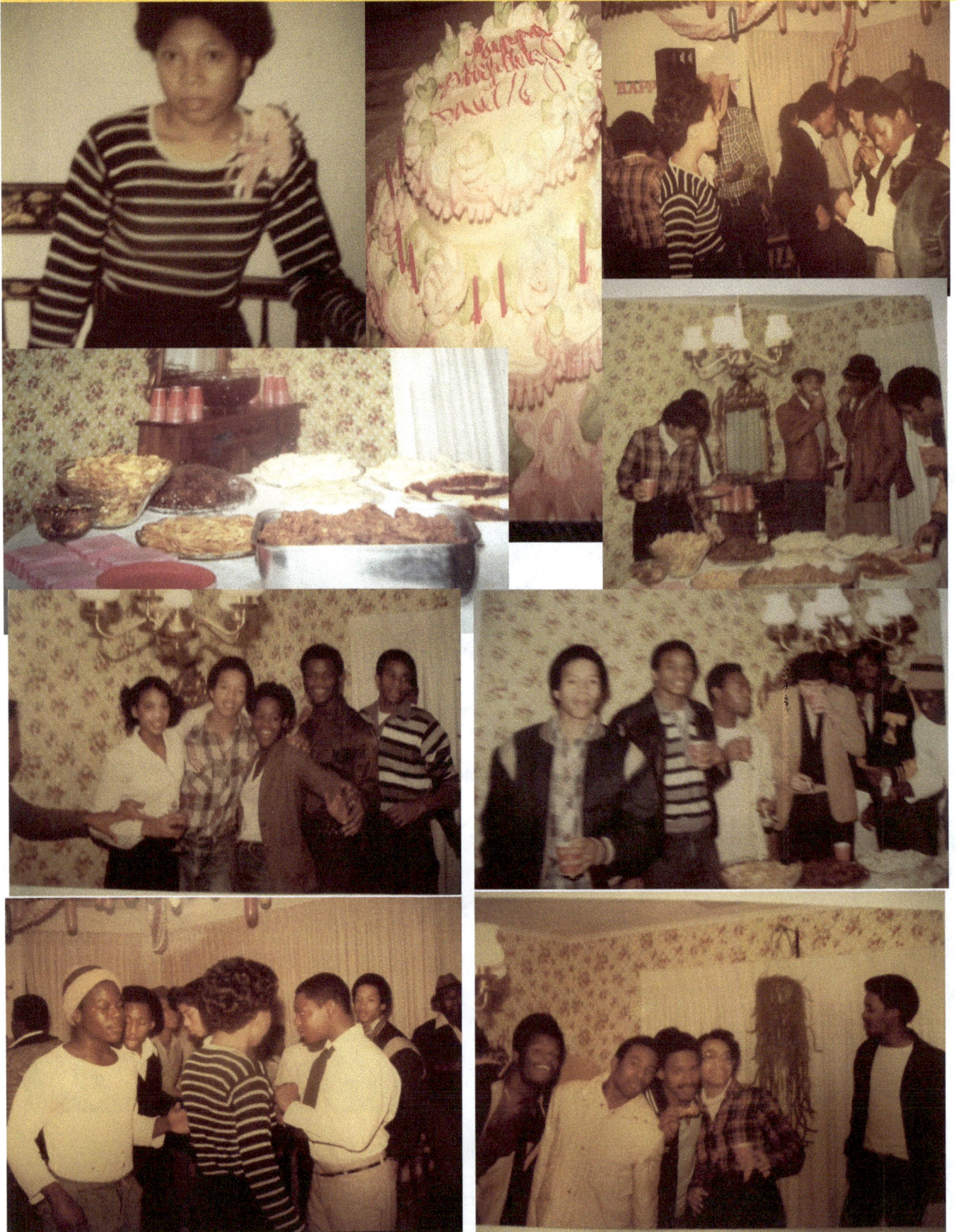

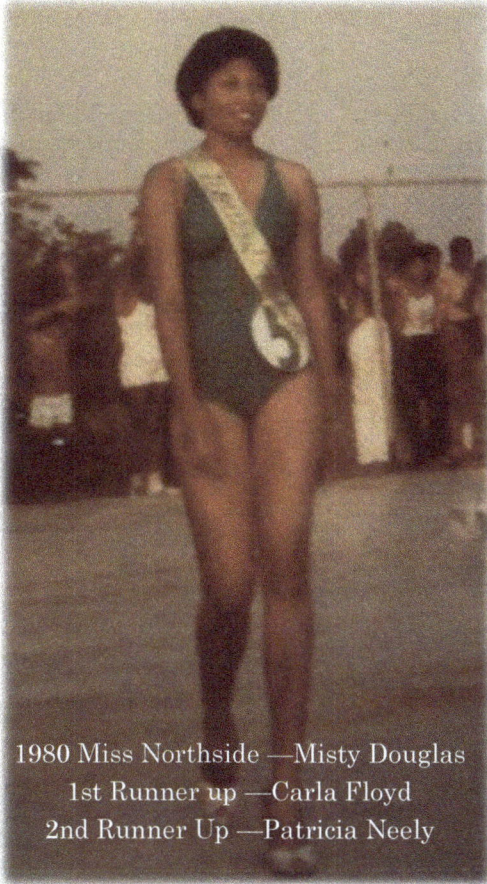

1980 Miss Northside —Misty Douglas
1st Runner up —Carla Floyd
2nd Runner Up —Patricia Neely

MISS NORTHSIDE ~

Our neighborhood beauty pageant
In the summertime
Was quite an event to see
In my 10th grade year, I decided,
The Miss Northside crown
Was waiting just for me.
I bought a stunning bathing suit
And did my stomach crunches
Advice from everywhere on how to win
Came to me in bunches.
In my high heels, around the house,
I practiced my stallion walk;
And considering the question and answer period;
I practiced how I'd talk.
For my talent, I did a ballet dance,
And I must say very well;
In my eyesight, compared to me,
The competition paled.
Our big night finally came,
And we strolled around the pool;
The lights were bright
And the crowd was wild
But, I remained absolutely cool
As it turned out,
I didn't get that winning Miss Northside cup
But, I considered it just as well,
I got 2nd runner up.

Patricia Neely-Dorsey

My Magnolia Memories and Musings - In Poems @2012

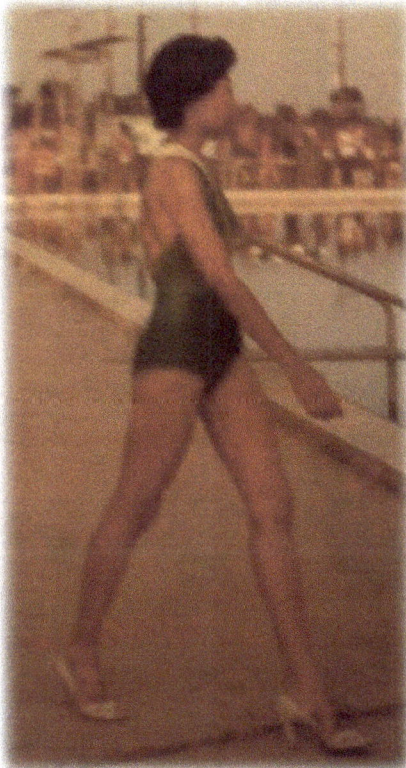

Miss Northside Pageant July 1980

EVERYONE in the Northside Community of Tupelo remembers the MISS NORTHSIDE PAGEANT

The Miss Northside Pageant was a "MUST SEE" event in the Northside /Park Hill Community for over 20 years. As one friend, Sameul Young, put it ...."It was the "Miss America of the Hood" It was held during 4th of July week from the 60's to the mid/late 80's.

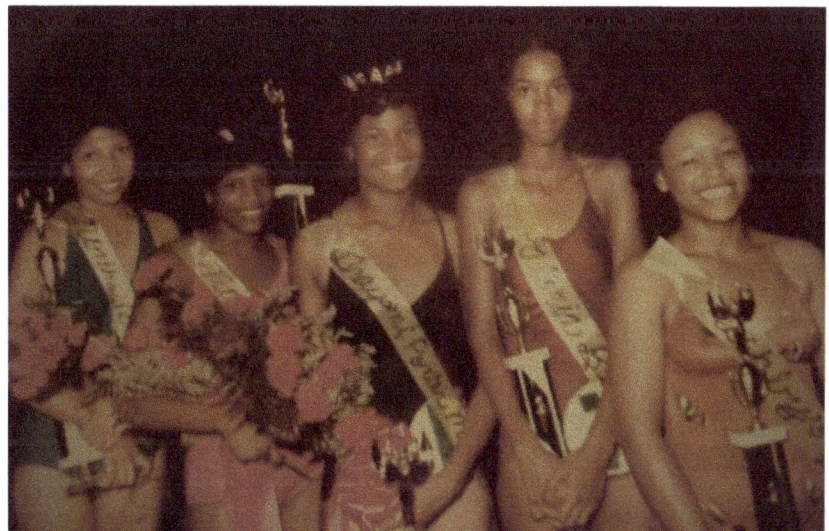

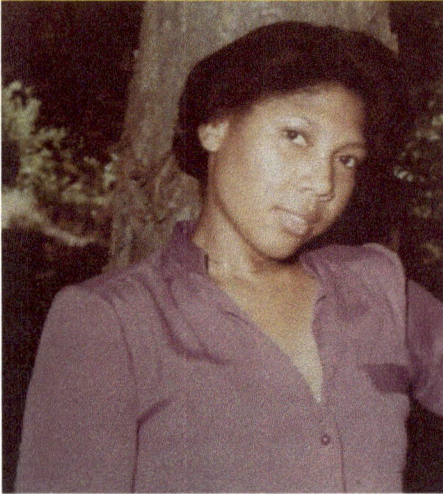

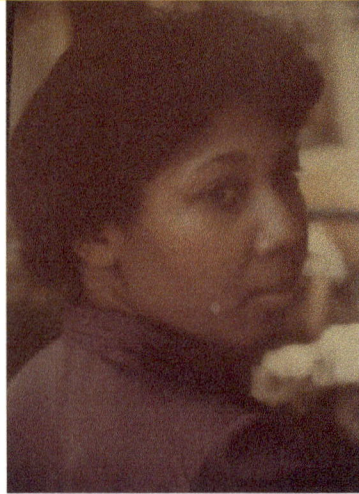

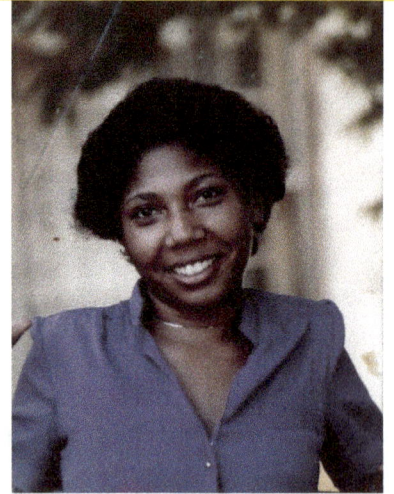

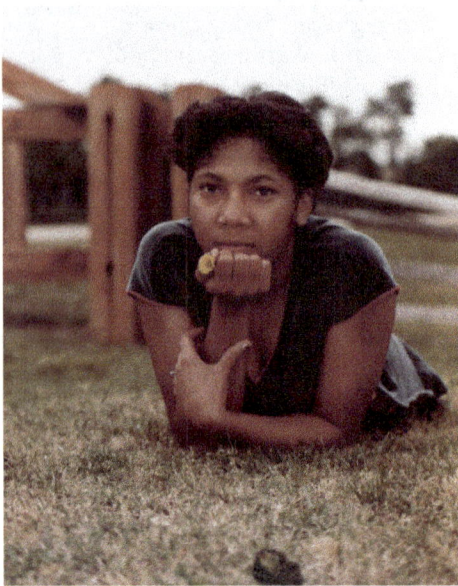

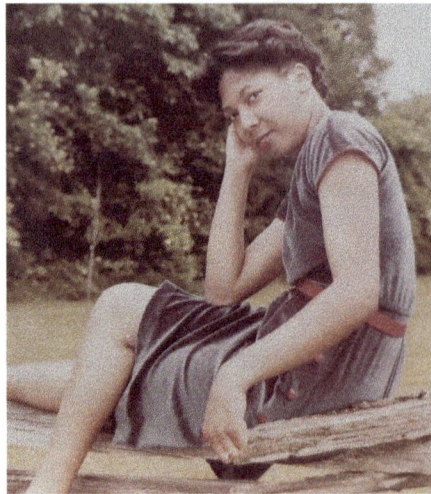

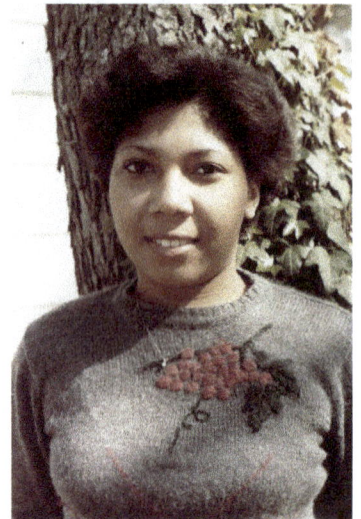

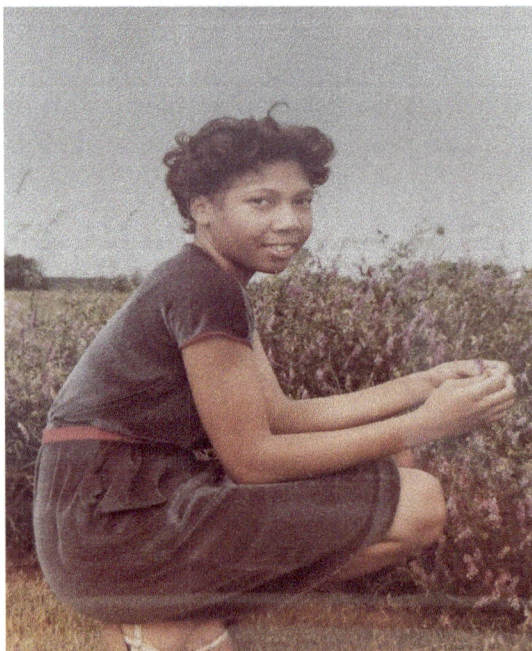

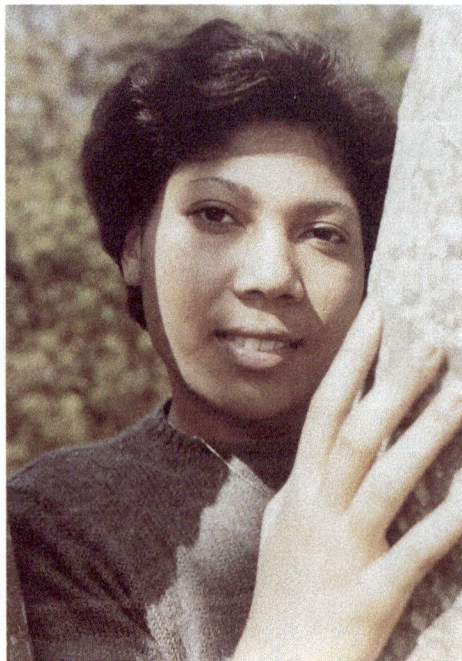

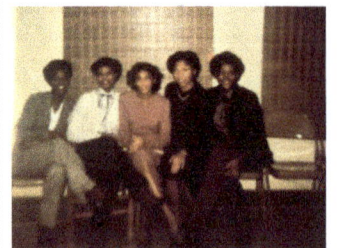

Photos by Larry
"Rob" Barnes

Northeast Mississippi **Daily Journal**

September 26-27, 1981

Page 12

Mississippi Debutante Cotillion

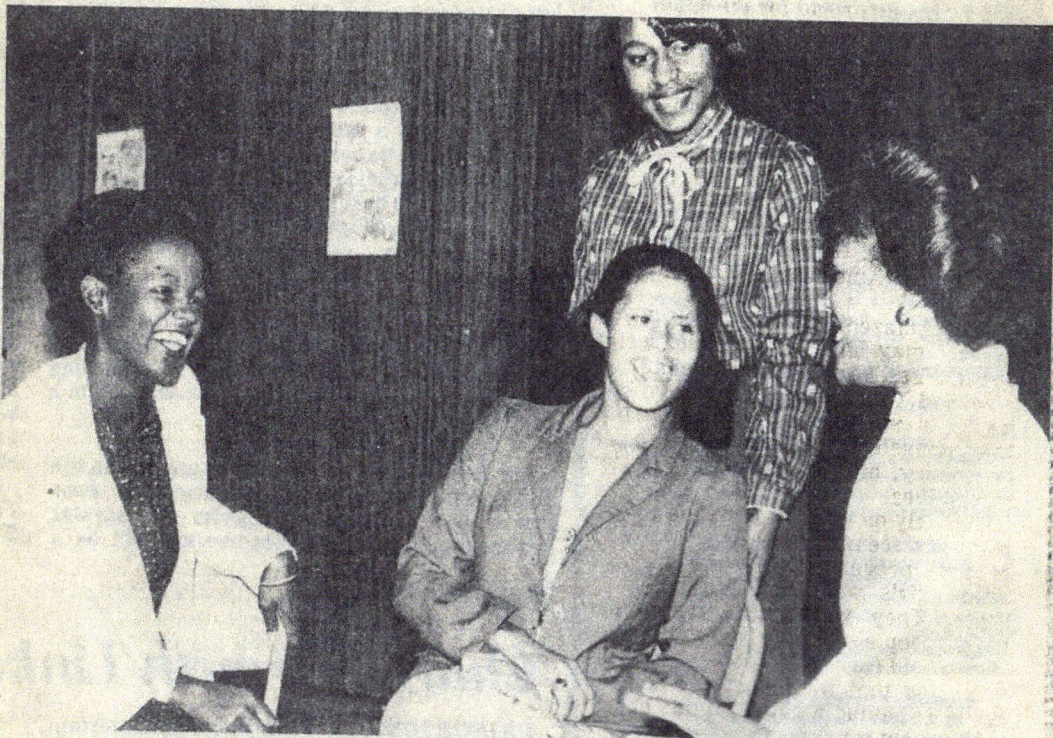

Photo by Susan Carroll

DEB TALK — Debutantes relax after last weekend's career forum. The next thing on their mind? The cotillion of course! Seated from left are Patricia Turner, Debra Scales and Kathryn Patton. Standing is Bonnie Mitchell.

The second meeting was a charm clinic that highlighted, makeup, etiquette, wardrobe planning and social grace. In mid-August the group went to Atlanta, had a private luncheon with Andrew Young and Martin Luther King III and later attended a campaign party for Young's bid as mayor of Atlanta.

Earlier this month, the debs had a tea and last weekend attended a career forum chaired by prominent members of the community. A luncheon followed.

The reaction among schoolmates was mixed. "At first maybe, some of them thought we were trying to be better than them," said Miss Neely. "But it was open to everybody and now I think more girls are going to want to join next year."

Black cotillions are prominent social events in large metropolition areas such as Atlanta and Dallas, Mrs. Williams said. The local group has tried to follow a basic pattern the larger towns have found successful.

"We're looking at it now on a long-term basis," Mrs. Williams said. "A lot of times mothers don't have the time to spend with their daughters to go places and do some of these things.

"If this catches on, girls will look forward to the cotillion. They'll see it as an incentive," she said.

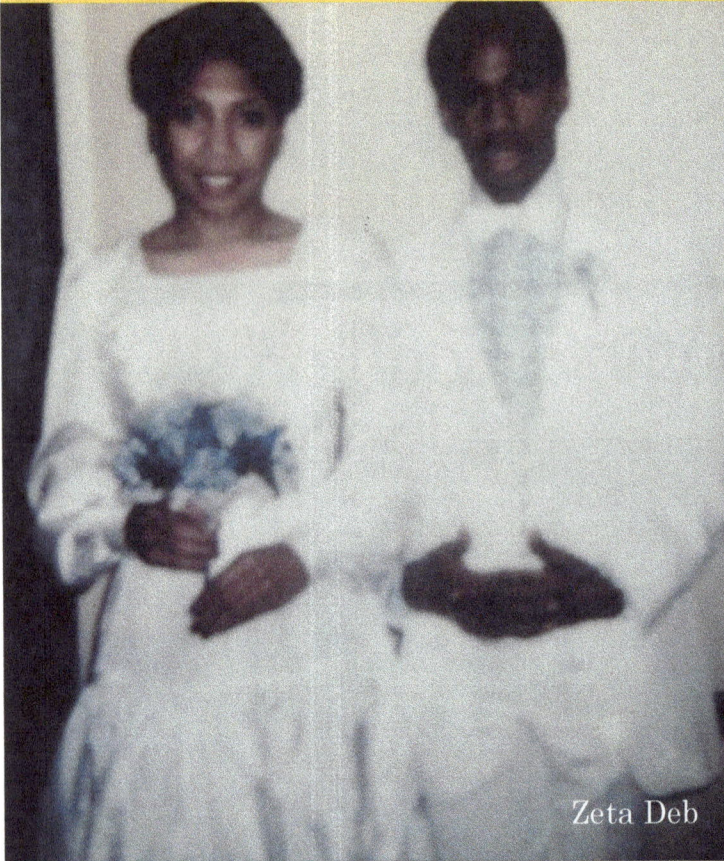

Zeta Deb

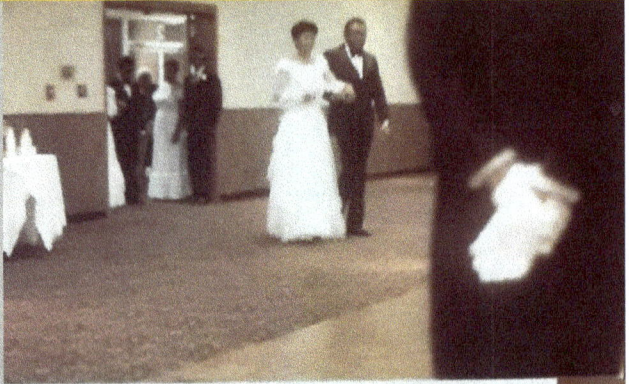

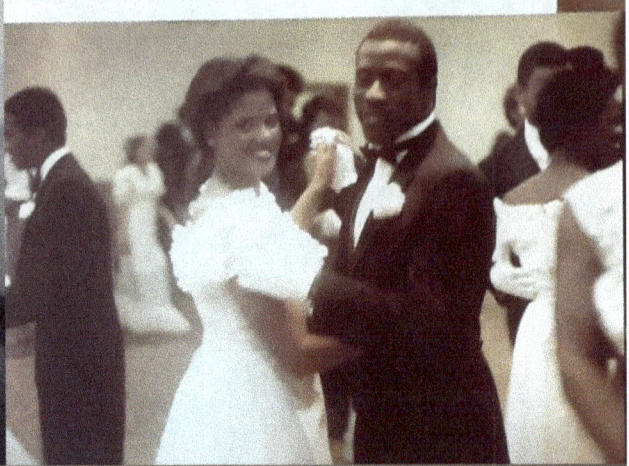

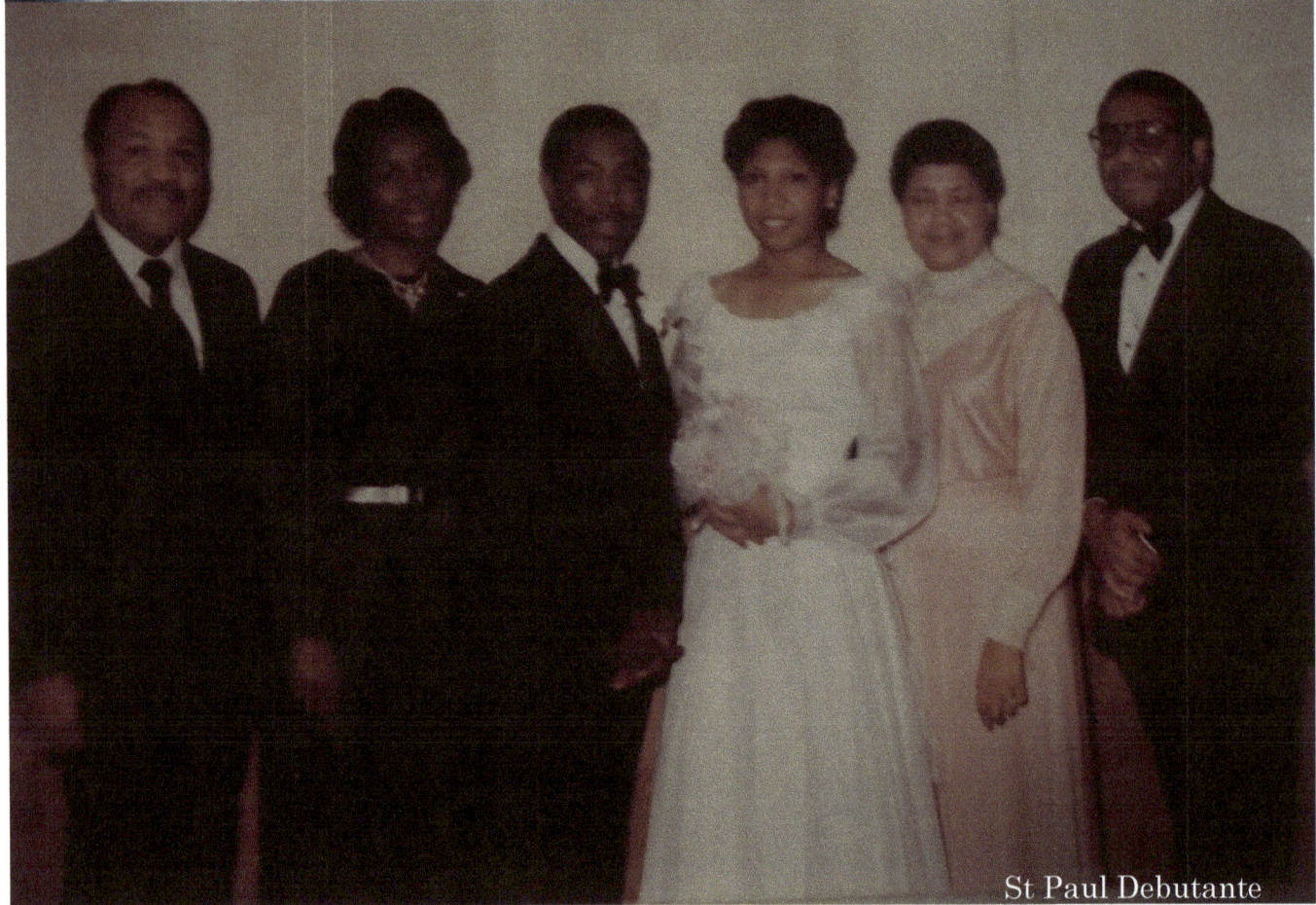

St Paul Debutante

COLLEGE

BOSTON (Language Barrier)

In my eighteenth year, I went off to Boston
To finish up with school;
I packed my things and headed north,
To enter the college pool.
There was one thong I soon found out,
The language was not the same;
If I wanted some very simple thing,
They's have some strange , new name.
When I wanted a milkshake , plain and clear,
"Frappe" was the name they had;
"What's going on" I'd think out loud,
"Has all the world gone mad?"
They'd say the word was "tonic"
When I wanted a soda pop ;
I really couldn't believe my ears
This madness had to stop.
Whenever I would order food,
It seemed that just to eat,
I needed some kind of interpreter;
For it was such a feat
But, regardless of the name they'd give,
I'd say it the southern way,
And I'll bet those folks remember it still,
To this very day.

2008 Patricia Neely Dorsey

TOO COLD FOR COMFORT

When I went off to school in Boston,
I realized why Southerners have a slower pace;
When the weather's not so frigid out,
There is no need to race.
When the weather's nice and toasty ,
You can take time to slowly walk;
When you don't feel you'll freeze to death,
With your friend, you can casually talk.
Northerners don't really know what it is ,
To take a leisurely stroll;
They're always rushing here or there,
'Cause the weather's just too cold.

2008 Patricia Neely-Dorsey

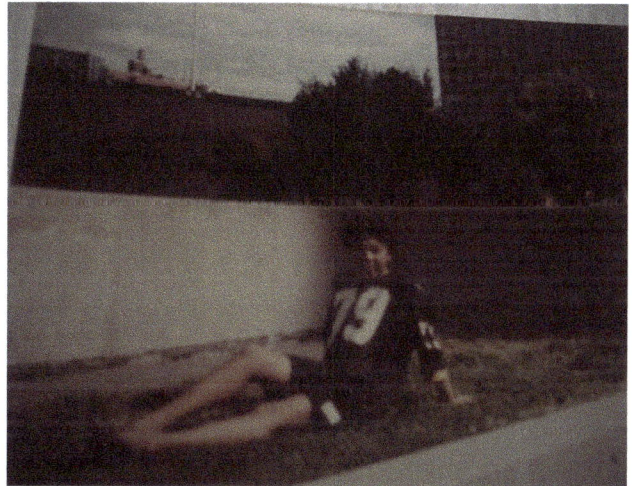

First Day on Campus Boston University

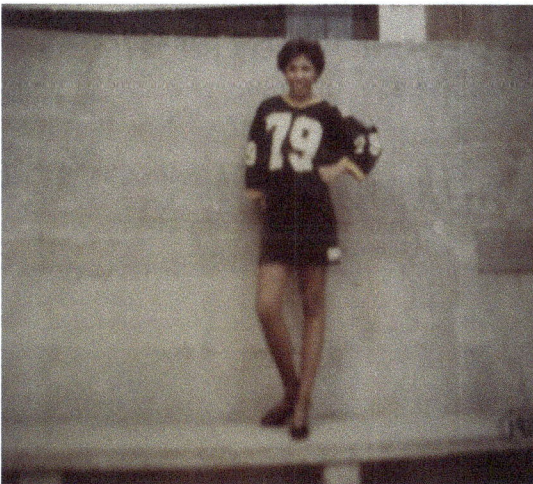

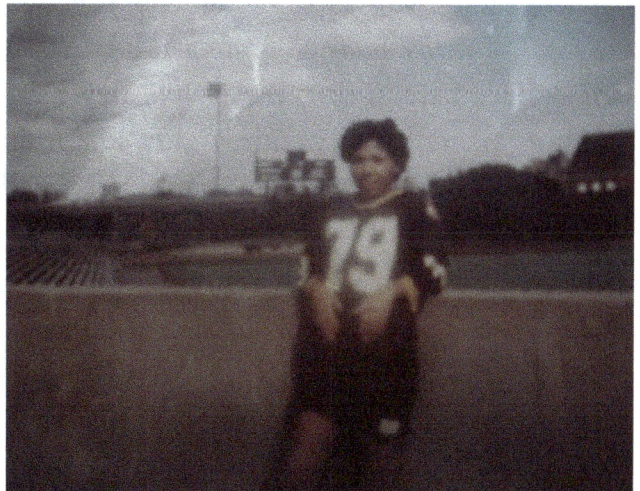

FACEBOOK POST May 6, 2023

Looking through pictures and papers in preparation for the book collaboration between me and my Mom, I ran across a letter that I had written to my Dad the Fall semester of my senior year of college. I have often said in my speaking engagements how grateful I am that my parents wanted me to go away(out of state) for college, so I could experience something new and different from my upbringing and how this made me appreciate Mississippi SO MUCH more. The poems that finally poured out of me years later (in my 40's) began with this deep, new appreciation of my home state. In a portion of the letter I wrote: (Fall 1985- Boston University) It is great being a senior. I'm really savoring each experience this year. I kind of see things in a different light. You know I miss you and Mom a lot and think of you often. I could never express how grateful I am to have parents like you. I could never have asked, hoped for or dreamed of a better life than you have provided for me. Thank you so very much for giving me the opportunity and allowing me to attend B.U. I have grown so much socially, intellectually, and spiritually. More than anything, B.U. has taught me much about life.

Things are not always fair, right , just and lovely but it's just life. Each day here is a learning experience. My stay at home this summer was very pleasant. I had a great time! It's unbelievable how much more I appreciate home and you and Mom now! Mississippi is beautiful- warm, relaxing, leisurely, bright, sunny, comforting and lots of goodies all rolled into one. Oh, I know it has drawbacks but doesn't everything...almost. I could not have grown up in a nicer place. I went on to write.. My classes are going OK. I love political Science class But ,statistics is a headache(I hate math almost as much as I hate Rats...if that is possible) You know, I had never seen a RAT until I came here! Now, it on an every day occurrence ...or ORDEAL!)

Years later I would write ... MY MISSISSIPPI M y Mississippi I s always home to me S he's warm, charming and alluring S he's the queen of hospitality I 've loved her from my earliest days S he's in my fondest memories S he's in my heart, in my soul and such a part of me; I love to share her beauty People often misunderstand Pleasures abundantly abound, I n my dear magnolia land . 2013 Patricia Neely-Dorsey P.S. It's amazing to me when I read the letter, that I had to leave Mississippi to have the opinion /revelation that "Things are not always fair, right , just and lovely " I lived a very charmed life. It's amazing also that I had never seen a rat until I had gone to Boston...and I mean RATS! (HUGE !) To this day, I still have only seen one since I left Boston. And that one was nowhere NEAR the size of the ones I saw there!

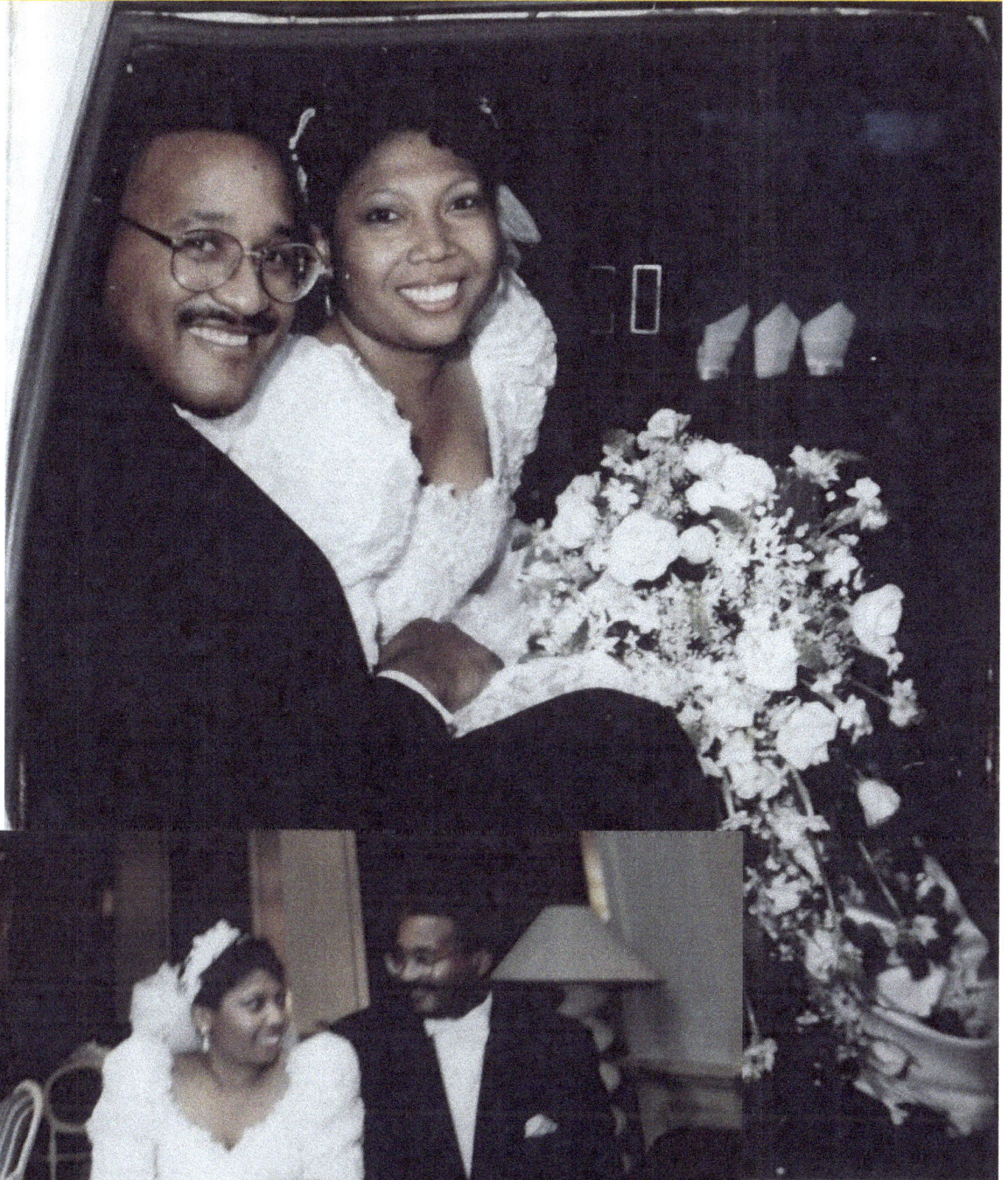

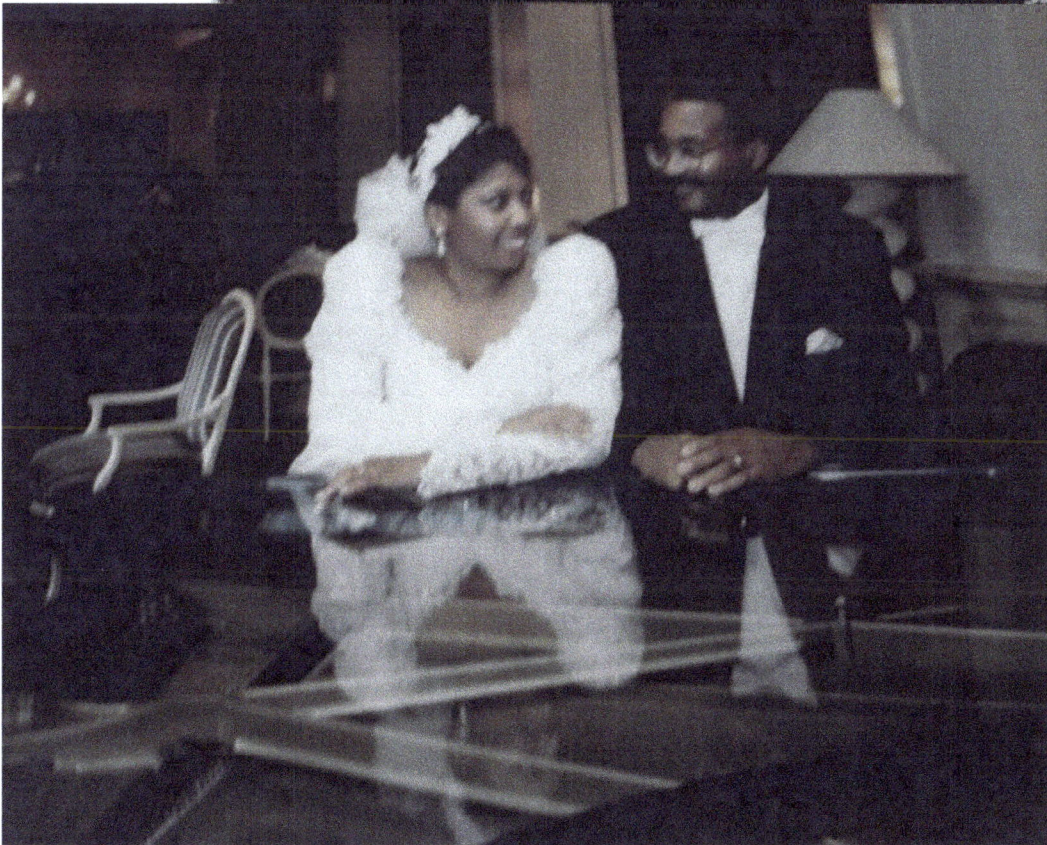

9-11-93
Boulevard Church of Christ, Memphis, Tennessee, Is it time yet???
Every time I look at this picture I smile. I wanted peach roses for my bouquet Ultra
Traditional Southern Mom said No! No! It turned out I really liked the white.

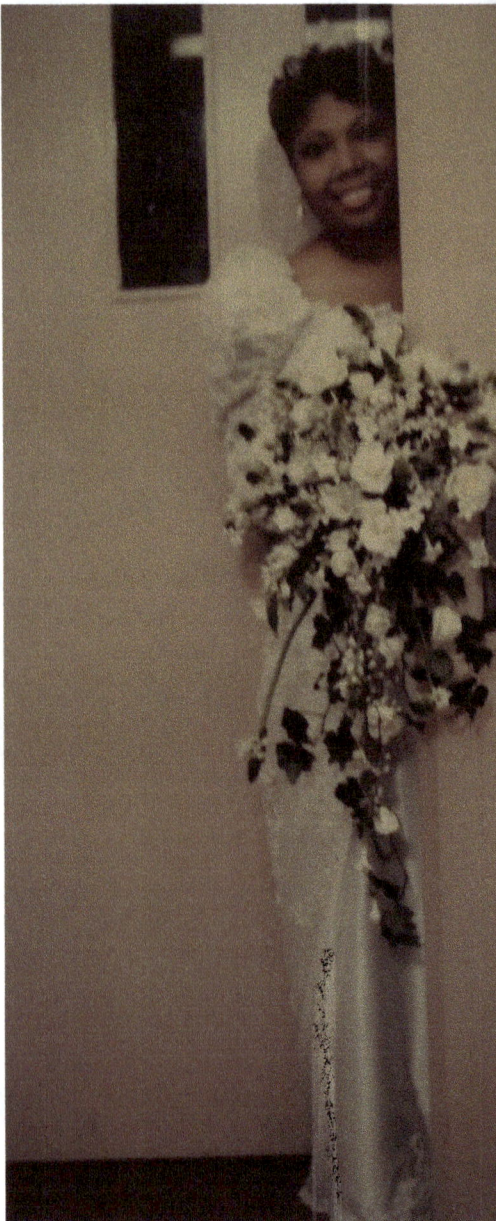

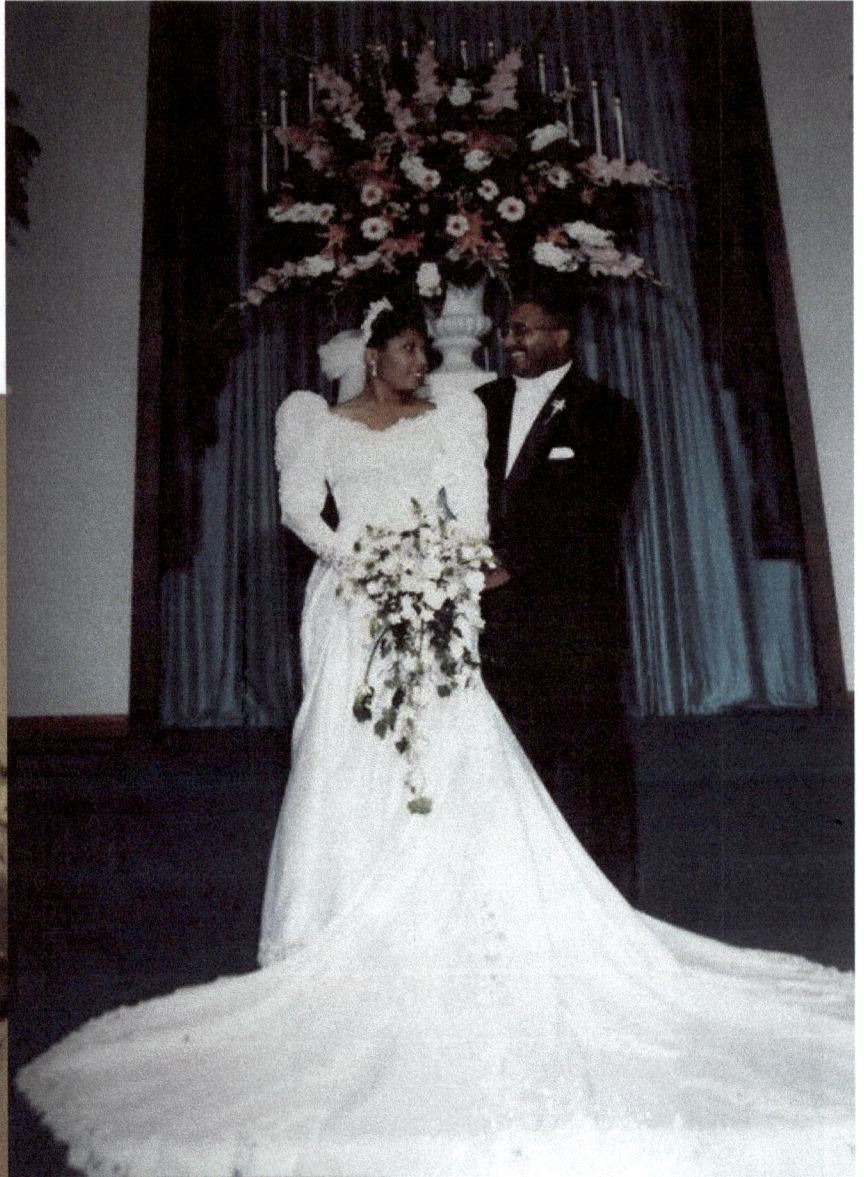

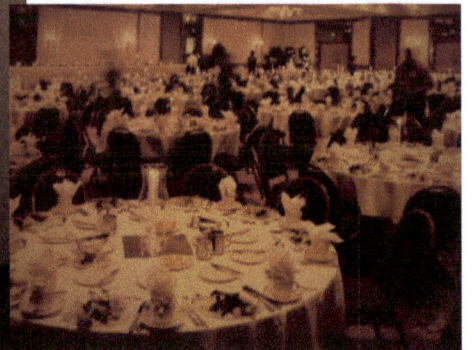

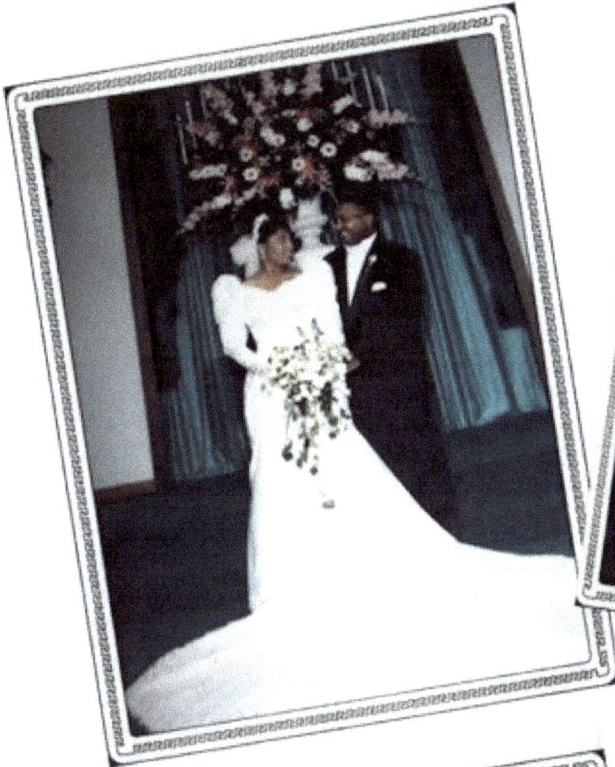

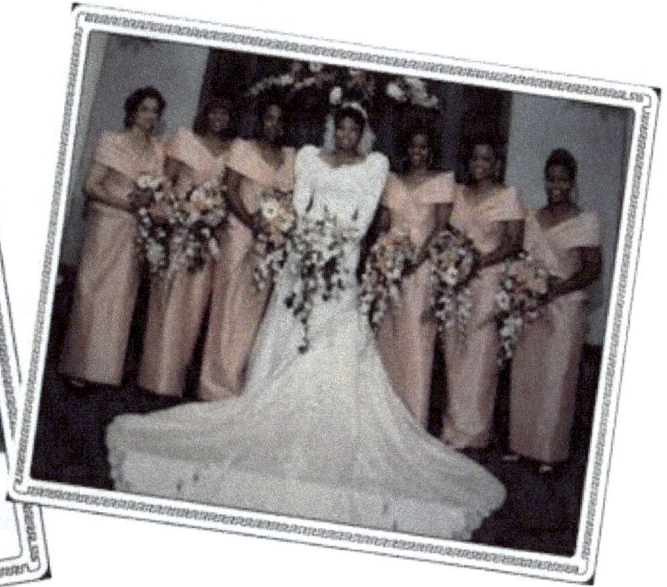

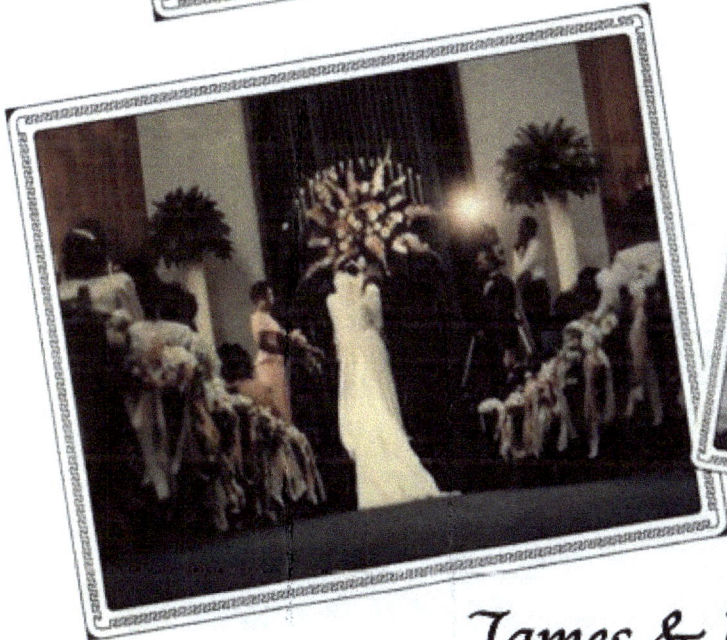

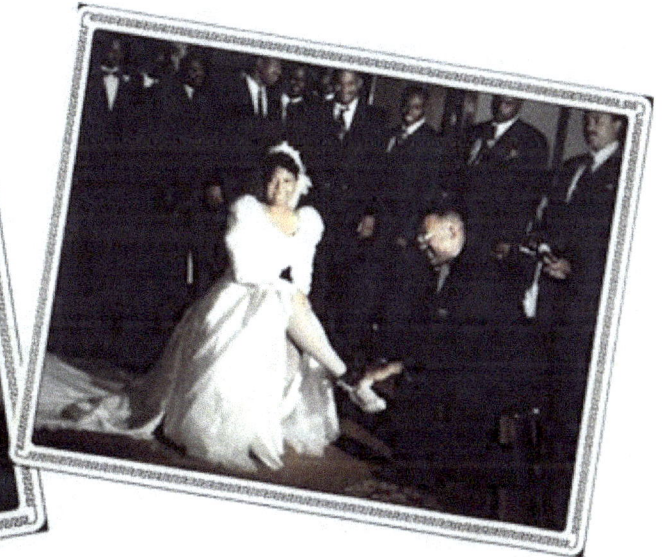

James & Patricia
9-11-93

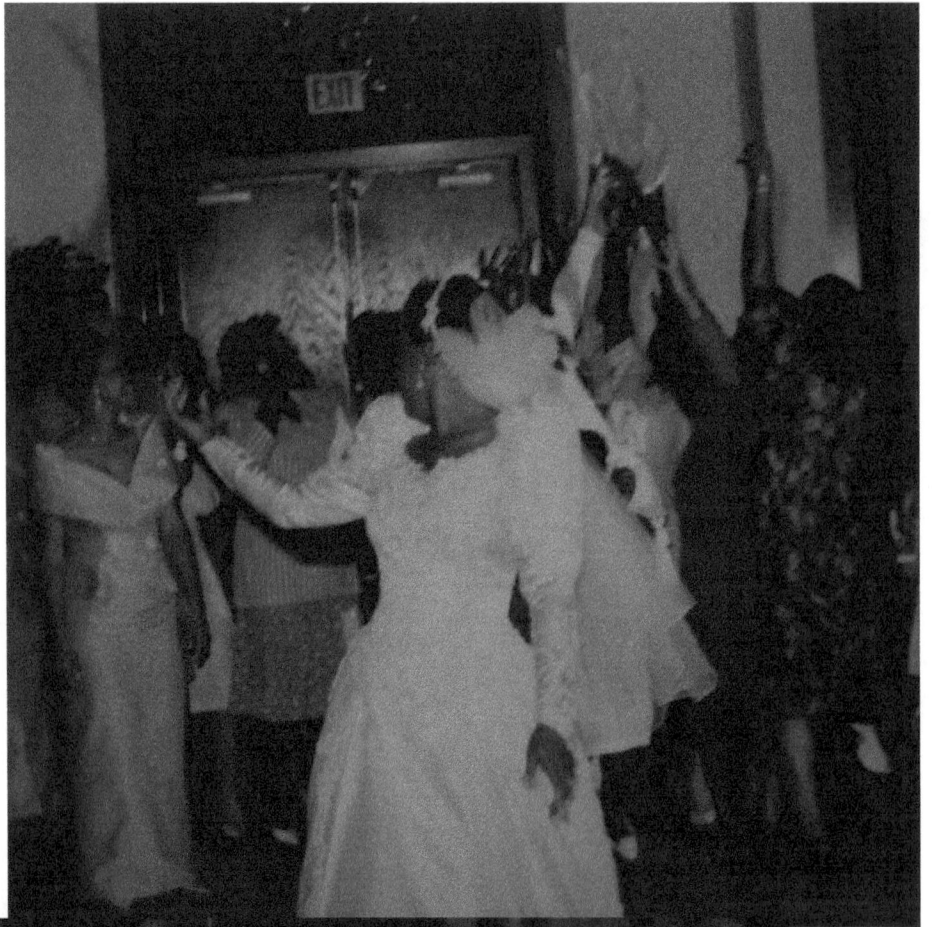

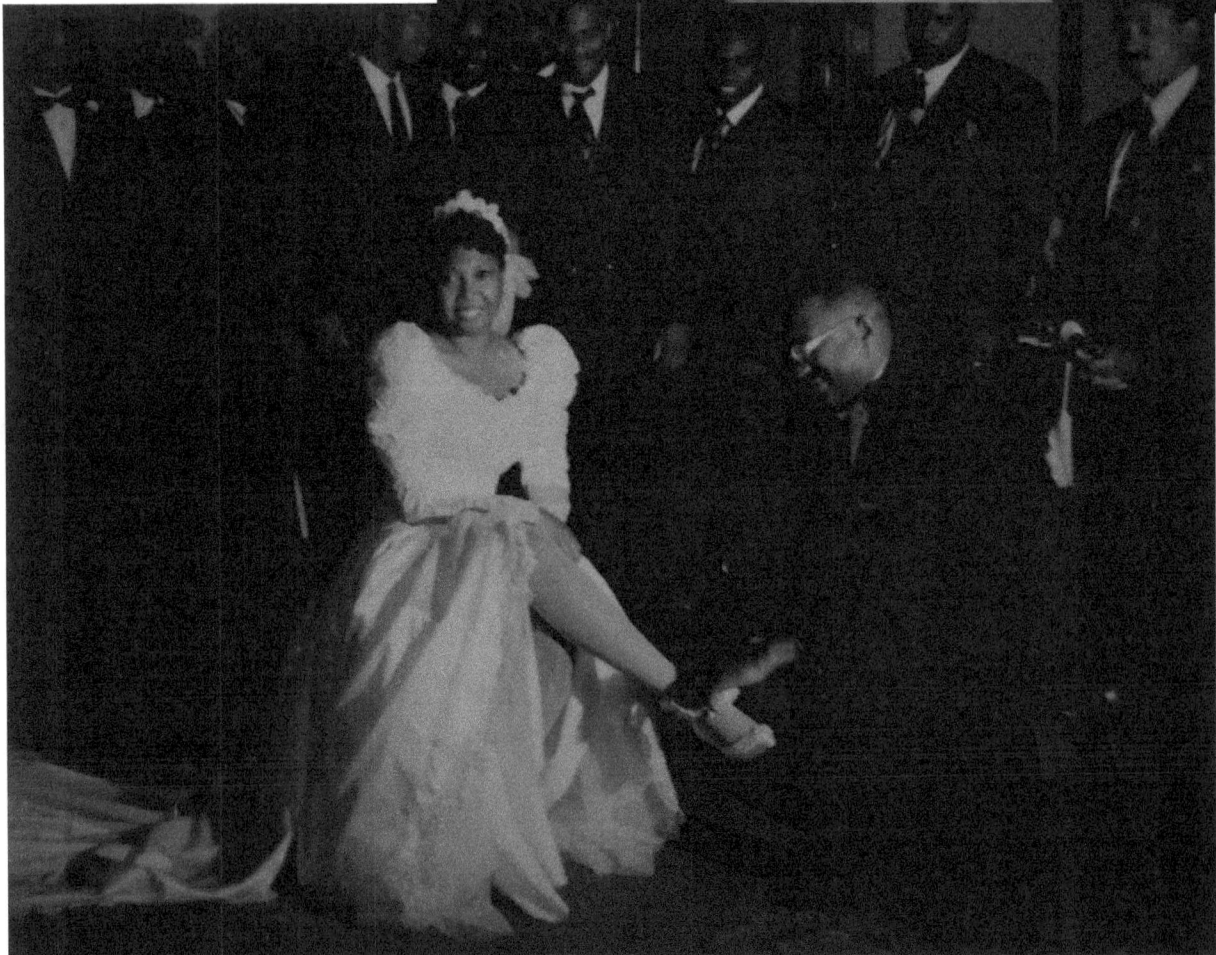

Bride *Patricia-Neely* DORSEY

My husband . James, and I were married on September 11, 1993 at the church of Christ on Elvis Presley Boulevard in Memphis , Tennessee, We met on a blind date, introduced by a mutual friend. Years later, I even wrote a poem abut it , called "The Hookup". It's in my first book "Reflections of a Mississippi Magnolia".

The first date was, AWFUL ! (LOL) I actually told him that he wasn't my type and I meant it !
But, of course, over 25 years later, it seems , I was wrong. He was definitely a God choice. God sent him to me to help me and complete me in ways that I never even knew I needed.

James has all of these OTHER "anniversary" dates for us (anniversary of our first phone call, anniversary of our first date, anniversary of the date we got our marriage license, ect.) These are dates that he quizzes me on every year. and dates that I NEVER remember !!!

Unfortunately, and sadly, terrorists made my wedding anniversary day one that I (and practically all Americans) will never forget ..9-11.

YOUR WEDDING

DRESS STORY

On September 11, 2001 thousands of Americans lost their lives in a terrifying , terrorist attack on U.S.soil. Although, we celebrate a joyous occasion on 9-11, it is always bittersweet.

About my dress, all that I knew was that I wanted lots and lots of beads and sparkle. I wanted lots of BLING ! I wanted a magical Cinderella dress. As soon as I saw the dress, I knew it was The One !I think that it was the 3rd or 4th dress that they brought me. I was beyond thrilled ! It absolutely "spoke" to me and called my name ! I immediately said, "Yes" to the dress!

I wanted to look and feel like a princess, so I chose a tiara style headpiece to go with my princess dress. Every time I look at my pictures I smile . All of these years later, I still think that I chose the perfect dress for me, a dress to match a fairy tale wedding and fairy-tale life. I wanted peach roses for my bouquet, to match my bridesmaids. But, my Ultra Traditional Southern Mom said No ! No ! No !

It turned out I really liked the white. Mother always knows best, Right?

JET Magazine

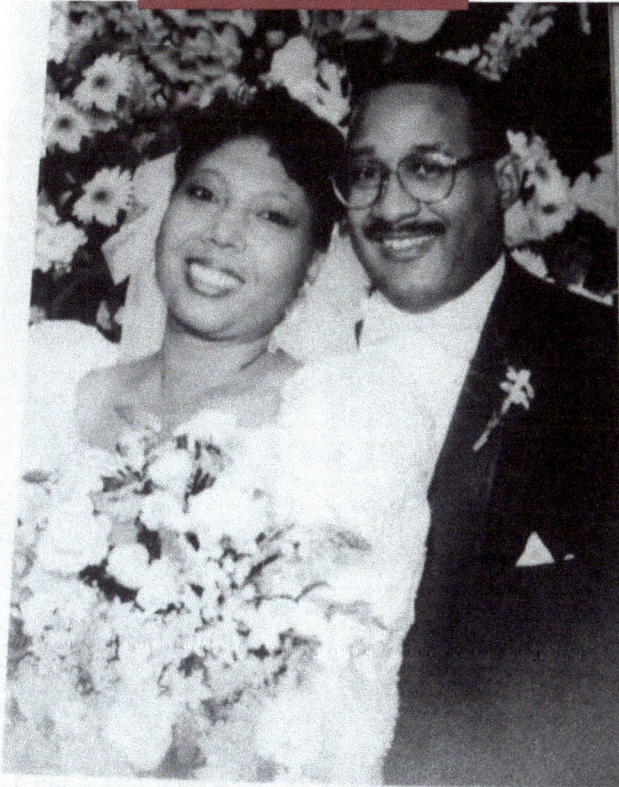

▲ **Perfect Pair:** After meeting on a blind date, Patricia Neely and Rufus Dorsey Jr., recently wed at Elvis Presley Boulevard Church in Memphis. The bride, a Boston University grad, is a mental health counselor with the Shelby County (TN) Dept. of Corrections. The man who won her heart is a graduate of David Lipscomb Univ. and is a claims rep with the Social Security Administration in the city.

THE HOOK UP

A very close friend of mine,
Called me up one day ;
And said "I have the man for you ,
You must meet him right away."
She said, "He attends church regularly,
And his contribution is good, too,
I just know I've found the man,
The perfect one for you.
"Blanche, I said, I think, I'll pass,
I don't believe in blind dates;
There has to be something amiss,
I think that I'll just wait."
"Does he have a car and a job?"
Does he live with his mother?"
If he filled out an application
For sex would he check OTHER?"
She said, "Come on, just trust me,
I wouldn't steer you wrong ;
I know you'll fall in love with him,
And I'll be singing your wedding song."
"O.K.. O.K. . I'll meet him,
But, don't expect anything at all;
One date is all I'll commit to,
And, yes, you can tell him he can call.
A long story short, we had the date,
And it didn't go very well;
I was very much a tyrant,
But by his response, you'd never tell.
At the end of the evening, to my surprise,
He asked for a second date;
I couldn't believe the confidence,
"Wow , he'd make SOMEONE a good mate."
Well, now it's been fourteen years
And guess what?
We're still together.
Sometimes what we think we want
Doesn't really even matter.

Patricia Neely-Dorsey

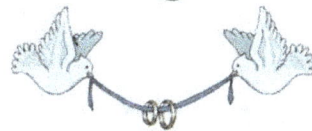

Reflections of a Mississippi Magnolia - A Life in Poems © 2008

201

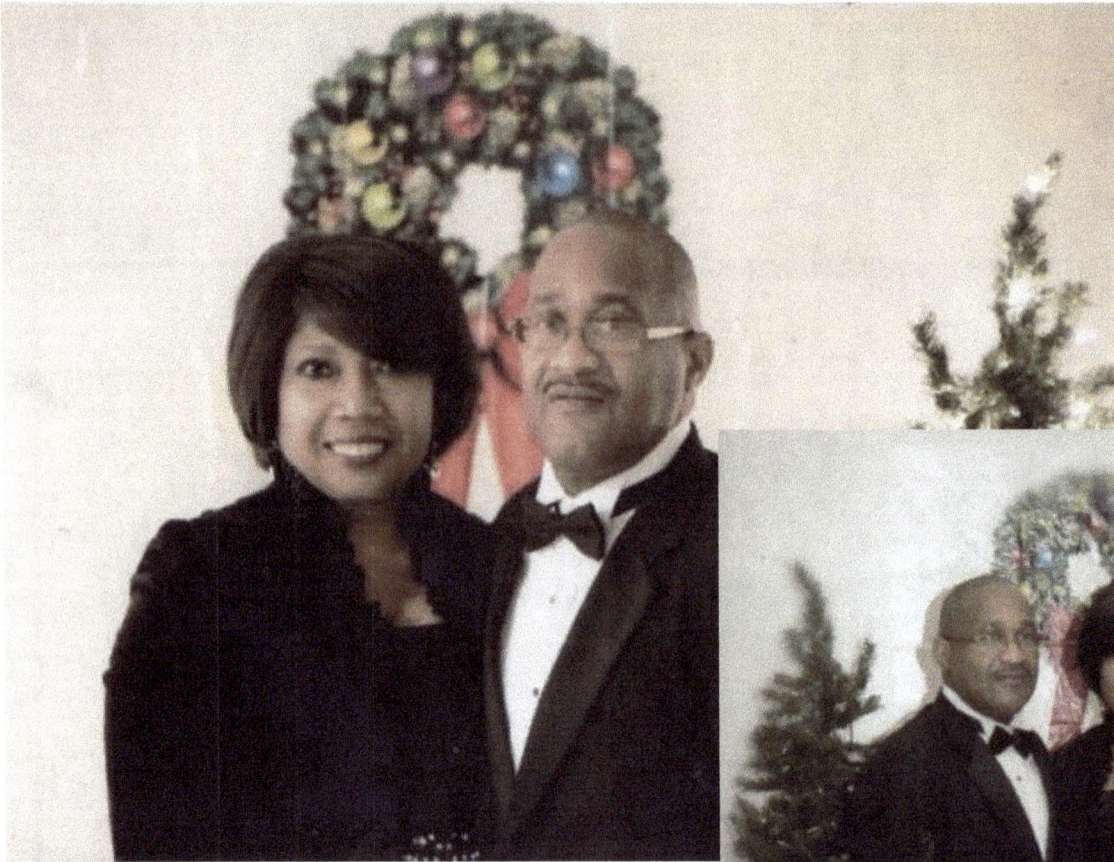

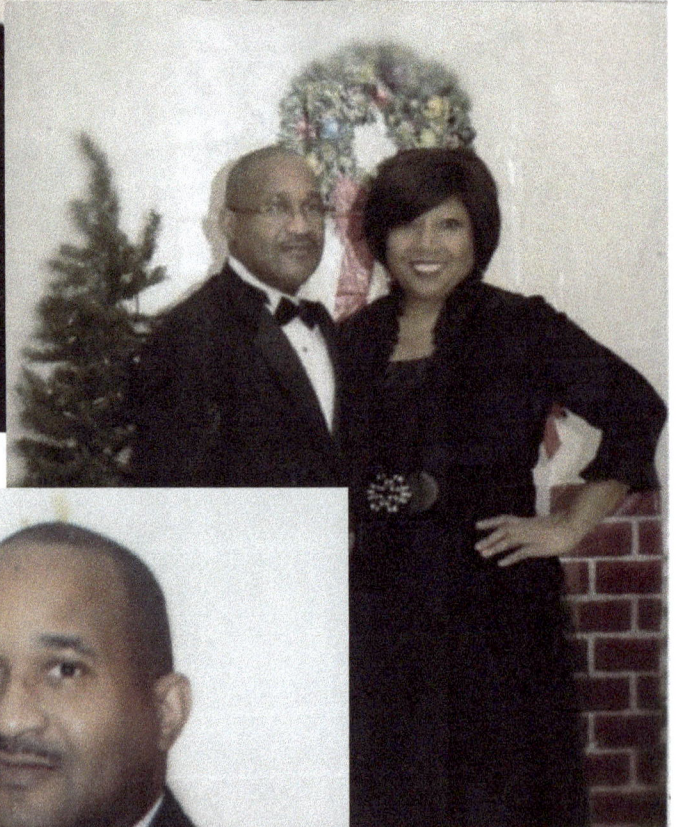

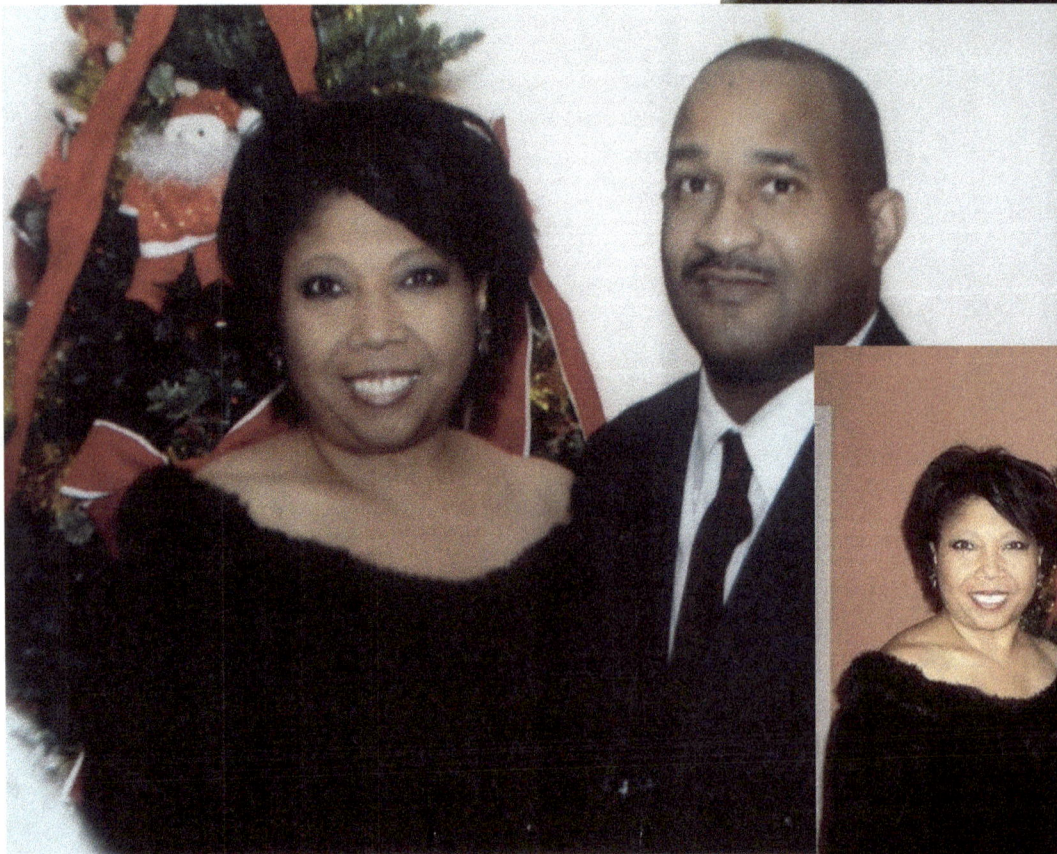

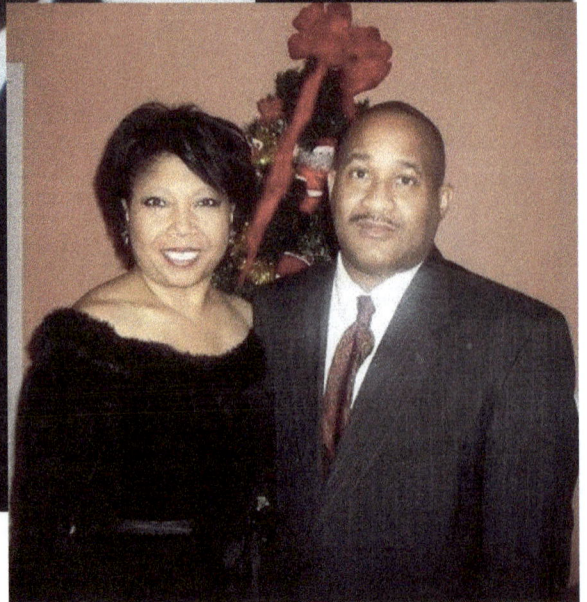

Photos by Leundra Tucker

I am always amazed and overwhelmed with thankfulness to God for seeing fit to bless me with such a charmed life. There are people that have and have had much more money than I have, They have been more places and had more adventures. But, I can not think of one that would have been the life that I wanted to live , a life that I felt was so perfect for me. It's just the way I see it in my own little bubble. I remember some of the arguments that Hubby and I would have in the first few years that we were married. Somewhere , in the argument he would inevitably say the words. "Everybody hasn't had the perfect life that you have had." Everybody doesn't have a fairy tale life ." "You just see things through rose colored glasses" My reply always: " You gonna let me ain't you ??!!!!" (I'm like..,Please!!!What you mad about it ???) Anyway, I said that to say this. To me ..It has been a wonderful life , whether it is because of rose-colored glasses or not.

Life could not have given me more. I would think all of the time, probably since I was in my thirties If I died tomorrow, there is no way I could say that I didn't had THE BEST life ..being owed nothing! You have to stick with me here because I am just rambling through my thoughts. It kind of eventually all connects together. And if not, it's just the random ramblings of a truly grateful person ..of the little things. So..I was driving my Dad to his scheduled doctors appointment. (of course ,my Mom came along as always) Somehow, I got on the subject of the 3rd grade reading test and how so many students failed the test ..and how sad that is to me. From there we started talking generally about reading, I was telling Dad how sad it makes me when people say they don't read or don't like to read and even worse don't have time to read . I was telling him about an incident recently when someone told me they didn't like to read . I grabbed my stomach and told her "Stop ! Stop ! Don't say it ! You are making me ill ! " I promise I had a physical reaction to it. My Daddy was laughing at me as usual! I told her : "Don't say another word about it, because I'm gonna start thinking differently about you !"She laughed! But I was TOTALLY serious!

Anyway , I started telling my Dad how thankful I am that I have loved reading from such an early age and can't imagine anything different. So I told him how thankful I was that he was always encouraging me to read the classics and how I was so totally prepared in 9th grade when we studied Great Expectations and Dickens works . I told him it was a breeze because I knew all of it because of how he would drill me after each book. I said I knew it all !. He laughed ! (He is always laughing at me) I told him I am so thankful of how he was always on me to learn things like that. So he out of the blue says. Yeah like that leaf collection we did together and you got an A+ (That was 10th grade Biology) I said Yes Yes, exactly like that ! I think we were supposed to find 25-30 leaves to find and describe in our little book. I think I had at least double that in my collection . Plus all of the wonderful explanations that he gave me as we collected them I even wrote about that in a poem. It was amazing to me that he still cherished that in his heart and mind (just like I do) I think it is amazing that I still have both of my parents to ride around with and talk about things like that .(86 and 83)...parents who have been married over 60 years .

It might seem like a little think, But it's not to me. I have led a sheltered life in so many ways and so many ways not . I have taken tap lessons and ballet lessons and piano lessons and violin lessons .and can't do any of them well! When I graduated from high school my parents said I could choose anywhere I wanted to go to college (that I got in) ANYWHERE. At 55, have never had a broken bone, I have never had a surgery . I take no medications. I have never been admitted to the hospital overnight except to have a baby . That "baby" has not given me an ounce of real trouble in his 20 years I can count on one had how many times he has even ever been really sick or even thrown up..no broken bones... hospitalizations. no life and death kind of situations or serious drama (at least to me) Hubby often asks me how many times I have ever bought soap or toilet paper,or tooth paste or bubble bath and things like that, since we have been married. I guess it is kind of a trick question but the answer is somewhere around. NEVER. He does that I know for all f these "charmed things in my life , it could all change tomorrow! And , I would have no cause to complain , because I have been given more than my share of the good. If there is no other message that I can convey with my life except to let God know and my parents know that I have been truly thankful and grateful ,it is enough .

FABULOUS FAMILY

Patricia Neely-Dorsey

Patricia Neely-Dorsey is a 1982 graduate of Tupelo High School in Tupelo, Mississippi. She received a Bachelor of Arts degree in Psychology from Boston University in Boston, Massachusetts. After living in Memphis , TN for almost 20 years, working in the mental health field, Patricia moved back to Tupelo in August 2007. Her first book of poetry, Reflections of a Mississippi Magnolia-A Life In Poems was published in February 2008. Her second book of poetry, My Magnolia Memories and Musings- In Poems was published in February 2012. Her third book "Mississippi In Me" was published in January 2017.

Through her poems, the author attempts to give a more positive view of Mississippi and the South, rather than all of the negatives usually portrayed. One of Patricia's poems "Country Living " is included in a German high school textbook , currently being used in teaching English as a Foreign Language . In 2015 , Patricia received a proclamation in her honor from Governor Phil Bryant declaring her as an Official Goodwill Ambassador for the state. The same year, a resolution was passed by the House of Representatives commending her work in promoting positive images of Mississippi through her poems. Patricia's poem , "Meet My Mississippi" was up for consideration as the official state poem in the 2016, 2017, 2018 and 2019 legislative sessions. The poem is now a best selling children's book , with the same title . (Published 2018) (Liberation's Publishing)

Patricia was the host of a talk show "Meet My Mississippi Authors and Artists" on the Hill Country Network. Several of Patricia's Mississippi poems were included on t-shirts in the Southern Belle T-shirt Company line in her continuing efforts to Promote a Positive Mississippi . Patricia is member of Alpha Kappa Alpha Sorority Inc. Patricia lives in Tupelo with her husband James. They have one son James Henry , a 2022 graduate of The University of Mississippi

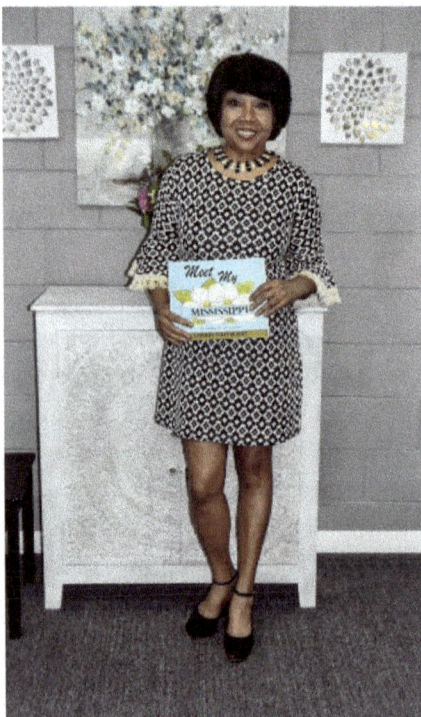

I Love Mississippi

Poet Patricia Neely Dorsey's mission in life is to get others to love Mississippi as much as she does. Now she's reaching an even wider audience with her inspiring words through a new line of Southern Belle T-shirts that feature lines from Dorsey's recently published third book of poems.

"The people who wear them are sharing the great things I see in this place even if they never pick up a book of my poetry," she said. "In my poems, you see that love for the family and community connections here, the core values, the beautiful landscape and the country living."

This is not the first time Dorsey's poetry has made news statewide. In 2015, Gov. Phil Bryant named her an official goodwill ambassador to the state because of her writing.

8 INVITATION TUPELO | *February 2018*

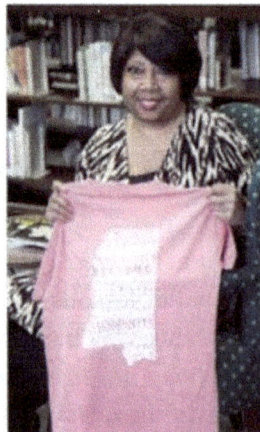

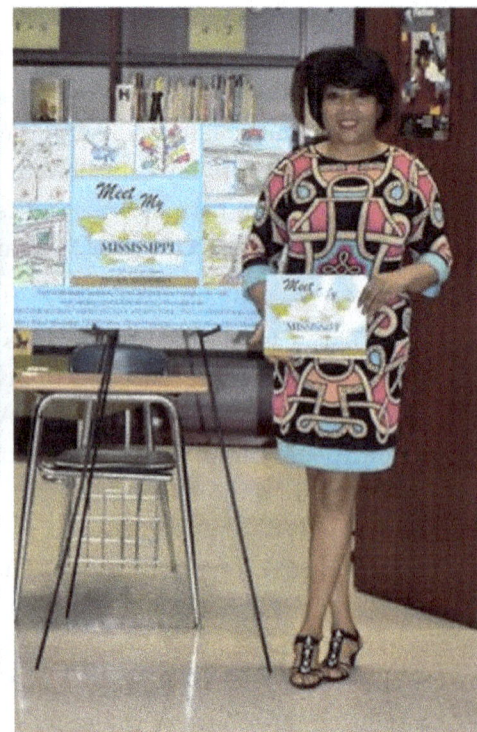

Elaine Kilgore Neely

Elaine Kilgore Neely was born in Mantee, Mississippi to Alton Odessa Kilgore and Julia Buckingham Kilgore. She says that some of her fondest memories were of her early days in Mantee living with her parents, grandparents and siblings up until age 5 , when her father moved the family to West Point. She attended Mary Holmes private school from elementary through high school . She always made excellent grades and enjoyed participating in school plays , where she most often landed the lead roles. One of her favorite roles was playing Meg in Little Women.

During high school she was voted Most Intellectual and Best Actress in Who Who's. At Mary Holmes, she met the love of her life, James Neely. They married on April 19, 1954 in Columbus, Mississippi , when she was 19 years old. She graduated from Mary Holmes Jr College in West Point, MS. and received her Bachelor's Degree in Elementary Education from Tennessee State University in Nashville in 1960. She graduated Cum Laude and had the highest grade point average in her department . She was a member of Kappa Delta Pi Honorary Society in Education and a member of The Meharry Wives Club, where she says she gained invaluable knowledge and instruction on how to support her husband in his chosen career of medicine.

He graduated from Meharry Medical College in 1960. The couple lived in El Paso, Texas and Belleville Illinois during her husband's military service in the Air Force, where he was a flight surgeon and earned the rank of Captain. She enjoyed those years, immensely. During those years her two children Brian and Patricia were born. After returning to Mississippi, she taught in the Tupelo School System at Green Street ,George Washington Carver and Pierce Street in the elementary grades. She has always been very proud to be from a family of educators. Her paternal grandmother , her father and her mother were school teachers. She touched countless young lives with her caring manner in the classroom. Before teaching at Pierce Street Elementary, she served as secretary of the PTA for several years. She was cub scout leader and girl scout leader. She was a member of the Ladies Waymakers Club which was devoted to mentoring young girls in the Northside community. She was a member of the W.A Zuber Reading Club and Bridge Club. She coordinated and directed countless weddings during the 60's and 70'sand never charged the lucky brides for her services. She has always been known as the ultimate hostess and homemaker.

She has also always been known for her grace and elegance. She is a very proud Life Member of Alpha Kappa Alpha Sorority, Inc. She was a devoted wife to Dr. James Neely for 66 years, before his death in 2020. He said that this marriage was one of his greatest accomplishments. She considers it one of hers. She is an avid , voracious reader and a passionate advocate for healthy lifestyle habits. She has been a vegetarian for over thirty years. When asked what she thought her gift was/ is. she said: Being Compassionate.

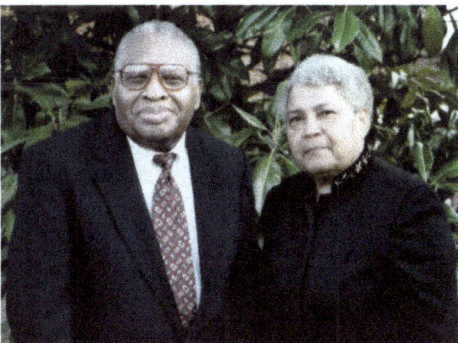

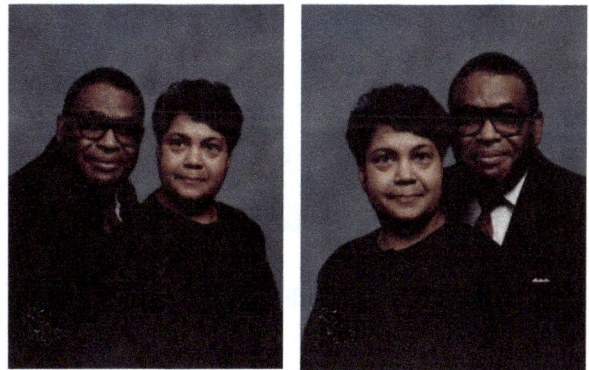

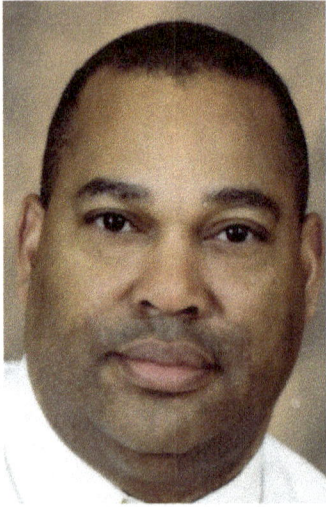

Brian Henry Neely

Brian Neely is a 1979 graduate of Tupelo High School. He is a 1983 graduate of Boston University with a B.A. degree in history, and a 1987 graduate of Southern Methodist University School of Law. After graduation from law school, Brian H. Neely landed a highly competitive clerkship with the United States District Court for the Northern District of Mississippi in Aberdeen, MS. He worked there until he joined the United States Marine Corps. During his Marine Corps service, Brian H. Neely was promoted to the rank of Captain and served during Operation Desert Shield/Desert Storm as a Casualty Coordinating Officer.

After leaving the military Brian H. Neely worked as an associate attorney for the prestigious Lake, Tindall law firm in Greenville, MS until he decided to return to his hometown of Tupelo, MS. In 1994, he engaged in the practice of law as a sole practitioner in Tupelo. While practicing law he served as Lee County Prosecuting Attorney in 2003, where he was responsible for the disposition of all misdemeanor cases for the county. He also served as Youth Court Prosecutor during this time.

Brian is a 2018 graduate of City University of London with a Masters in Law. Brian currently serves as Assistant District Attorney - First Circuit Court District of Mississippi for the counties of Alcorn, Itawamba,

September 2019...
Sister- in -Law Shari Long Neely posted: My husband presided over his first meeting as Chair of the Prosecutors Section of the Mississippi Bar today.

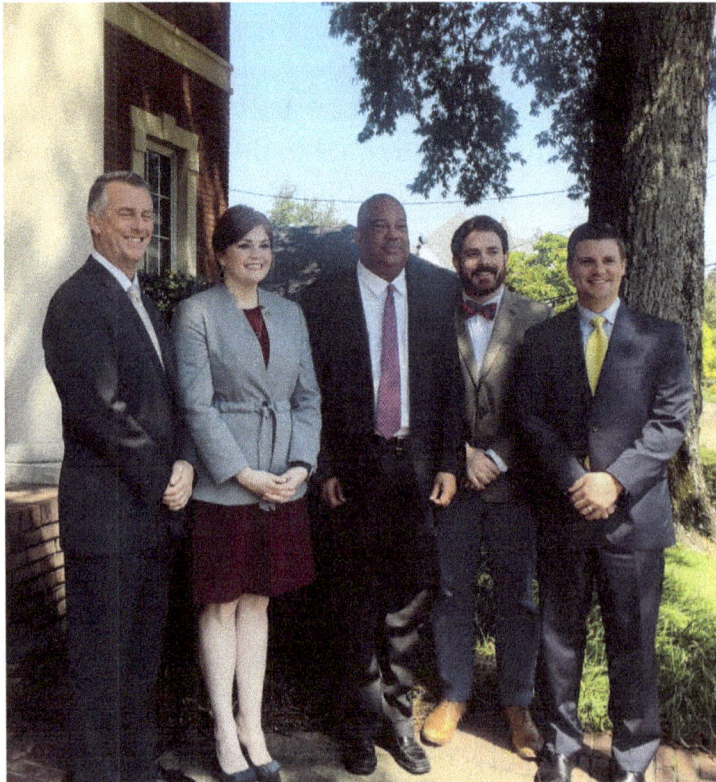

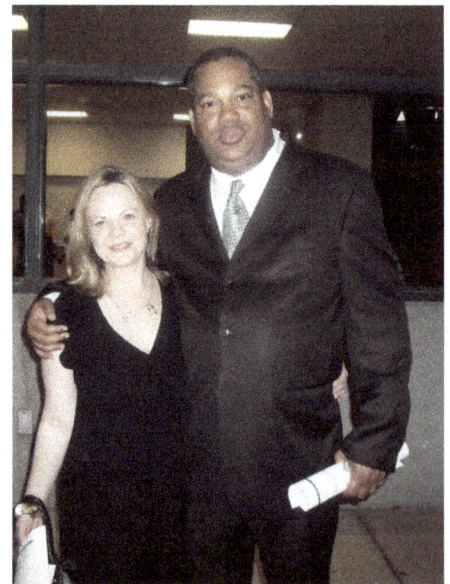

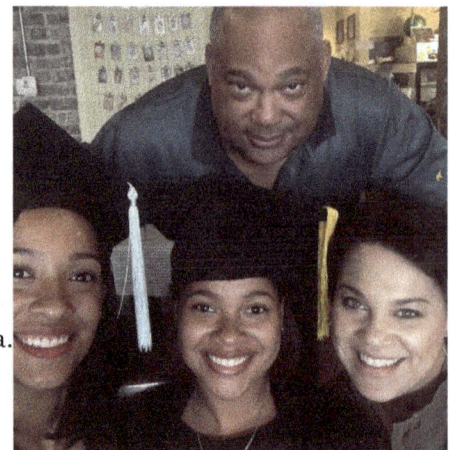

Brian has three daughters: Ivy Elainea, Julia Charmaine and Lesa Patricia.
Brian has five grandchildren- Zakary , Dash , Alana , Prince and Sterling .
Brian is married to Shari Long Neely.

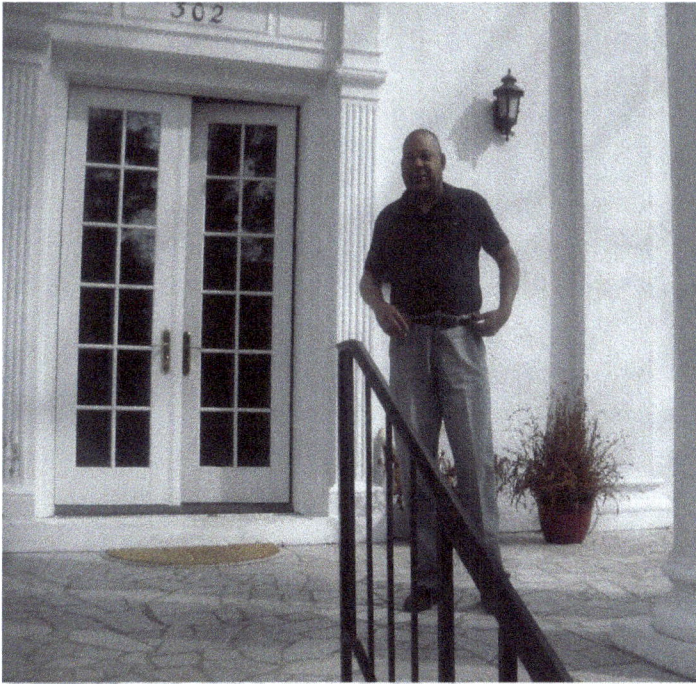

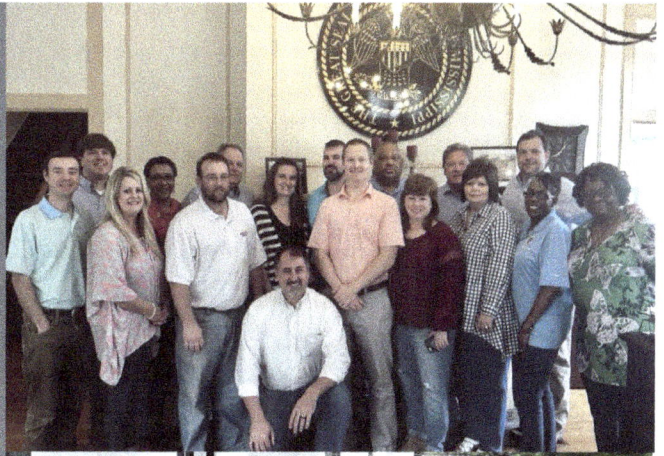

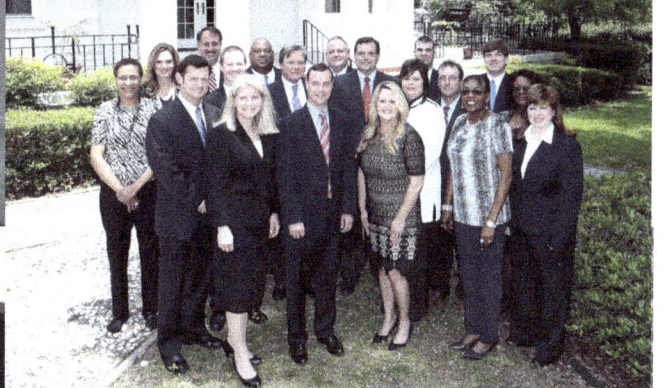

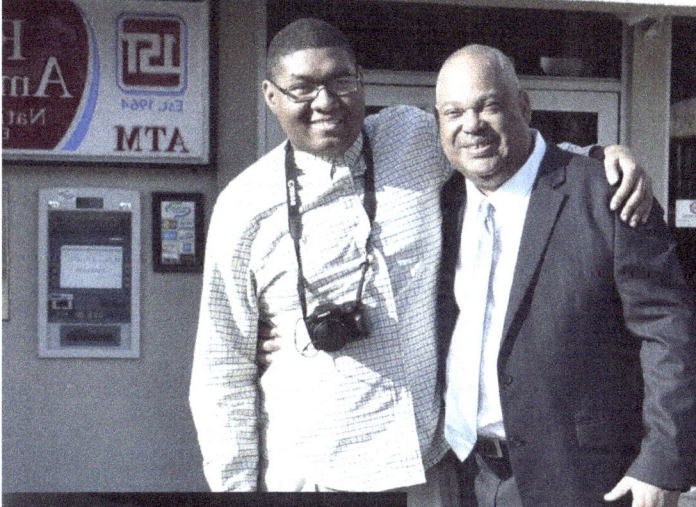

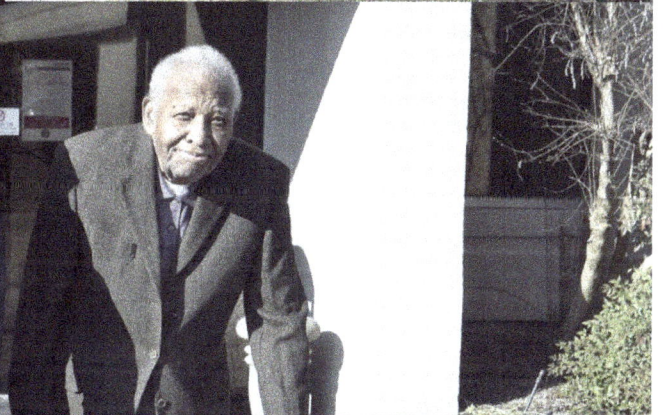

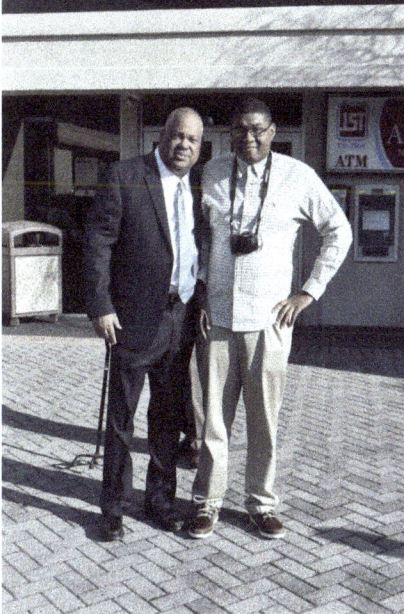

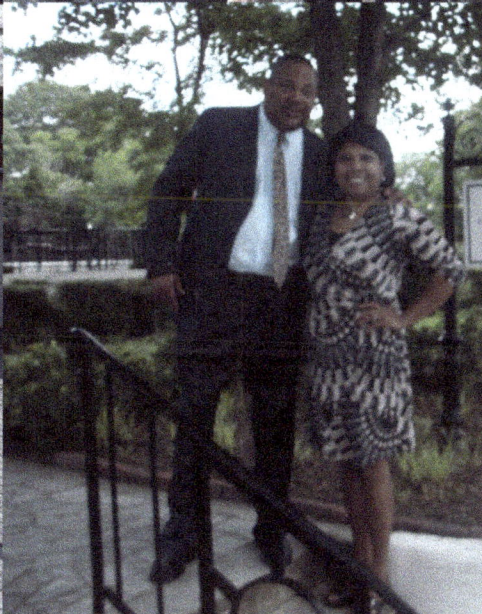

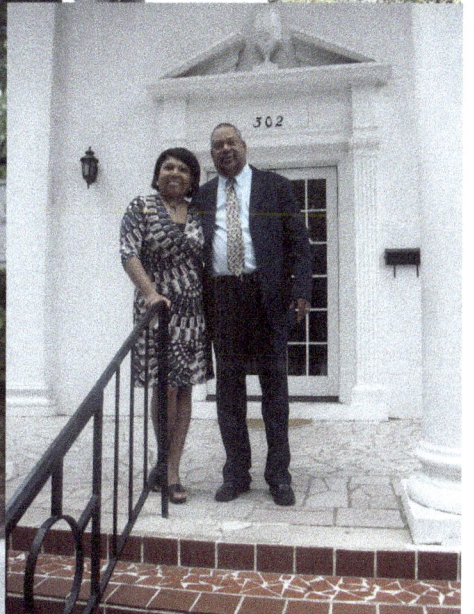

James Henry Neely M.D.

Dr. James Henry Neely was born in West Point, MS on August 8, 1932 to the union of Robert and Missouri Neely. He attended Mary Holmes College High School where he was the editor of the school newspaper, secretary of the senior class, president of the Athletic Club and member- at- large of the Student Council. He received his Bachelor's degree in 1955 from Kentucky State University, formerly Kentucky State College, in Frankfort, Kentucky with a major in chemistry and a minor in math and French.

He received his Doctor of Medicine degree in 1960 from Meharry Medical College in Nashville, TN. After graduation he entered the United States Air Force, where he earned the rank of Captain and served as a Flight Surgeon stationed in El Paso, Texas and in Belleville, Illinois. After an honorable discharge from the military in 1964, He relocated to Tupelo to set up his medical practice, upon the encouragement of the late Dr. Walter A. Zuber. He was the first African-American doctor to have full hospital privileges of admitting and treating patients at the North Mississippi Medical Center. He diligently served his community in medical practice for 35 years, until his retirement in 1999.

He was a member of Trinity United Presbyterian Church in West Point. Dr. Neely was a member of Alpha Phi Alpha Fraternity, Sigma Pi Phi Fraternity and a Life member of the NAACP. He held memberships in numerous other organizations, including The National Medical Association, The Black Business Association of Mississippi and the Henry Hampton Elks Lodge. In the 1970s, he served as a member of the Board of Directors of Community Development Foundation (CDF) and as a member of the Northside Beautification Committee, along with Mr. Ulysses Mayhorn and Mrs. W. A. Zuber. A project that he was very proud of was the planting pink crepe myrtle trees along North Spring Street (between Jackson Street and Franklin Street) in Tupelo, which still bloom beautifully each year.

Dr. Neely was honored with numerous awards during the course of his notable career, including: Mississippi Medical and Surgical Award - Practitioner of the Year (1982) Alpha Kappa Alpha Sorority Inc. Nu Sigma Omega Chapter- Distinguished Service Award Meharry Medical College Distinguished Service Award for 25 years of service (1985) The Black Business Association- Legend Award for Outstanding Community Service (1999) UNCF Tupelo Lee County Committee- Recognition Award for Outstanding Dedication and Leadership in the field of Medicine. Magnolia Bar Association- Harriet Tubman Award (2001) The Committee for King Dr. Martin Luther King Jr.- Drum Major Award (2001) He was married to the former Elaine Kilgore of West Point for 66 years. He said that this was one of his greatest accomplishments. He departed this life on June 23, 2020 at the Baptist Memorial Hospital in Oxford, Mississippi.

A tribute from Ronnie Agnew June 2020

They were the same age, Dr. James Henry Neely and my mother, both born in 1932. As far as she was concerned, he was the only physician in the world. The absolute best part: We had the privilege growing up of living next door to Dr. Neely, his lovely wife Elaine, and Brian and Pat, the kids who are the 10th and 11th children of my rather large family. We were a true family, just as close as any family could be. Mom passed away years ago. And Dr. Neely, who has been a part of my life all of my life, left us yesterday, June 23, 2020. You should read about Dr. Neely. His life's accomplishments would fill pages. But I will leave his long resume to you, in hopes that you will find it and read it. I will say that he was the first African American physician with hospital privileges at North Mississippi Medical Center in Tupelo. He was a military officer. An Alpha Phi Alpha man. And so much more. To the Agnew family, he was just Doc, a West Point, Miss., native who stayed in close contact with his country roots through us. He allowed my daddy to build a pig pen on his property, and on every hog-killing day, he would show up without fail to get a bag of cracklings. He allowed my dad to put a sizable garden on his property and took great joy in retrieving fresh vegetables from it. Doc loved my family and we loved him back. Each time when I return home, driving down Beech Springs Road, I always turn my head in hopes of a Doc sighting.

As a doctor, Doc probably could have used some business lessons. He had paying customers. But for those who couldn't pay, he would always look the other way. He loved the practice of medicine. It was more important to him than money. He would expose us to his brilliance without even knowing it. And he would openly show us his humanity by being a regular man who did regular things, although everything about him was extraordinary. My family has lost one of its champions. Brian and Pat have lost a father. Mrs. Neely has lost her husband of 66 years. And America has lost one of its brightest, most compassionate minds. A big part of my life passed away Tuesday. A big part of Mississippi history did, too.

—Ronnie Agnew
June 2020

As an insurance agent, for most of my life, I met Dr. J. H.. Neely when he first opened his office in Tupelo because I wrote most of the professional liability insurance for all the doctors in Tupelo and the insurance for the hospital also. He was a nice man, and I knew from the very start that he would fit in with the Tupelo Spirit that most of us here in Tupelo embraced.

The Tupelo Spirit is that special feeling we have here in Tupelo that means every person is important, and every person has something to add to our community to make it better. And that we all work with a sense of cooperation toward making Tupelo a better place for everyone. The results of that cooperation over a long period of time are evident in many places all around town.

Over the years I came to know his family as well and especially his daughter Patricia as she began to be active on social media. She would go to yard sales, estate sales, and thrift shops and buy things very cheaply. And then she would post her purchases on her social media page showing how wonderful they were as standalone objects or as clothing outfits. At that time she was just laying them out on her bed and photographing them and I suggested to her that she might like to model the clothes that she was buying as it would make her posts much more interesting. And as we all know, she took my advice, I always look forward to seeing her in her latest outfit. She has certainly adopted the Tupelo Spirit with her poetry and her writings. Her poem, Meet My Mississippi is known by almost everyone in the state. And along the way, I met her brother, Brian, who is an attorney here in town and found him to be an interesting fellow as well. I would run into him often when eating lunch at The Stables. All of the Neely's have made their mark on Tupelo, in a very good way. Patricia and her mom will continue making their mark with this new book, Fabulous Life. Let the Neely's example encourage you to embrace the Tupelo Spirit.

Jim High
Columnist Lee County Courier

2nd Place in the Daily Journal 2008 "Celebrating Dad" Fathers Day Essay Contest?
It read in part like this,

When I think of my father, Dr. James Henry Neely, , I think of the term "Renaissance Man" Some common definitions of that term include one who is versatile with many interests and talents, one who is well-educated and who excels in a wide variety of subjects, fields, a universal , well-rounded man, or a man of many accomplishments . All of these descriptions apply to my exceptional, extraordinary dad.

My father was born in West Point, Mississippi, on August 8, 1932, to Robert and Missouri Neely. Coming from a time and place that often offered very adverse, even hostile conditions for an African -American male, he still excelled. My dad attended Mary Holmes Jr. College High School and was the editor of the school newspaper, secretary of the senior class , president of the Athletic Club and member -at-large of the Student Council He attended Kentucky State College ..now University He made house calls to those in the more rural parts of the county who could not readily come in to see him at his office.

Many of his patients could not afford to pay him for his services , so he accepted whatever means that they had available in exchange. I remember knocks at the door on Saturdays or Sundays with deliveries by patients of fresh vegetables from their gardens , freshly gathered eggs from their chicken coops or freshly cut or cured meats from a recent hog killing.

My father certainly did not perform his job for the money. He truly had a great love for his profession and a burning desire to help people, especially the poor, underprivileged: and disenfranchised. He continued to make house calls well into the 80's and 90's , which was practically unheard of . My father retired from practice in 1999, following a stroke , after serving the community for almost 35 years.

Aside from all of his professional accomplishments, my father is a man who loves the arts. During my childhood he would frequently recite poetry to me and later in my teens, he would frequently quiz me different classic books such as "Great Expectations" , making sure I knew the things he thought I should know about them. My father is humorous and witty, he cooks and he likes to garden. Every year, he plants his small garden in the backyard where he and his only grandson, my son, James Henry Dorsey, 9, spend countless hours discussing the mysteries of the universe. This is the one person in all the world to whom this extraordinary man takes a back seat- because Henry is ALWAYS right and has the answer to EVERYTHING -he thinks, and his extraordinary granddad LET's him think it.

SECOND PLACE

'My Father – A Renaissance Man'

When I think of my father, Dr. James Henry Neely, I think of the term "Renaissance Man."

Some common definitions of that term include one who is versatile with many interests and talents, one who is well-educated and who excels in a wide variety of subjects or fields, a universal, well-rounded man, or a man of many accomplishments. All of these descriptions apply to my exceptional, extraordinary dad.

My father was born in West Point, Miss., on Aug. 8, 1932, to Robert and Missouri Neely. Coming from a time and place that often offered very adverse, even hostile, conditions for an African-American male, he still excelled. My dad attended Mary Holmes Jr. College High School and was the editor of the school newspaper, secretary of the senior class, president of the Athletic Club and member-at-large of the Student Council.

He attended Kentucky State University, formerly Kentucky State College, in Frankfort, Ken., where he received his bachelor's degree in 1955 with a major in chemistry and a minor in math and French. There he became a member of the distinguished Alpha Phi Alpha Fraternity, the first African-American collegiate fraternity.

My father says he cannot remember ever wanting to be anything but a doctor. He received his Doctor of Medicine degree from Meharry Medical College in Nashville, in 1960. Soon

Dr. James Henry Neely

after, he entered the United States Air Force where he earned the rank of captain, and served his country as chief of an Air Force flight medical section.

In the summer of 1964, he moved to Tupelo to set up practice. He was the first African-American doctor in Tupelo to receive full hospital privileges of admitting and treating patients. My dad was a true "country doctor." He

Turn to RENAISSANCE on Page 2D

My Daddy, MD

Whenever Daddy signs his name,
he always writes M.D.,
so everyone will know,
that he belongs to me.
For M.D. means "My Daddy",
or something just the same.
And that is why he always
puts these letters in his name.
Some letters in his name are
small, but these are not,
you see. He always makes them
big like that because he's so proud of me.
Jay MacDonald (Happy Mann)

Dr James Neely was a one of a one of kind doctor. I can recall him coming down in a little community in Frisco Alley making house calls. Some of those house calls were not paid visits. He treated my whole family and countless others. My grandmother would only see Dr. Neely, no other doctor could treat her. He was attentive to his patients, especially the senior citizens. Any day any time of night. It was not to late for him. There are certainly very few others like him.. He was a Treasure . All I can say is well done thy good and faithful servant.

Mrs. Neely is a very special jewel to her community. Alongside every good man is a good woman.

—Jessi Hooper

COUNTRY DOCTOR

My Dad was a country doctor,
And I have such memories galore;
I even remember the house calls,
As he literally traveled 'round door to door.
Sometimes, on Saturday mornings,
When I was just a young thing;
My daddy would let me go with him,
As he did all his doctoring.
He'd have his black bag in one hand,
And his stethoscope wrapped 'round his neck;
He was most definitely the captain,
And I was his first man on deck.
We traveled way deep in the country,
And there were always such sites to see;
Believe you me, I noticed them all,
Down to the last bumblebee.
I'd always meet really kind people,
As I stayed by my daddy's side;
He'd always give my introduction,
As he stood there beaming with pride.
Many of the people had no indoor plumbing,
And most of them were all very poor;
So my daddy would let patient's pay him,
With whatever it was they'd procure.
Sometimes, he took brown eggs or slab bacon,
Fresh vegetables, hams and the like;
All of this was so amazing to see,
For me as such a young tike.
The old women, he'd always call "young lady",
But old and young all addressed him as sir;
We'd make so many stops on our journey,
I'm quite surprised that it's not all a blur.
I remember learning about all these people,
And all of the crops that they grew.
Each time, I'd learn something different,
Each time, I'd learn something quite new.
My eyes would grow wide with excitement,
As I saw all the animals and stock;
We'd see so much beautiful scenery,
As we'd drive to the next door to knock.
My dad had such a busy schedule,
I can't imagine how he got it all done;
All I remember is I loved tagging along,
And all I remember is fun.
Copyright 2008 Patricia Neely-Dorsey

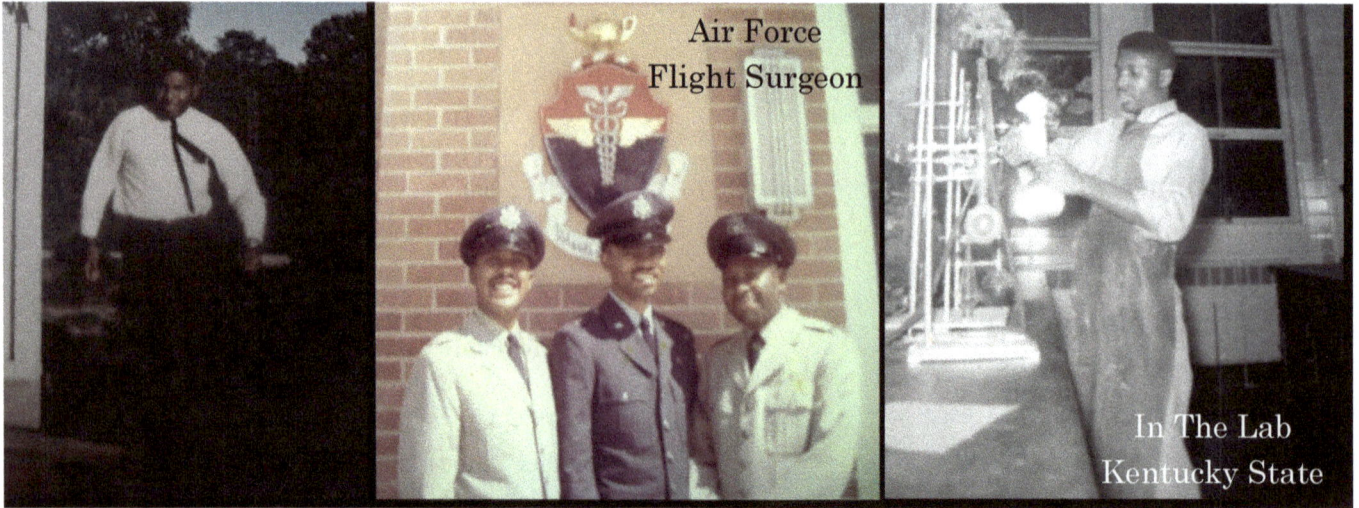

Air Force
Flight Surgeon

In The Lab
Kentucky State

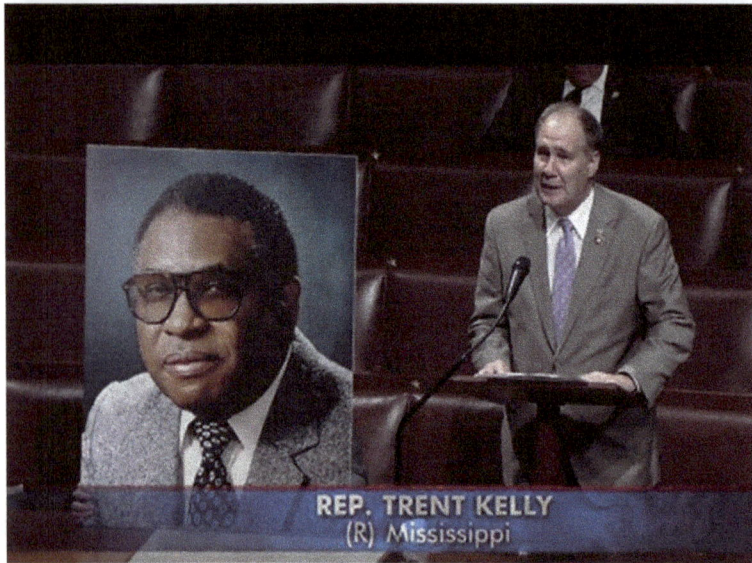

REP. TRENT KELLY
(R) Mississippi

Tribute to my Dad on the House floor (Washington, DC) on June 29, 2020 by Representative Trent Kelly

from Representative Trent Kelly's Facebook page :

It was an honor to pay tribute to Dr. James Henry Neely on the House Floor. The West Point native passed away on June 23. Dr. Neely lived a life we should all admire a life of public service. His accomplishments are many, proof of the great strides he made for generations to follow.

Dr. Neely's legacy will always be his family. He was married to his wife, Elaine, for 66 years. Brian Neely, Dr. Neely's son, is a friend and mentor who served as an assistant district attorney in my office. I am thankful to know this great family.

Graduating from Meharry

Alpha Man

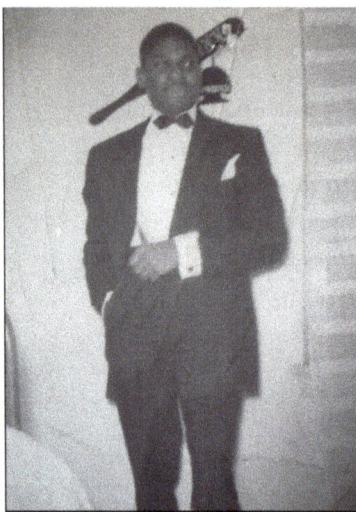

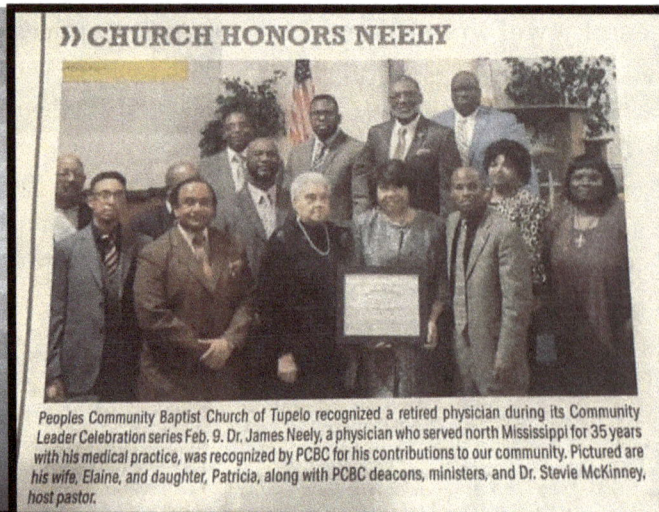

» CHURCH HONORS NEELY

Peoples Community Baptist Church of Tupelo recognized a retired physician during its Community Leader Celebration series Feb. 9. Dr. James Neely, a physician who served north Mississippi for 35 years with his medical practice, was recognized by PCBC for his contributions to our community. Pictured are his wife, Elaine, and daughter, Patricia, along with PCBC deacons, ministers, and Dr. Stevie McKinney, host pastor.

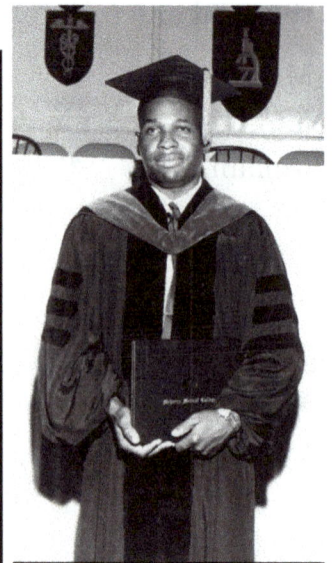

Legendary doctors Dr. James Neely and Dr. John Elliott remembered

Daily Journal July 2020

 from the article:

Dr. James Henry Neely and Dr. John Pascal Elliott Jr., two legendary doctors who changed the Northeast Mississippi community within both the medical field and as community leaders, passed away last week. Both men started practicing in Tupelo the same year – 1964 – and passed away within one day of each other, with Neely passing June 23 at the Baptist Memorial Hospital in Oxford and Elliott passing June 24 at his Tupelo residence. Loved ones and colleagues remember them as great doctors and better men.

"That's just how my dad was. He wasn't going to accept second class status from anybody. He wouldn't accept second class status for his patients, he wouldn't accept second class status for the members of his community, anybody," Brian Neely said. A brilliant doctor, James Neely received patients of all racial and socioeconomic backgrounds, and his patients trusted him fiercely. Former colleague Dr. C.K. White, a retired obstetrician-gynecologist and past chief medical officer for North Mississippi Health Services, remembers James Neely as someone who served patients regardless of if they could pay. The two men had a running joke about how often when James Neely sent patients to White, patients would still follow up with Neely to receive his professional opinion.

Legendary doctors Dr. James Neely and Dr. John Elliott remembered

By Danny McArthur Daily Journal   Jul 5, 2020

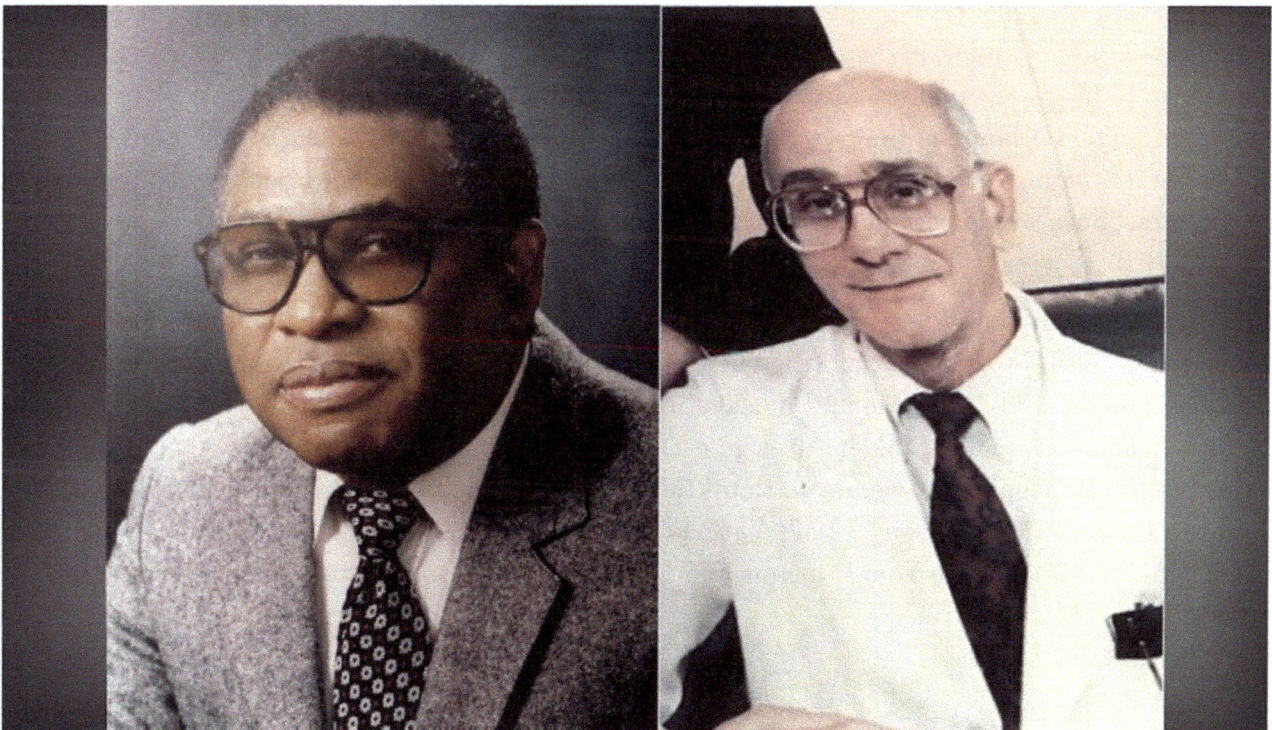

FACEBOOK POST: November 26, 2013

Say it!!! "I love you." "Thank you." "Please." It makes all the difference

I just saw this on a status update, and it really struck me. Expressing our love and gratitude verbally is really very important. Everyone loves to HEAR that they are loved and appreciated. I think that I will write a blog post about this and share one of my stories. Everyone who knows me personally knows that I was a VERY spoiled, pampered princess growing up .and VERY much a daddy's girl. I am always saying jokingly that I didn't even know I had a mother until I was in my teens. Actually, I have the most extraordinary mother that anyone could image, but as a child, in my mind, everything in my world centered around my Daddy, In my mind, he could do no wrong, and he could do everything!

I followed him everywhere. We were like two peas in a pod. We would go fishing together, pick figs together, watch The Flip Wilson Show every Thursday night together with me sitting on his lap and play tickle games every Sunday morning. He took me to get my ears pierced at McRae's Dept store .and was all over the lady telling her how to do it right! LOL!!! We had an almost unbreakable standing weekly date to eat Chinese food from my favorite Sun Kai Restaurant, in my teens. He helped me to gather and identify all of the leaves for my 10th grade leaf project...and of course I got a 100. He taught me to love poetry. I would sit by the sink while he shaved, and he would recite his favorite poems for me. If you've read my first book of poetry, Reflections of a Mississippi Magnolia, you might think it's all about him! LOL!

Every other poem seems to have something to do with my Daddy! But, surprisingly, with all of this I never HEARD my father SAY " I Love You" until I was an adult! Actually, it's not all that surprising, in that he was "old school". He was from the generation that believed in showing their love or concern by providing and taking care of your needs and not so much so verbally. I never really thought about it, at all, until I was probably in my late teens and early twenties. When I moved to Memphis, and was about 24 or 25, I just started to be more keenly aware of how important family is and how much I wanted my parents to know how much I appreciated, loved cared for them. I wanted them to hear me say it, too. It might have had something to do with seeing some of the very terribly dysfunctional families that I would come in contact with, in my work in the mental health field. I made it a point to say " I Love You" at the end of every conversation. I don't remember exactly what his response would be. but it was probably something like just. OK.

One day, at the end of one of our phone conversations, I said. Aren't you going to tell me you love me, too? It really took a lot of nerve for me to say that ... and I think it took him by surprise. But, of course, he said I love you .and the barrier was broken. Just like that. From that day on, until this day, I say it all of the time and he says it right back, without any hesitation It's very natural. I love hearing it and I think he does too. During this Thanksgiving season when we all are thinking about the people that we are so thankful for ...don't forget to SAY the words to go with the sentiments. (I think I tell my son " I Love You " at least 4 or 5 times a day!) Get used to saying those words. Thank You and I Love You. It means a lot! You won't have to ever regret words left unsaid.

MEET MY MISSISSIPPI

William Faulkner's Sanctuary
Eudora Welty's home state
Elvis Presley's birthplace
The bulk of the Natchez Trace;
Choctaw Nation native land
Rolling hills of the Chickasaw Band
Sprawling beaches along the Gulf Coast shore
One blues man's Crossroads and inspiration for more;
Like Albert, B.B., Bukka, Howlin' Wolf,
Little Milton and Muddy Waters who came to the fore
There's farm raised catfish, Delta tamales,
Vardaman sweet potatoes, seafood galore
And warm front porch welcomes with a wide open door
Creative muse for Barq's, Stetson, Peavey, Viking
And Henson's famous green frog
And "Where The Southern Crosses The Yellow Dog"
An abundance of history, tradition and folklore
With Ruins of Windsor, Vicksburg Battlefield
Emerald Mound, Grand Village, Ingomar, Winterville
and Pharr Mounds to explore
You'll find an authentic Dentzel carousel merry go round
Where Jimmie Rodgers fathered a unique country sound
Conway, Charley, Tammy and Marty came down the line
Along with Bobbie Gentry, Faith Hill, and young LeAnn Rimes
She's the place where Coca Cola was bottled for the very first time
And Pine-Sol invented to combat dirt and grime
A Mississippi native, few would guess,
Was the innovative mastermind behind Federal Express.
The first heart transplant and first lung transplant were performed right here
Where Dr. James Hardy stepped in, when others had fear.
For football legends, you don't have to think twice,
There's Brett Favre, Archie Manning, Walter Payton and Jerry Rice.
More Mississippi greats, amazingly,
include Jerry Clower, Ruby Elzy, John Grisham
James Earl Jones, Willie Morris, Tennessee Williams,
Mary Wilson, Oprah Winfrey, Morgan Freeman,
Ida B Wells, Medger Evers and Leontyne Price
She's a ride down the Mighty River on the American Queen
And some of the most beautiful countryside that you've ever seen
She's music and melodies and the mockingbird's songs,
By valor and arms and faith ever strong;
She's magnolias blooming around Jackson's capitol dome
With the buzz of the honeybee
And sweet scent of the honeysuckle
That forever say "home"
She's a land of cotton
Where the white tailed deer roam
Since December 10, 1817
Our 20th state
"Go Mississippi "
The Hospitality State
Roll On Mississippi
You're a true State of Grace.

by Patricia Neely-Dorsey

MY MISSISSIPPI

M y Mississippi
I s always home to me
S he's warm, charming and alluring
S he's the queen of hospitality
I 've loved her from my earliest days
S he's in my fondest memories
S he's in my heart, in my soul and such a part of me;
I love to share her beauty
P eople often misunderstand
P leasures abundantly abound,
I n my magnolia land .

2013 Patricia Neely-Dorsey

MISSISSIPPI

In the heart of Dixie,
Perfumed by
The sweet, fragrant smell of magnolias
and serenaded with
The melodious songs of the mockingbird,
Lies a true Queen of the South.
Her name is Mississippi .
I don't know how to explain this place,
Except to say that she "speaks" to me.
The rocks, the flowers, the birds and trees
Speak to me.
They sometimes whisper,
And sometimes they shout;
But always they say,
This is where you belong."

2012 Patricia Neely-Dorsey

MADE IN MISSISSIPPI

Along with...
Syrupy, sweet hospitality
Down home , Delta blues
And beautiful Magnolia girls;
Strong family values,
Unbreakable bonds,
And lifelong memories
Are Made in Mississippi

2012 Patricia Neely-Dorsey

MADE IN MAGNOLIA

I'm Made in Magnolia
I'm Mississippi strong
I'm so proud to say
Mississippi's home:
I'm Made in Magnolia
It's my heart and my soul
The joys that she's brought me
Will never grow old ;
I'm Made in Magnolia
And it's not hard to see
Mississippi, forever and always,
Lives inside me.

2013 Patricia Neely-Dorsey

IF MISSISSIPPI'S IN YOU

If Mississippi's in you
It'll always be that way;
It matters not how far you
Or how long you stay.
If Mississippi's in you,
It always plays a part;
In how you live and move and breathe,
And in every notion of the heart.
If Mississippi's in you,
It's in you through and through;
It's in in who you are and how you be,
And it's in everything you do.
If Mississippi's in you,
There is some special glow;
A different something down inside,
That all the home folks know.
If Mississippi's in you,
It'll always be that way,
From the time you enter in the world,
Till in the grave you lay.
Every true Mississippian,
Can surely have it said;
I'm Mississippi born,
I'm Mississippi bred,
And when I die,
I'll be Mississippi dead.

2008 Patricia Neely-Dorsey

A MISSISSIPPI HOME

Lots of Cooking
Lots of Eating
Lots of Friendly Neighbor Greetings
Lots of Praying
Lots of Singing
Lots of Sunday-Go-To Meetings Lots of Love
Lots of Laughter
Lots of Front Porch Swings
Lots of Stories
Lots of Memories, Lots of Sweet, Simple Things

Patricia Neely-Dorsey is one of the most genuine and down-home sweet individuals that I have ever met. When I say, "met", I would have to disclose that we have actually never met in person. The history of our friendship or sisterhood as we describe it goes back over 11 years. She first reached out to me on Facebook because she had seen some graphics that I had created for a mutual friend. I am a watercolor artist, and also a graphic artist. Patricia asked if I would be able to illustrate some of her poetry. I said certainly. My efforts have not had monetary compensation. Knowing the good and positive that Patricia sends out in the world is enough pay for me.

Over the years, I have also illustrated her fashion sense. She calls that, "Diva on a Dime". This woman can hunt down a bargain and layer herself in an outfit that one would swear must have cost hundreds. If someone were to ask me to describe Patricia, I would tell them...."She is heartfelt with a fierce passion."

In the beginning of knowing Patricia I could tell she was passionate about wanting to change the preconceived ideas that people had about her beloved home state of Mississippi. That has never wavered or changed. I would say she is the state of Mississippi's biggest cheerleader and ambassador. I am really looking forward to this book, because I sincerely believe that the apple, Patricia, did not fall far from the tree. Under the guidance of both of her loving parents, the late Dr. James Henry Neely, and Mrs. Elaine Neely, we will learn what nurtured her down-home sweet charm into the drive and dedication of anything she puts her mind to.

Over the past few years, Patricia has directed that passion to bring out the best in herself in a physical and mental sense. She and her Mother are showing the world, if we can do this, you can too.

—Debra Estep

One can experience Mississippi in many ways ... a taste, a scent, a sound, a feeling, and no one conveys the beautifully unique FEELING that is Mississippi more than Patricia Neely-Dorsey. I love the memories from my own life experiences that come flooding back when reading Patricia's poetry. Her ability to take readers to places that they remember well AND to places that they've never even been is a perfect fusion of where one has been and where one wants to go, bringing memories of the past and anticipation for the future together.

As a local director for the Mississippi Miss Hospitality program, I always give the young women who participate in our local representation a copy of Patricia's Meet My Mississippi book. They can learn so much about people, places, and things to appreciate in Mississippi. They have read the book to students around the state.

Patricia's words make readers feel the Mississippi Hospitality. If there was a Mississippi MRS. Hospitality, It would certainly be Patricia. She is a gifted ambassador for this state. Her hospitality shines bright in her words. We were friends on Facebook before we ever met in person, and when we finally did meet, I saw a woman whose desire to be a light for Mississippi shining even more brightly. She is the "real deal." She loves Mississippi more than anyone I know, and that FEELING permeates through every word in her work. The best writers make you "feel." Patricia Neely-Dorsey's words will reach up from the pages to give you a Mississippi hug ... and that is a GREAT feeling.

—Jennifer McNeal

Patricia Neely-Dorsey One of the best benefits of establishing The Mississippi Club has been getting to know dozens of interesting Mississippians, and Patricia Neely-Dorsey is one of the most interesting Mississippians that I have met! When I started The Mississippi Club, which is an online gathering place for Mississippians to explore Mississippi people, places, and events, I had no idea there was someone else just as determined as I was to expose the goodness of Mississippi. Patricia's positive promotion of Mississippi had already far exceeded my efforts and was a great inspiration to me. Because of her genuine devotion to her home state, she had been given the title of Ambassador to Mississippi, by Governor Phil Bryant in 2015. I cannot think of any other Mississippian more fitting to be an ambassador for Mississippi. Patricia's love for the magnolia state shines through in her published books of Mississippi poems, her children's illustrated book titled Meet My Mississippi, and her daily outpouring of Mississippi facts and trivia on social media. Until disrupted by COVID, she also put the spotlight on other Mississippi authors and other notables by broadcasting live interviews on the Hill Country Network.

In addition to being an avid spokesperson for Mississippi, Patricia Neely-Dorsey is quite an expert at finding high-end fashion at thrift-store prices. Her "Diva on a Dime" venture has hundreds of followers and is an inspiration to women around the south and beyond. Some have even asked advice on how to thrift-shop for themselves. One of the things I have observed about Patricia is that she is consistent and persistent. Whatever she puts her mind to, she will do it. Her recent successful decision to lose weight by changing her eating habits and patterns shows what a strong and determined person she is. She is genuine and does her very own thing. And you can bet money that whatever her "thing" is, Mississippi will be involved somewhere, somehow. If I could give out titles, I would dub Patricia "Mississippi to the Bone."

It is truly a pleasure to know such a positive and upbeat Mississippian as Patricia Neely-Dorsey

Rosalin Grace May 2023

I started working with Patricia Dorsey (yes I called her by her first and last name) in Memphis in 2001. I found out that she was from Mississippi. I was also born in Mississippi. Patricia talked about Mississippi all of the time. I started introducing her as that Mississippi Magnolia. She kept us laughing and always had me shopping for shoes.

We would frequent a wonderful discount shoe store near our job. She would, also, go to thrift stores daily and always find some really cute things. There were several thrift shops in walking distance to our office.

When she started writing and sharing her poems, in 2007, they were all about Mississippi and the love she had for Mississippi . She had some really beautiful poems. I was so excited when she published her first book and surprised to see that she gave me credit for inspiration of the title ,Reflections of a Mississippi Magnolia because of my title for her. Although she no longer works with me I am still excited to have worked and know a celebrity.

—Tekela Cooper Coleman

God's plan for our lives has no expiration date and we must respect HIS timing. Miss Patricia, I am so happy to see you fulfilling this dream project with your lovely mother, Mrs. Neely; how awesome!

It is a wonderful time to express how much I appreciate you and acknowledge that what began as an "Inherited Friendship" has truly evolved into a " Familyship". .I honor it and am proud of you.
Keep Living..Keep Staying Alive..Keep Showing Up..Keep On!!!

—Yvonne Jackson Roberts

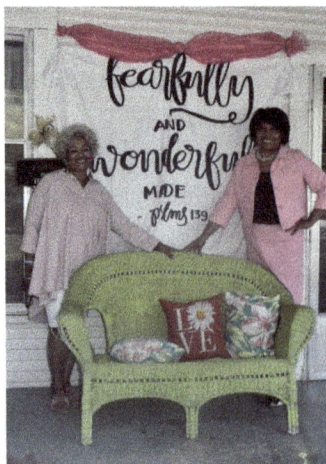

As R. J. Lee, Mystery Writer, I have interacted with Patricia Neely-Dorsey on many occasions over the years. We have been on panels together at Mississippi Library Association Conventions and at other venues. Patricia supports the positive aspects of her home state, including writers, actors, artists, singers, and general go-getters in every category. Her children's book, MEET MY MISSISSIPPI , truly belongs in every library in the state. And it wouldn't hurt one bit if libraries in other states offered it because it presents an entirely different picture of some of the accomplished people who live here and their achievements.

—Robert Kuehnle

I met Patricia (Neely at the time) Dorsey many years ago. We worshiped together at the Boulevard Church of Christ for many years. I learned a little latter that we have something in common… we are both native Mississippians!!! Pat, (if I'm allowed to call her that) always struck me as quiet, reserved and very articulate. The more I got to know her, the more I realized that she wasn't really quiet. She is an extremely intelligent and observant person. I remember that she loved to dress, but mostly in black or neutral colors (Smiles). I don't remember her as a flashy dresser. She was always well put together and was the epitome of sophistication. She still exemplifies that same classy sophistication.

We don't see each other much these days because she and James moved back to her favorite state, Mississippi. We still communicate via Facebook. I believe I have all her books of poetry except maybe one. She will have to confirm what I'm missing. Her books are proudly displayed for anyone to read or browse through when they are a guest in our home. I'm proud to say they are not stuck on a bookshelf. I'm so very proud of Pat and her writing accomplishments.

I admire this classy lady and I've always considered her to be a dear friend. I extend blessings and much success to her and her mom on their new book project, Fabulous Life.

—Genevia Jackson

A Letter to My Best Friend Patricia E. Dorsey

Patricia, do you remember… When we first met at Boulevard Church of Christ. You had recently relocated to Memphis and you were looking for a church home. Wow, I remember that was over 30 years ago. Remember how Sister Peggy Rapier called you "Virginia Slims" and gushed over your legs in those pumps and pencil skirts. I can still hear her say "If I had those legs I wouldn't be in Church." You wore 2 piece suits and pumps every Sunday. Your fashion style was Elle Woods (Legally Blonde) before Reese Witherspoon made her famous. I remember your desire to live for him.

Remember operation "Boyfriend/Husband"? Girl, can you say "Thelma and Louise" without the mayhem and driving out the cliff in the end. We were like day and night; but our end goal was the same, to find a suitable mate in the Lord. Thinking back, our method was ahead of the times. Remember the polaroid camera and handwritten letters and cards. Now there's Facebook…I had fun snapping all those pics, and reading those letters and cards you mailed out. I remember how we grew closer to God in prayer, and how we put our trust in him. We Thank You Father God for James Rufus Dorsey! Your Wedding was Gorgeous and a true labor of LOVE!

Remember our Spiritual journey as Sisters-in-Christ…Those Ladies Retreats, Teachers' Workshop, The Ladies Day Programs, Friday Night Potluck, Gospel Meetings and the Willing Workers Committees. Those years of serving the Lord, the spirit of cooperation and fellowshipping with the saints will always be near and dear in my heart. To God be the Glory. I remember you being right there. Don't ever stop singing "Because He Lives". Remember how we encourage one another as Wives and Mothers. You were right there when we adopted Dasmine…and I was your biggest cheerleader (besides James) for squeezing out Henry. Thanks to God, our Kids are grown, graduated from college and doing well. Life is leading us still in different directions. I will always remember how you taught me to step- out on faith trusting God and to follow my dreams. Although we are separated by miles, my Love for you remains deep within my heart. Sisters-in-Christ/Best Friends Forever,

Brenda Garrison

I am very passionate about Promoting a Positive Mississippi , especially to the youth of our state. I want to EDUCATE the world that there is more to Mississippi than all of the negatives usually portrayed. I want to EMPOWER our children with knowledge that will help to instill a sense of pride in our state. I want to EQUIP our children with knowledge that will help to combat all of the negative images that they are constantly bombarded with. I want to ENLIGHTEN all to a new way of thinking about Mississippi. I want to use my poem "Meet My Mississippi " to help to teach the children of our state (and people of all ages) some important things about Mississippi in a way that can be easily understood , remembered and recalled.

The state song, the state motto, the state tree the state bird and the state capitol , the state insect are all included in the poem..along with other famous landmarks and people of Mississippi. Many of the students (and adults) that I have run across don't know the state motto or the state song or that Pine Sol was invented in Mississippi or that Coca Cola was first bottled in Mississippi . Learn about these things and MUCH MORE in the "Meet My Mississippi " children's book !

I am so thrilled to be able to offer an amazing book that can help foster a love for reading, a love for poetry and a love for Mississippi from a young age ! I see my poem being used in as many ways as a teacher or educator can think of with an underlying theme of gaining more knowledge about the state. I would like to see it used poetry units, for reading lessons , lessons in research and geography , in Mississippi studies and Mississippi Writers classes, and general social studies , music lessons on Mississippi born musicians and music types born in Mississippi. I would love for it to be the inspiration for murals and other works of art. The directions in which the poem /book can be taken are endless. Read and enjoy the poem and amazing illustrations. in the Meet My Mississippi children's book ! Re-read with more attention to the interesting facts on the signs and in the notations. Do further research on the people and historic locations Then....ROAD TRIP !!! HELP PROMOTE A POSITIVE MISSISSIPPI WITH THE MEET MY MISSISSIPPI CHILDREN'S BOOK ! ORDER YOUR COPY TODAY ! ORDER A COPY FOR A TEACHER OR CHILD THAT YOU KNOW!

The Textbook edition is perfect for Mississippi Studies classroom use and homeschooling! AVAILABLE ON AMAZON. WHOLESALE AVAILABLE FROM LIBERATIONS PUBLISHING West Point, MS.

Contact nicole@liberationspublishing.com

No Mississippi child should be without this book!

Adapted from the poem Meet My Mississippi by Patricia Neely-Dorsey, the Meet My Mississippi children's book is an EXCELLENT EDUCATIONAL TOOL AND FUN LITERARY TOUR GUIDE FILLED WITH INTERESTING FACTS ABOUT MISSISSIPPI, it is a wonderful way to share love and knowledge of Mississippi across generations. KNOW More About Mississippi, LEARN More About Mississippi and LOVE More About Mississippi with the Meet My Mississippi children's book! SPREAD MISSISSIPPI LOVE ACROSS GENERATIONS! GREAT FOR ALL AGES!!

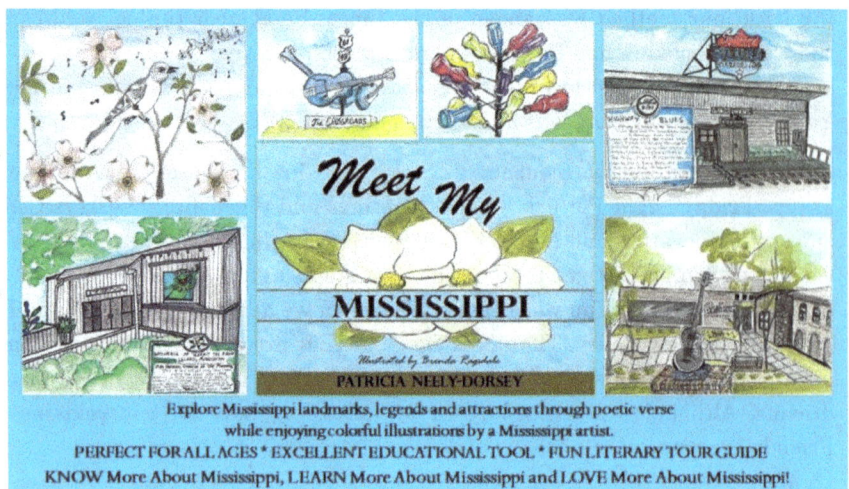

Explore Mississippi landmarks, legends and attractions through poetic verse while enjoying colorful illustrations by a Mississippi artist.
PERFECT FOR ALL AGES * EXCELLENT EDUCATIONAL TOOL * FUN LITERARY TOUR GUIDE
KNOW More About Mississippi, LEARN More About Mississippi and LOVE More About Mississippi!

My Friend Pat Dorsey, Mississippi's Goodwill Ambassador- March 20, 2015 by Ronnie Agnew

We grew up together, running through pastures and filling hot summer days with adventures only young, fearless minds could imagine. We lived all of 15 minutes from downtown Tupelo. But as far as we were concerned, our little piece of earth afforded us quiet respite from the city kids.

We had open fields and muddy creeks. We had wild imaginations that fueled creative ventures, tempered by the stern guidance of older siblings who took seriously their job of ensuring we stayed within boundaries. Our world was simple and we liked it that way, protected it with everything in us from outside sources threatening any measure of complexity. We'd pick fresh vegetables out of the garden and keep a dash of salt on hand to accompany fresh tomatoes plucked off the vine.

I learned the beauty of writing on that patch of land. Our explorations took us to the lake one day and to the makeshift baseball field the next. We would chase stubborn horses through open pasture land in futile attempts to catch them in their domain. The place of my youth taught me the power of observation, of taking it all in, of descriptively assembling thoughts that have lasted a lifetime. Sometimes they escape from my memories in a rush; sometimes in a trickle.

I'm far from alone in the "taking it all in" department. My dear friend Patricia Neely-Dorsey has done that and then some. It was emotional for me as the governor's office, at the urging of State Rep. Randy Boyd, recently honored her with the Goodwill Ambassador Award for accentuating the positive in Mississippi through her poems. Her work is a biography of my life. We have a shared experience that serves as a tether that binds us together with each word she eloquently pens. No matter how far we stray away from each other, our days of running barefoot through country fields, barren and undeveloped, inevitably pushes our memory back to where we started. While she often writes of the past, the towns, communities, cities and neighborhoods continue to provide an infusion of new stories that Pat is poised to tell. Endless are the stories in Mississippi, and relentless is Pat in her desire to tell them.

djournal.com
Northeast Mississippi Daily Journal

Lifestyle » Accentuating the positive: Patricia Neely-Dorsey spreads love for Mississippi

Accentuating the positive: Patricia Neely-Dorsey spreads love for Mississippi

Posted on March 9, 2015 by M. Scott Morris in Lifestyle

Adam Robison | Buy at photos.djournal.com
Patricia Neely-Dorsey's ongoing support for Mississippi has earned official notice from Gov. Phil Bryant and the Mississippi House of Representatives.

221

www.ingramcontent.com/pod-product-compliance
Lightning Source LLC
Chambersburg PA
CBHW080418030426

42335CB00020B/2493